AF540669

HOSPITALS IN COMMUNITY HEALTH CARE

HOSPITALS IN COMMUNITY HEALTH CARE

(Encyclopaedia of Hospital Management—12)

DR. S.L. GOEL

Professor of Public Administration (Retd.),
Panjab University, Chandigarh
Editor, Indian Journal of Public Administration, IIPA, New Delhi
Former Member, UGC, Former Member Distance Education Council
Former Member All India Board of Management, AICTE
Member, Executive Council, IIPA, New Delhi.
Former Vice-President, IIPA, New Delhi.
Emeritus Fellow, University Grants Commission
Former Director, State Bank of India (Local Board) Chandigarh
Former Director, National Horticulture Board, Ministry of Agriculture,
Government of India, New Delhi.

and

DR. R. KUMAR

MBBS, MS, Ex. PGI
President, Chandigarh Ophthalmological Society, 2000-01,
Columnist on Health Education and Management,
Advisor on Health Care and Medical Tourism,
Member Tourism Advisory Forum,
Chandigarh Administration, Chandigarh

DEEP & DEEP PUBLICATIONS PVT. LTD.

F-159, Rajouri Garden, New Delhi-110027

HOSPITALS IN COMMUNITY HEALTH CARE
(Encyclopaedia of Hospital Management—12)

ISBN 978-81-8450-227-5

Typeset by S.S. COMPOSERS
3190, Mohindra Park, Shakur Basti, Delhi-110034.

Printed in India at MAYUR ENTERPRISES
WZ Plot No. 3, Gujjar Market, Tihar Village, New Delhi-110018.

Published by DEEP & DEEP PUBLICATIONS PVT. LTD.
F-159, Rajouri Garden, New Delhi-110027.
Phones: 25435369, 25440916
E-mail: ddpbooks@yahoo.co.in • ddpubs@gmail.com
Showroom:
2/13, Ansari Road, Daryaganj, New Delhi-110002 • Telefax: 23245122

Contents

Preface

One of the very important functions of hospitals at all levels is to enlighten community members for preventive health so that they can lead a decent and healthy life. In all research and teaching hospitals, community medicine department is set-up so that doctors besides clinical knowledge may be made aware of the preventive services to people to keep them informed as to how they can keep themselves healthy. However, in practice, doctors pay scant attention to it. We thought it desirable to write a separate volume on essential matters which community medicine must focus. World Health Organisation has stated that 75 percent diseases are preventable while 25 percent are curative. Still, community medicine department in a hospital is neglected. In order to focus the desired attention of hospital authorities, policy-makers and planners on community health services, we are covering some topics which are basic to good health in the community.

On the one hand developing countries are spending negligible amount on health services while on the other, the money available is allocated to set-up institutions, e.g. hospitals, health centres, etc. What is the impact of all these developments? Spending more and more on curative services neglecting preventive and health education services.

Improvements in the health status of a population cannot be achieved simply by expanding and developing the health services. The prevention and control of disease and the promotion of health require a concerted effort for the improvement of human well-being as a whole. In this task, what has been defined, as "Health Care" has to be supported by improvements in the social and economic infrastructure, and contributions from various sectors other than health.

Certainly there has been a broad understanding of the linkages between health development and development in other sectors. The health experience of the industrialized countries has contributed significantly to this understanding. We know that the major causes of sickness and death arising out of a large cluster of diseases associated with poor sanitation, illiteracy and 10°Y levels of income were effectively controlled in these countries well before the discovery of antibiotics and other spectacular curative "breakthroughs." The control of diarrhoeal diseases, tuberculosis and a wide range of communicable diseases was primarily achieved through far-reaching improvements in the urban infrastructure, housing and environmental sanitation, through the changes in health behaviour which accompanied higher levels of education and literacy, and through the improvement in nutritional status as incomes and living standards steadily rose. The positive outcome in health was, therefore, the result of an intersectoral effort. (See Appendix 1, CHCMI, at the end of the book).

The more recent experiences of a few developing countries illustrate even more dramatically the way in which health forms part of an integrated process of development. These countries have been able to achieve high levels of life expectancy and have shown remarkable progress in reducing infant and maternal mortality and comparatively low levels of income. The state of Kerala, with per capita incomes well below the average for India as a whole, enjoys a health status—as measured by life expectancy, infant mortality and other health indicators—which is well above the rest of India.

Intersectoral linkages which combine increased family income, education, and effective health services targeted to the most high-risk groups can yield positive improvements in health conditions. At the same time, there is a growing awareness that the failure to take account of the implications of macro-economic policies and projects on the environment and on health can have serious negative consequences for national health goals. What Latin America and the Caribbean have learnt from the economic and adjustment crisis is that understanding the nature of intersectoral linkages and promoting mutually productive intersectoral cooperation are not merely desirable; they are essential to the achievement of both Health for all and economic development objectives.

More than ever before, the experts responsible for planning national economies are recognizing that a country's health forms part of an integrated process of development. The experience of the world's industrialized countries showed that diseases associated with poor sanitation, illiteracy and poverty were eventually controlled, not by spectacular medical breakthroughs, but by improvements in urban services, housing and the environment, higher levels of education, and better diets.

The moral for all the world today is that the health sector cannot do it alone! Many other ministries, services, institutions, official and unofficial bodies, and all levels of administration down to the community and the family must become involved in health.

So the drive towards the goal of Health for All by the year 2010 can only be inspired and fuelled by concerted intersectoral action. Our graphic model suggests only the eight elements included in WHO's definition of Primary Health Care: education about health, proper nutrition, safe water and basic sanitation, maternal and child care including family planning, immunization, prevention and control of locally endemic diseases, appropriate treatment of common diseases and injuries, and provision of essential drugs.

But these symbolize a huge range of factors to which other sectors besides health must contribute if all people are indeed to attain a level of health that will permit them to lead a socially and economically productive life. 75 per cent of the diseases are preventable. Inspite of this realization all money is being spent on curative services. In most developing countries the resources available for health care delivery and services are severely limited, often amounting to less than two per cent of the gross national product because other priorities are more demanding or more politically attractive. The tendency, in turn, is for health education to be given a low priority rating in the health care services of those countries, most attention being paid to providing hospital care-and-to a lesser extent-to preventive medicine. It is unfortunately not appreciated that every form of health service should have a relevant health education component.

Thus, if we really want to build effective and efficient health services there is a need of strengthening health education services independently as well as a part of all the health services. Health education can solve a great number of health problems.

High morbidity and high mortality particularly among children result from low priority accorded to health education. Many diseases can be averted if proper education is given to the people. Without the understanding, active cooperation and involvement of all members of the community and a knowledge and motivation on their part of how to obtain the most from the health services provided, whether preventive or curative, much of the time, money and effort invested in these services can be lost.

Dr. H. Mahler is very critical about the inability of health workers in contemporary society to influence those social and environmental factors, which truly determine public health. He states:

"There persist widespread negative attitudes among health professionals towards the health care of the poorest strata in the rural and urban populations in the developing countries. Most of these attitudes imply-with a repetitiveness of an old gramophone record caught in a narrow, arrogant, condescending and indifferent groove that these poor people are too apathetic, too superstitious, too illiterate to benefit form the health care potentially available to them. Health professionals and those who train them should be much more radical in accepting a social responsibility for the health needs of the people in these poor rural and urban communities so that they can act as agents for change."

National Health Policy has also emphasized the importance of health education. The recommended efforts, on various fronts, would bear only marginal results unless nation-wide health education programmes, backed by appropriate communication strategies are launched to provide health information in easily understandable form, to motivate the development of an attitude for healthy living. The public health education programmes should be supplemented by health, nutrition and population education programmes in all educational institutions, at various levels. Simultaneously, efforts would require to be made to promote universal education, specially adult and family education, without which the various efforts to organize preventive and promotive health activities, family planning and improved maternal and child health cannot bear fruit.

The authors are of the view that Health Education should form an integral part of any medical education and training programme for all categories of personnel. The medical and health personnel must be given rigorous training in the art and science of health education, health communication and information, education and communication to develop a first rate health system.

The book "Hospitals in Community Health Care" covers the principles, methods and philosophy of the theory and practice of Community Health Care. Contents reflect the coverage. It is hoped that the book would be useful to academia, researchers, medical practitioners and general public.

Chandigarh

S.L. GOEL
R. KUMAR

Environmental Health

A GOOD ENVIRONMENT IS THE KEY TO HEALTH AND DEVELOPMENT

Environment has been defined by Webster's New Collegiate Dictionary as "the aggregate of all the external conditions and influences affecting the life and development of an organism."

T.N. Chaturvedi in his Editorial to *IJPA*, July-Sept. 1989 (Special Number on Environment and Administration) rightly sees the intimate relationship between human beings and nature since times immemorial. To quote: "Man, since his origin, has lived in harmony with Nature through the ages, holding Nature in awe and reverence. The Vedas, folklore and scriptures of different religions, faiths and beliefs also speak of the need for harmony with the universe, which is the habitat not only of man but also of all animals, birds, insects, plants and vegetation. The mutually supportive role of all living things is often mentioned as a crucial factor for a balanced social and harmonious existence. The ecological balance is inherent in the very process of creation. Everywhere, the seers, poets and thinkers, through the ages, have referred to the need for living in harmony with environment. In fact, the Taitariyopanishad looks at the relationship between man and his environment in its totality and stresses complete harmony and interdependence between them in order to attain real prosperity."[1]

Dr. Hiroshi Nakajima, Director-General of World Health Organisation, sounded a warning alarm about degradation of this planet in his Article "A Wounded Planet."[2] He rightly visualises that it is now increasingly evident that more and more diseases stem from the degradation caused by man to his own environment. The potential harmful effects of industrial development on our global ecosystem are now better known. Ozone layer depletion, acid rain, climate change, chemical pollution are some examples of the man-made wounds to our planet.

Water and Sanitation

Water supply and sanitation are accepted as basic needs. Urban water supply and sanitation are areas critical to the quality of life, people's health and environmental protection. They affect the productivity in the towns and cities which contribute significantly to the national development. While water supply has received greater attention, sanitation has been comparatively neglected. Inadequate sanitation leads to degradation of environment and serious health problems of water-borne and vector-borne diseases. It is, therefore, necessary that both water supply and sanitation are treated together as issues in environmental health.

We are at a turning point; warnings of the damage to our health and quality of life are growing louder. An increasing number of people are acting to stop the degradation of our environment.

Sixty years of Indian Republic especially in the urban areas, are under great stress and strain. The degradation of our environment has to be arrested immediately otherwise it would have long-term impact on the quality of life of future generations. ...We should also take this opportunity to educate our children regarding the importance of the preservation of our environment. Dr. Wilfried Kreisel also elaborates the aspects of environment which affect health of mankind.[3]

"How can we make environmental health a more potent force to serve people faced with growing threats to their health? How can our improving environmental health technology be better used to foster positive health? I know of no country-developing or industrialized in which this issue is not urgent and important. I know of many countries in which it is critical."

The remarkably wide range of environmental concerns include the international problems of acid rain, the greenhouse effect, and depletion of the planet's ozone layer. It includes national concerns with medical wastes disposal, radioactive and toxic wastes control, transportation accidents, health aspects of urbanisation and traffic, occupational health and safety, and air and water pollution. It also includes local concerns over inadequate water supplies and sanitation facilities, water quality, clean air, solid wastes management and finding a balance between the economic incentives of development and a decent quality of life. In the report on Our Common Future, the World Commission on Environment and Development (sometimes called the Brundtland Commission) pointed out that the situation is getting increasingly critical.

WHO, South-East Asia Regional Office Declaration on 'Health and Development in the South-East Asia Region' in the 21st Century mentions that significant differences exist between the environmental problems of rural and urban areas.[4] In rural areas, poverty, unsafe drinking water, inadequate excreta disposal, combined with contaminated food and illiteracy, are responsible for a majority of illnesses. Poor ventilation, coupled with the use of poorly-designed cooking stoves, causes severe indoor air pollution and health problems, particularly in children and infants. With the intensification of agricultural activities large quantities of pesticides and herbicides are being applied without taking adequate precautionary measures. (See Appendix 4, Village Health and Sanitation Committees).

In urban areas, on the other hand, environmental problems are the result of rapid and massive population migration from rural to urban areas and of uncontrolled industrialization. Municipal services are unable to keep pace with the urban growth, like providing adequate water supplies, sewerage and sanitation. Overcrowding, inadequate housing with poor ventilation and absence of protection against rain, heat and cold add to the stresses and dangers of urban living. Industries are often located in and around urban areas with uncontrolled disposal of wastes. The Bhopal gas tragedy in India over a decade ago is an example.

Of course, there are other major environmental concerns such as deforestation, global warming, ozone depletion, cross-border movements of hazardous products and other forms of environmental degradation. Protection of the environment and of health endangered by environmental hazards comprises a very large and important international public policy agenda. In developing countries the problems are doubly difficult because of the immediacy of local environmental threats as well as the larger regional and global issues.

ENVIRONMENTAL ADMINISTRATION IN INDIA: GENESIS, GROWTH AND LEGAL FRAMEWORK

As stated in India 1999 — A Reference Manual published by Ministry of Information and Broadcasting, in the beginning of the Fourth Five Year Plan, problems and issues centred around environment, this resulted in the establishment of the National Council of Environmental Planning and Coordination in 1972 at The Department of Science and Technology. Another empowered Committee as set-up in 1980 for reviewing the existing legislative measures and administrative machinery for ensuring environmental protection and for recommending ways to strengthen them. On the recommendations of this empowered committee, a separate Department of Environment was set-up in 1980 which was subsequently upgraded in a full-fledged Ministry of Environment and Forests in 1985 to serve as the focal point in the administrative structure of the Government of India for the planning, promotion and coordination of environmental and forestry programmes. The state department of environment, Central and State Pollution Control Boards, the Botanical and Zoological Survey of India. the Forest Survey of India, the National River Conservation Authority (formerly Central Ganga Authority), the National Afforestation and Eco-development Board, the Indian Council for Forestry Research and Education, the Wildlife Institute of India, the National Museum for Natural history, etc. are the Ministry's partners in carrying out environmental protection activities.

Prevention and Control of Pollution

The policy statement on Abatement of Pollution, adopted in 1992. provides instruments in the form of legislation and regulation. Fiscal incentives, voluntary agreements, educational programmes and information campaigns to prevent and control pollution of water. Air and land, since the adoption of the policy statement, the focus of activities has been on issues such as promotion of clean and low waste technologies, waste minimization, reuse/recycling, improvement of water quality, environment audit, natural resource accounting, development of mass-based standards, institutional and human resource development, etc. The whole issue of pollution prevention and control is dealt with by a combination of command and control methods as well as voluntary and regulatory, fiscal measures, promotion of awareness and involvement of public.

Central Pollution Control Board

The Central Pollution Control Board (CPCB) is the national apex body for assessment, monitoring and control of water and air pollution. The executive responsibilities for enforcement of the Acts for Prevention and Control of Pollution of Water (1974) and Air (1981) and also of the Water (Cess) Act, 1977 are carried out through the Board. The CPCB advises the Central Government on all matters concerning the prevention and control of air, water and noise pollution and provides technical services to the Ministry for implementing the provisions of the Environment (Protection) Act, 1986. Under the Act, effluent and emission standards in respect of 61 categories of industries have been notified.

Education, Awareness and Information

Priority is accorded by the Ministry of Environment and Forests to promote environmental education, create environmental awareness among various age-groups and to disseminate information through Environmental Information System (ENVIS) network to all concerned. Special emphasis is given to non-formal environmental education through seminars/symposia/ workshops, training programmes, eco-camps, audio-visual shows, etc. The Ministry has been organising a National Environment Awareness Campaign (NEAC) since July 1980. As a part of this campaign, 19 November to 18 December every year is observed as the National Environment Month. The main themes for the 1997-98 campaign were Pollution Prevention and Control, and Conservation and Plantation of Trees for Environmental Protection. A large number of organisations have been granted financial assistance by the Ministry to organise various activities for creating environmental awareness. The Ministry also provides financial support for setting up eco-clubs at schools and for production of films on environment.

A new scheme, Paryavaran Vahini, was launched in 1992-93 to create environmental awareness and to ensure active public participation by involving the local people in activities relating to environmental protection.

Paryavaran Vahinis are proposed to be constituted in 194 selected districts all over the country which have a high incidence of pollution and density of tribal and forest population. The Vahinis also play a watch-dog role by reporting instance of environmental pollution, deforestation, poaching, etc. They function under the charge of District Collectors, with the active cooperation of the State/Union Territory governments. This scheme is entirely financed by the Ministry of Environment and Forests.

International Cooperation

The Ministry of Environment and Forests functions as a nodal agency for United Nations Environment Programme (UNEP), South Asia Cooperation Environment Programme (SACEP) and International Centre for Integrated Mountain and Development (ICIMOD), International Union for Conservation of Nature and Natural Resources (IUCN) and various international agencies, regional bodies and multilateral institutions.

India is signatory to the following important international treaties/ agreements in the field of environment: (i) International Convention for the regulation of Whaling, (ii) International Plant Protection Convention, (iii) The Antarctic Treaty, (iv) Convention on Wetlands of international importance, (v) International Convention on International trade in endangered species of wild flora and fauna; (vi) Protocol of 1978 relating to the international convention for the prevention of pollution from ships, (vii) Vienna Convention for the protection of the ozone layer; (viii) Convention on Migratory Species; (ix) Basel Convention on trans-boundary movement of hazardous substances; (x) Framework convention of climate change; (xi) Convention on conservation of biodiversity; (xii) Montreal protocol on the substances that deplete the ozone layer; and (xiii) International Convention for Combating Desertification.

Environmental Legislation

Major legislations directly dealing with the protection of environment are the Wildlife (Protection) Act, 1972, the Forest (Conservation) Act, 1980, the Water (Prevention and Control of Pollution) Act, 1974, the Water (Cess) Act, 1977, the National Environment Appellate Authority Act, 1977, the Air (Prevention and Control of Pollution) Act, 1981, the Environment (Protection) Act, 1986, the Public Liability Insurance Act, 1991 and the National Environment Tribunal Act, 1995. The Constitution (Forty-second Amendment Act of 1976) gave Parliament the power to enact laws on virtually any entry in the State list, and through Article 253 brought environmental regulation under the Concurrent List.

India has increasingly institutionalized its environment concern after the United Nations conference on Human Environment at Stockholm in 1972, to serve as a guideline to the governments, both Central and State, Article l48A was added to the Directive Principles of State Policy in 1976, which said, "The state shall endeavour to protect and improve environment and safeguard the forests and wildlife of the country." In a new chapter entitled 'Fundamental Duties', Article (51Ag) imposed a similar responsibility on every citizen to protect and improve the natural environment including forests lakes, rivers and wildlife and to have compassion for living creatures. Supreme Court of India has held whenever a problem of ecology is brought before the Court, the Court is bound to bear in mind Art. 48A of the Constitution.

ENVIRONMENT VIS-A-VIS DEVELOPMENT

Nature and Scope of Environmental Health Programme

Meaning

Environmental health refers to the ecological balance that must exist between man and his environment in order to ensure his well being. The deterioration of the human environment through the population explosion, pollution of air and water, and other disruptions of the ecological balance pose a major international health hazard and a serious challenge. Professor J. Logan, in a paper published in *American Journal of Tropical Medicine* in 1960, was able to show that environmentally transmitted diseases were responsible for the sufferings of 500 million people every year particularly among infants and children.[5] The UN Secretary-General's report on problem of the human environment sounds a similar ominous note: "If current trends continue, the failure of life on earth could be engendered and thus, it is urgent to focus world attention on these problems which threaten humanity in an environment that permits the realisation of the highest human aspirations."[6]

The close relationship that exists between an unhealthy Environment and the economic condition of a community was pinpointed by a panel of experts which met in 1971 to discuss the environmental problems of the developing countries. "Poverty and the very lack of development", these experts said, "constitute an essential environmental problem in the developing countries. They recommended an attack on the problems of inadequate water supply, poor housing, sanitation, nutrition and widespread disease as prime targets in an effort to improve the environment of millions of people, and to lay the groundwork for their economic betterment."[7]

Ninth Five Year Plan (Draft) also warns about the bad consequences of poor environment on Health. Environment can allot human health in many ways. Deficiency of iodine in soil, water and foodstuffs is the cause of iodine deficiency disorders. Excessive fluoride content in the water is the cause of fluorosis. Environmental degradation may affect air, land and water. Pollutants may enter the food chain. All these may enter human body through various portals and affect the health status. Rapidly growing population, urbanisation, changing agricultural, industrial and water resource management, increasing use of pesticides and fossil fuels have all resulted in a perceptible deterioration in the quality of environment and attendant adverse health consequences. Environment pollution due to developmental activities are increasingly becoming the focus of concern. The interactive interdependence of health, environment and sustainable development was accepted as the fulcrum of action under Agenda 21 at the Earth Summit in Brazil in 1992. Environmental health in its broader perspective would have to address the detection, prevention and management of:

(i) existing deficiencies or excesses of certain elements in natural environment;
(ii) macro-environmental contamination of air, land, water and food; and
(iii) disaster management,

Aspects of Environmental Health

The environment can be defined as an aggregate of all the external conditions and influences affecting the life and development of an organism. Human Environment means everything that is experienced by man and it is the total nature of this experience that determinesthe quality of life. According to Roggers, "the environment appears to possess two main avenues by which it may reach man and affect man health; it may act upon his body as a material agent or it may act upon his mind and emotions as non-material agent, although sooner or later this may very well produce a material effect.[8] The effect of both is the pollution of environment. Prof. Samuel Halter, Professor of Public Health at the University of Brussels defines pollution as "the presence in the ambient environment of chemical. physical or biological factors capable of inducing disturbances in the normal physiology and functioning of human organs.[9]

We can classify the environmental factors impinging on the health of the people as follows:

(a) Physical, Chemical and Biological factors.
(b) Social, Economic and Cultural factors.
(c) Ecological, Economic and Aesthetic factors.
(d) Individual human system.

All these agents in the environment interact with one another and produce the favourable or unfavourable impact on the health of the people.

MEANING AND ROLE OF ENVIRONMENTAL HEALTH ADMINISTRATION

Environmental Sanitation Administration is an activity of diagnosing and controlling the environmental factors which exercise or may exercise a deleterious and unhealthy effect on the physical, social, and mental life of the people. The Draft Five-Year Plan (1978-83) has rightly mentioned: "The

Chart 1.1

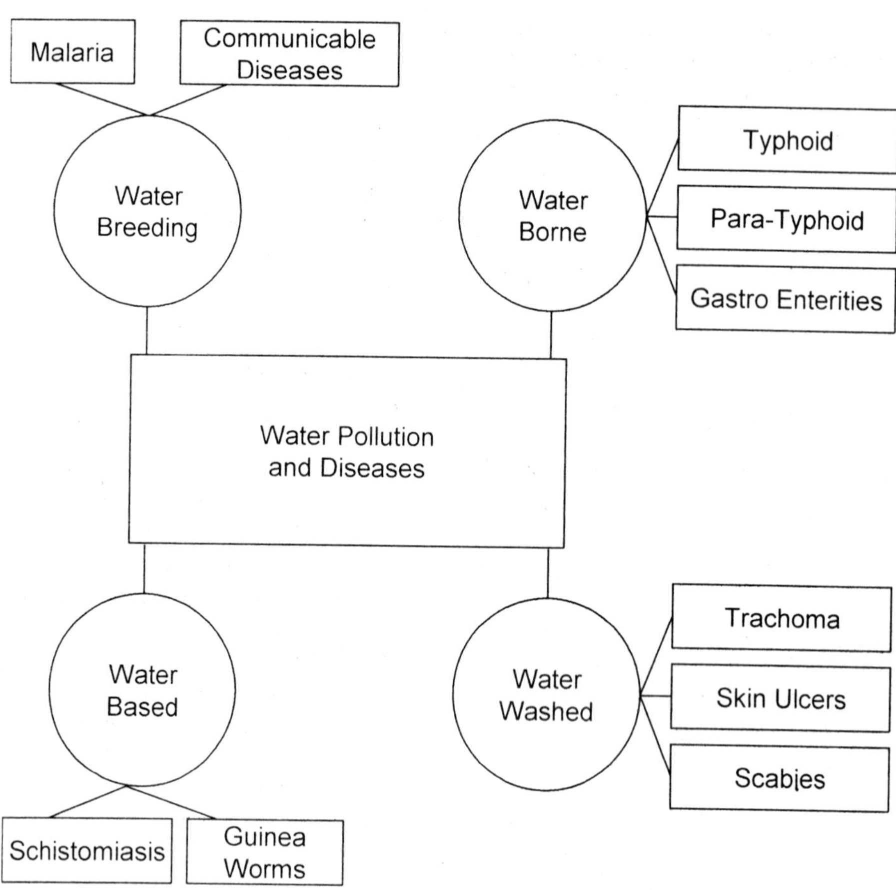

essence of sound environmental growth lies in a happy blend of the realisation of the physical out limits to the exploitation of environmental resources and the inner limits to human needs and aspiration.[10] Environmental health administration is quite complex and complicated owing to the complexity and diversity of the socio-political and institutional arrangements in which the programmes are implemented and the complexity, multiplicity of the physical, biological, social and economic factors that they must take into account. The objective of the environmental sanitation administration is to plan thoroughly to change favourably the environment itself and modify the interaction of human beings with the environment so that the people can enjoy a good quality of life. The administration of environmental programme is not within the purview of any single discipline but presents a challenge to many disciplines. The administrators responsible for such programmes must plan to attack the unfavourable factors in concert with one another. We may mention some of

CHART 1.2

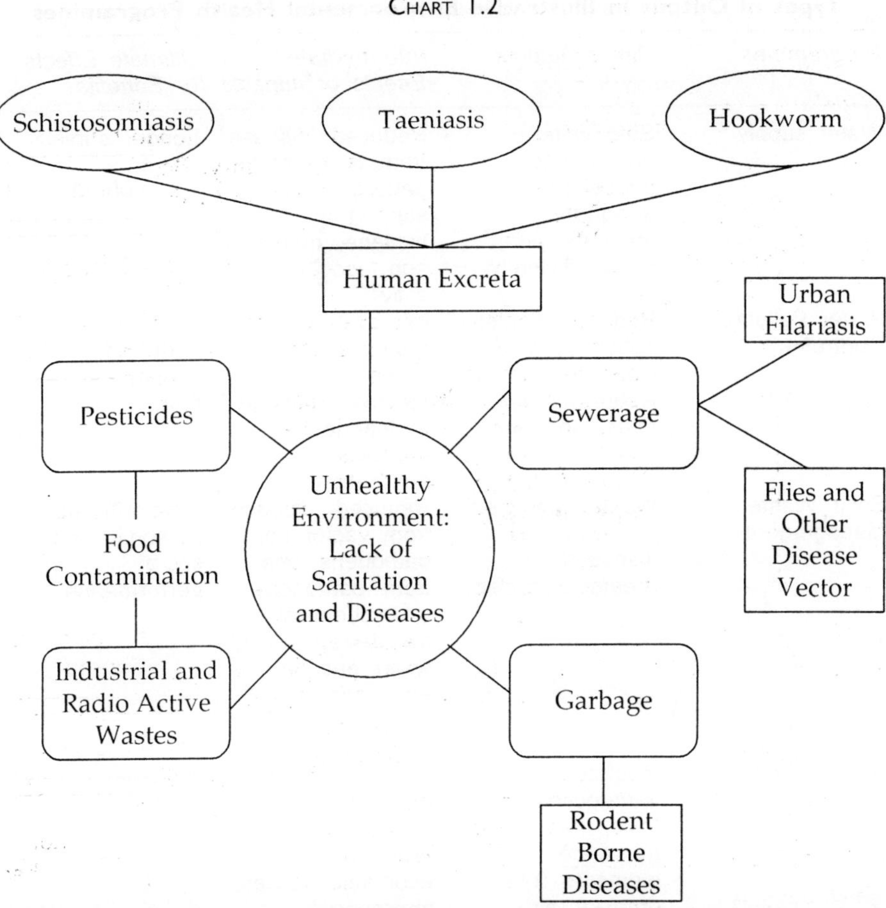

the important areas which need the immediate attention of the planners, policy-makers and administrators to solve these impending problems—potable safe water supply and water pollution, solid wastes management. air pollution control, occupational health, food, sanitation, urban planning and housing, slum clearance, soil erosion, noise pollution., etc. The administration must define in the geographical context the magnitude of each problem, its relationship with others and the benefits expected. direct outputs, intermediate effects or impacts and the ultimate effects or benefits. Some of these have been indicated in the form of a Chart (see Chart 1.2). The administration of environmental health programmes are very expensive and complicated. In order to translate the benefits of such programmes to the society, the administrators must ensure that the progmmme:

(a) receives acceptance and support;
(b) achieves the desired objectives and results;
(c) links its efforts with those of other health and socio-economic development programmes; and

Types of Output in Illustrative Environmental Health Programmes

Programmes	*Direct Outputs*	*Intermediate Effects or Impacts*	*Ultimate Effects or Benefits*
Water supply	Safe water provided to households in adequate amounts and used efficiently	Reduced disease from water borne pathogens; support to hygiene, nutrition and economic activity	Longer survival
Water Pollution Control	Reduced contamination of (used water returned to) watercourses, seas, soil and food	Improved water resources for human use; reduced damage to marine life; improved aesthetics	Less disability, suffering impairment and pain
Solid Wastes Management	Wastes confined, removed and disposed of (treated recycled)	Reduced disease from vector borne pathogens and from pathogens and chemicals transferred to air, water and land; economic gains; improved aesthetics	More efficient personal and social performance
Air Pollution Control	Reduced introduction of toxic, irritant and nuisance elements into ambient air	Reduced death, disease and discomfort; reduced economic losses; improved aesthetics	Improved quality of life
Occupational Health	Reduced physical/chemical hazards in work environment, through primary and secondary disease prevention services	Reduced illness, trauma and poisoning; safer work environment; improved working conditions and productivity	Socio-economic development
Food Sanitation	Food safeguarded against contamination in production, processing, delivery, preparation and consumption	Reduced disease and death from pathogens and toxins in food; enlarged markets; improved aesthetics	

Source: WHO: Public Health Paper, No. 59, p. 113.

(d) accomplishes its work economically, with a minimum waste of money and other scarce resources.[11]

We may now take up two important aspects of environment, i.e. water supply and sanitation which affect health development in a big way.

Environment Health Promotes Public Health which is defined as follows:

Public health is one of the efforts organized by society to protect, promote and restore people's health. It is the combination of services, skills and beliefs that are directed to the maintenance and improvement of the health of all people through collective or social actions. The programmes, services and institutions involved emphasize the prevention of disease and the health needs of the population as a whole. Public health activities change with changing technology and social values, but the goals remain the same; to reduce the amount of disease, premature death and disease produced discomfort and disability in the population. (J.M. Last, 1983).[12]

Water Supply and Sanitation

Safe water and improved sanitation are a necessary condition for better health. and there can be no lasting improvement of public health without them. There is no denying the fact that inadequacy of sate drinking water. improper disposal of human excreta. solid and liquid wastes leading to unfavourable environmental condition have been the causes of many killer diseases.

Water is variously considered as life giving, life sustaining, purifying, a vital nutrient and essential for life. However, it can also spread disease and kill. Predictions are that drinking water is becoming a scarcer commodity. With ground water being used faster than it can be recharged, shortage of drinking water is likely to become an important problem in the future. Fifity percent of infant deaths are attributed to waterborne diseases. An estimated 1.5 million under five deaths occur in India every year, due to water related diseases, and approximately 1800 million person hours are lost annually in the country, due to same. It is estimated that poor quality and inadequate quantity of water accounts for about 10% of the total burden of disease in developing country situations, as in Karnataka state.[13]

M. Aktar has stated that inadequacy in the availability of safe drinking water, unfavourable environmental conditions and lack of personal hygiene have been the major causes of disease and disability among people. As per WHO statistics, 80 per cent of diseases in the developing countries are related to unsafe water supply and inadequate sanitation causing high child mortality, low life expectancy and poor quality of life. In India, more than one million children below 5 years die from dehydration caused by diarrhoea annually, while another 250 thousand are victims of tetanus. Poliomyelitis has been a cause of lameness among 170 thousand children per year. There is also a very high rate of occurrence of intestinal worms, particularly in West Bengal, Bihar, Orissa,

Andhra Pradesh, Tamil Nadu, Kerala and Maharashtra. The national goal to reduce child mortality from 146 per thousand to 125 by 1995 and 70 per thousand by 2000 cannot possibly be achieved without a significant change in the existing mortality/morbidity related to water and sanitation. Also important is to change the peoples' perception about the link between sanitation and health. According to a recent KAP survey in the country, 37 per cent people do not know/do not believe that exposed excreta can harm health. Outdoor defecation is not generally seen as a problem except in terms of inconvenience during rain night or winter and to women.

Y.N. Nanjudiah has stated that majority of the rural people practice open air defecation as the coverage of sanitation facilities has reached only a negligible population. For want of awareness on health on the part of users quite a large number of latrines are out of use or misused. Further, open air defection generally enjoys social acceptability. It is considered hygiene and wholesome and in tune with the nature and fresh air. At the same time toilet has a poor image. It is believed to be dirty and a breeding place for flies and mosquitoes. Social surveys carried out so far have highlighted that there is lack of knowledge regarding latrine, which can be summarised as under:

(a) Faecal-borne diseases can be prevented by using a latrine.
(b) Pathogenic microbes survive from days to years in the moist soil and may become wind borne.
(c) Social status and prestige can be attained by having a latrine.
(d) Constipation, particularly among rural women can be eliminated.
(e) Privacy can be achieved.
(f) Low cost sanitation options are available, and these can be maintained in an eco-friendly way.

Dr. H. Mahler, former WHO, Director-General, has rightly said that, "I am utterly convinced that the number of water taps per 1,000 population will be an infinitely more meaningful health indicator than the number of hospital beds per 1,000 population" Mr. Kurt Waldhelm, former UN Secretary-General also stressed that, the provision of safe water and sanitation does not merely mean happier, healthier citizens; it also means increased economic productivity. Nikolas P. Napulbow in his editorial "Water For All, a Human Right" has rightly said that, "water is a basic human need for health—indeed, for survival-and therefore it is not an exaggeration to call it one of the basic human rights. Without safe water and sanitation, there is no real development. A community ravaged by diarrheal diseases, dracunculiasis or schistosomiasis cannot look beyond its immediate problems towards social and economic welfare. Safe water is the doorway to health and health is the prerequisite for progress, social equity and human divinity."[14]

Infectious diseases resulting from water pollution can be classified into four groups, depending upon the ways in which their incidence can be lessened by improvements in water supply.

(1) "Water-borne" diseases are those in which infectious agent remains alive in drinking water, e.g. typhoid, paratyphoid, gastroenterities, etc. The incidence of these diseases can be reduced by the purification of water.

(2) "Water-washed" diseases include infection of the outer body surface, e.g., trachoma, skin ulcers, scabies and typhus, bacillary and amoebic dysentery and gastro enterities. The incidence can be reduced by augmenting water quantity.

(3) "Water-based" infections, i.e. schistosomiasis, guinea worms. The infection occurs when the skin is in contact with water or through drinking water.

(4) "Water breeding" or water promixity diseases are caused by mosquitoes or flies living near aquatic conditions.

The group of disease, in (1) called the faecal oral group are transmitted from person to person through water or food via the oral route. Breaking the faecal-oral route forms the basis for public health intervention for disease control. This is through a combination of good personal hygiene, increased water quantity, improved water quality, food hygiene and provision of sanitary facilties.[15]

There is probably no single factor that has a greater effect on the health, well-being and development of a community than the provision of ample and convenient supply of wholesome and good quality water. In towns and cities water supply is recognised as a basic necessity for industrial and commercial purposes; it is vital for the maintenance of public health and the prevention of epidemics. Dame Barbara Ward, President of the International Institute for Environment and Development, rightly observes that, "Water is everywhere, the key to human health. .... clean water is a key to human comfort, health and even survival."[16] Martin Boyer, Adviser, Drinking Water Programme, UNICEF has observed that "The provision of ample supplies of safe water and the sanitary disposal of excreta have a direct and far-reaching effect upon the health and well-being of rural populations. Indeed, it is believed that no other single measure can make a comparable contribution to the improvement of their health and standard of living. The choice of an appropriate technology depends on local conditions."[17] To quote WHO: "One hospital bed out of four in the world is occupied by a patient who is ill because of polluted water. Provisions of a safe and convenient water supply is the single most important activity that could be undertaken to improve the health of people living in rural areas of the developing world."

Kofi Annam, United Nations Secretary General says that the centrality of freshwater in our lives cannot be overestimated. Water has been a major factor in the rise and fall of civilizations. It has been a source of tensions and fierce competition between nations that could become even worse if present trends continue. Lack of access to water for meeting basic needs such as health, hygiene and food security undermines development and inflicts enormous hardship on more than a billion members of the human family. And its quality reveals everything, right or wrong, that we do in safeguarding the global environment.[18]

WHO estimates that as much as 80 percent of all diseases in the world are associated with water, Iain Guest (Geneva), a specialist in development topics submits that an astonishing number of people suffer from these water related diseases at any time, 400 million with gastro enterities, 160 million with malaria, 30 million with river blindness, 200 million with Schistosomiasis.[19] At the 1969 World Health Assembly, a delegate from the region (SEA) estimated that water-borne diseases accounted for 40 percent of all morality, and 60 percent of all morbidity in his country.[20]

I.V. Rajeshwar, ex-Governor of West Bengal in his article, "Endemic Problems defying solution" in *The Daily Tribune*, dated January 16, 2000 rightly says that Fifty-two years after independence even basic amenities like drinking water supply and unpolluted air are not available to most citizens. At present, water supply is available to 84.33% of urban population and 76.68% to rural population. However sanitation coverage is 49.91 in urban areas and 14.02 to rural areas.

Ninth Plan finds that the existing norms for rural water supply is 40 liters of drinking water per capita per day (LPCD) and a public stand post or a hand pump for 250 persons. Further, the sources of water supply should be within 1.6 km. horizontal distance in plains or 100 metres elevation distance in hills. For cattle in Desert and Drought Prone (DDP) areas, an additional 30 LPCD is recommended. Against this, the norm for urban water supply is 125 LPCD piped water supply with sewerage system, 70 LPCD without sewerage system and 40 LPCD in towns with spot sources. At least one source for 20 families within a maximum distance of 100 metres has been laid down.

As against these norms, the studies as on 1.4.1997 reveal that there were 61,724 habitations without any safe source of drinking water (called not covered habitation), 3.78 lakh habitations which were partially covered and 1.51 lakh habitations which had quality problems like excess fluoride, salinity, iron and arsenic, etc. Apart from the provision in the state plans for water supply, there are major Centrally Sponsored Schemes called the Accelerated Rural Water Supply Programme and the Urban Water Supply Programme for small towns with population of less than 20,000. In order to cover this backlog in rural drinking water supply, it has been estimated that approximately Rs. 40,000 crore will be required including the funds enquired for operations and maintenance and funds to tackle quality problems. Similarly, the estimates of investment required for full coverage of urban water supply is Rs. 30,734 crore.

Drinking water and sanitation improvements could reduce the overall incidence of infant and child diarrhoea by one quarter and cut total infant and child mortality by more than one-half. Country programmes are increasingly taking measures to improve water supply and sanitation within their primary health care programmes. Giuinea worm disease can be effectively prevented by providing safe drinking water and its global eradication is clearly possible within the next few years. As for schistosomiasis, some 60% reduction could be achieved by improving water supplies. Building latrines, giving health education and introducing selected drug therapy could reduce the prevalence even more.[21]

A great surge in the population of India's big cities, poses hug problems for safeguarding water supplied.

We suggest here the methods of conserving water supply:

- Integration of water and waste water management, coupled with health education for cost-effectiveness and promotion of preventive measures for health;
- Prospecting for water resources through state of the art techniques of remote sensing and geophysical surveys;
- Protection of water sources against pollution;
- Decentralization of water supply matching the required quality and quantity through waste recycle and reuse;
- Maintenance of the water distribution system. which can prevent up to 50% of the purified waste water from being lost; and
- Application of mathematical programming techniques with exact fluid flow relationships in the design of water and waste water systems. so as to ensure functionality and to conserve material and financial resources.

Lack of sanitation causes many diseases related to human excreta, sewerage disposal. Garbage and the use of pesticides and the industrial and radio active wastes. (See Chart 1.2). Following the suspected plague outbreak in the country during 1994 the Planning Commission constituted a High Power Committee on Urban Solid Waste Management in India under the Chairmanship of Member (Health). This committee undertake a comprehensive review of current situation of urban solid waste management. specially in cities with one million or more inhabitants and made recommendations for safe methods for collection, transportation of waste and suitable cost-effective. environmentally friendly methods for disposal of these wastes. Pilot projects exploring the dimensions of the problem and aimed at seeking realistic solutions were initiated during the Eighth Plan period. During the Ninth Plan period it is expected that many more cities will initiate programmes for the efficient methods of management of wastes generated and improve environmental sanitation.

In the Johannesburg Earth Summit it has been agreed to halve, by the year 2015 the proportion of people who do not have access to basic sanitation, which would include action at all levels to develop and implement efficient household sanitation systems, improve sanitation in public institutions, especially schools, promote affordable and socially and culturally acceptable technologies and practices, promote safe hygiene practices and integrate sanitation into water resources management strategies.

Sanitation is a broad term that includes disposal of human excreta, wastewater, solid wastes, domestic and personal hygiene, etc. Human excreta is the cause of many enteric diseases such as cholera, diarrhea, dysentery, typhoid, infectious heptatitis, and those based on worm infestation, etc. Studies reveal that over 50 infections can be transmitted from diseased persons to healthy ones by various direct/indirect routes from human excreta that cause nearly 80% of sickness in developing countries.

The health implications of this state of affairs as said are appalling. Improved hygiene and sanitation help reduce sickness from diarrhea considerably. Intestinal worms infect about 10% of the population of developing countries that can be controlled through better sanitation, hygiene and water supply. As per the WHO report globally 200 million people are infected with schistosomiasis, of whom 20 million suffer seriously. Basic sanitation facilities reduce the disease by up to 77%. Sanitation facilities help check transmission of many feacal oral disease by preventing human excreta contamination of water and soil. [22]

So far, the major focus has been on communicable disease burden due to poor environmental sanitation in urban areas and due to improper disposal of human excreta, garbage and waste water in rural areas and methods to tackle these. These efforts will be intensified during the Ninth Plan. In addition. efforts to reduce pollution and related non-communicable disease burden will also be strengthened. Efforts will be made to document the extent of the problem of environmental pollution and its impact on health status of the population through linkages between existing environmental monitoring data and data on health status of population living in these areas. Prevention and management of health consequences of environmental deterioration will receive increasing attention.

The Expert Committee on Public Health System had noted that major developmental activities in any field such as agriculture, industries, urban and rural development may result in environment changes which could have adverse health implications and recommended that health impact assessment may become a part of environmental impact assessment of all large developmental projects. The feasibility of making appropriate provision for health care of people involved in developmental activities and prevention and management of health consequences of developmental activities on the population living in vicinity of the project as a part of the project budget will be explored.[23]

Brian Appleton in his article, "Seven out of ten for Efforts" in the *World Health*, June 1988 clearly mentions that donors have agreed to collaborate globally and within individual developing countries, to ensure that water supply and sanitation programmes which receive external funding or technical assistance are based on the accepted Decade Approaches, namely:

- Complementary in developing water supply and sanitation;
- Strategies giving precedence to under-served rural and urban populations;
- Programmes promoting self-reliant, self-sustained actions;
- Community involvement in all stages of project implementation;
- Socially relevant systems that people can afford, using technologies appropriate to specific projects; and
- Association of water supply and sanitation with relevant programmes in other sectors, particularly with primary health care, concentrating on hygiene education, human resource development, and the strengthening of institutional performance.

Lori L. Heise in his article "Violence Against Women" in the *World Health*, Jan. 1993 clearly mentions that Seldom seen as a public health issue, violence against women is a significant cause of female morbidity and mortality around the globe. In the USA, for example, wife abuse is the leading cause of injury among women of reproductive age. Between 22% and 35% of women who visit United States emergency clinics are there for symptoms related to on-going abuse. But women in the USA share the reality of violence with women in virtually every other culture in the world. Data from developing countries reveal that one-third to over half of women surveyed report being beaten by their partner. Not uncommonly, beatings are part of a pattern of emotional and physical abuse that escalates over time. In Papua New Guina, 18% of all urban wives surveyed had sought hospital treatment for injuries inflicted by their husbands. A survey of one Caribbean island revealed that one in three women had been sexually abused as a child.

Wife abuse also provides the primary context for many other health problems. Again, research from the USA indicates that battered women are four to five times more likely to require physchiatric treatment and five times more likely to attempt suicide than non-battered women. And they are at increased risk of alcohol abuse, drug dependence, chronic pain, and depression. In one US study of the use made of health care, a history of rape and/or assault was a stronger predictor of physician visits and outpatients costs than were a women's age or other health risks such as smoking. Along with physical injury and emotional trauma, rape survivors run the risk of becoming pregnant or contracting sexually transmitted diseases including AIDS.

Violence poses a powerful obstacle to achieving other goals that are high on the development agenda. During pregnancy, for example, it threatens the goal of "Safe motherhood" for all women. Battered women run twice the risk of miscarriage and four times the risk of having a low-birth-weight infant.

Occupational Health (see separate chapter)

WHO recently proposed a global plan of action on workers' health 2008-17. The plan envisages development of a comprehensive approach to workers' health. Workers' health is determined by numerous factors, e.g. physical, chemical and biochemical exposures within the work premises. There are other factors, such as social determinants of health (e.g. occupational status, employment conditions, income, inequalities in gender, race, age and residence). Individual behaviour (e.g. individual risk-taking behaviour, physical exercise, sedentary work, diet and nutrition and unhealthy habits such as smoking and alcohol) influence the health of workers. Besides the above mentioned factors, access to health services is also important.[24]

Climate Change and Human Health

Over the last 100 years, human activities, particularly related to burning of fossils fuels, have released sufficient quantities of carbon dioxide (CO_2) and other greenhouse gases to affect the global climate. The atmospheric concentration of CO_2 has increased by more than 30% since pre-industrial times, trapping more heat in the lower atmosphere.

As a follow-up of the 2005 Mukteshwar, India workshop, the Regional Office continued to create awareness and stress the urgent need to address climate change issues at various WHO-sponsored seminars and workshops attended by health professionals. It is recommending to:

- Assess the national health sector's response;
- Strengthen the response capacity of the health sector by preparing for medical emergency response;
- Strengthen public health systems aimed at controlling vector-borne and water-borne diseases;
- Set-up an early warning sub-system by coordinating disease surveillance and climate monitoring activities;
- Reduce the risks of vector-borne and water-borne diseases by engaging and empowering local communities to implement integrated pest and vector management and to safeguard drinking water sources; and
- Raise stakeholder engagement by advocating and creating awareness, notably at the level of local communities.

Food Safety

- The Health Department must review and revise the regulations and legislative measures governing food safety. Regulations must include all food serving facilities including street vending. They must check and prevent adulteration and contamination of foods at various stages of production, processing, storage, transport and distribution.

- The Health Department should develop guidelines for the health check-up and immunization of food handlers against typhoid fever and hepatitis A.
- Control measures recommended include, training and certification of food handlers in restaurants, hostels, hotels, etc.
- Personal hygiene, adequate cooking of food—this needs to be part of the health promotion package for children, women and public in general. [25]

Chemical Safety

The headlong expansion of science and technology is constantly providing human society and the environment with more and more new substances. Different molecules are being created, tested, discarded or commercialized according to their usefulness or economic advantage. But little or no attention is being paid to the consequent risks for human or environmental health.

It is neither practical not economically feasible to evaluate the short and long-term effects of the vast number of chemicals which are being invented and re-invented! The objectives of this dynamic creativity are usually beneficial: to protect crops, to increase food stocks, to simplify household chores, to protect our health and hygiene. But . . . are all those new chemicals really indispensable? Does mankind really need to be swamped by so many new chemical compounds?

What used to be "chemical development"—the production of highly useful pharmaceuticals, anilines, antiseptics and pesticides—turned into a "chemical revolution", and is now on the way to becoming "chemical chaos." Too many substances and compounds are entering our homes, our working place, our environment and our bodies without our really knowing their risks and benefits, without a true evaluation of their usefulness and—worse still-without complete studies of their harmlessness for other forms of life.

Examples of the poisonings and chemical disasters that have resulted are legion. It took many years to realize that industrial and domestic use of flurochlorocarbon propellants in aerosols were contributing to the depletion of the ozone layer, with all its environmental consequences. Prolonged use of asbestos fibers have caused malignant measotheliomas (tumours) in exposed workers, Clinical studies of patients who took high doses of analgesics shows that certain renal insufficiencies were due to those apparently innocuous pharmaceuticals. All too late did medicine link. The drug thalidomide was responsible for the birth of children with deformed arms and legs. And the indiscriminate use of pesticides is still causing a high toll of Morbidity and mortality in some rural areas of developing countries. Long-term "hidden" tragedies such as Mina-mata disease in Japan or explosive chemical disasters such as Bhopal in India are other examples where a large human group falls victim to uncontrolled chemicals.

In the intervening night of 2nd/3rd Dec. 1984, a lethal gas known as Methyl iso-Cyanate (MIC) stored in the tank of the Union Carbibe pesticide factory at Bhopal escaped suddenly into the atmosphere causing death and injury to a large number of people of the Bhopal City. The leakage of gas occurred between 12.45 a.m. to 1.30 p.m. By 6.30 a.m. the entire area was clear. But by then, massive damage and suffering had been inflicted. More than 800 persons died during the first three days of the incident. Subsequently, the casualty figure rose to more than 7000.

GUIDING PRINCIPLES FOR AVOIDING CHEMICALS POLLUTION

The guiding principles of responsible care are:

- To recognize and respond to community concerns about chemicals and the operations.
- To develop and produce chemicals that can be manufactures, transported, used and disposed of safely.
- To make health, safety and environmental consideration a priority in planning for all existing and new products and processes.
- To report promptly to officials, employees, customers and the public information on chemical-related health or environmental hazards and recommend protective measures.
- To counsel customers on the safe use, transportation and disposal of chemical products.
- To operate the plants and facilities in a manner that protects the environment health and safety of employees and public.
- To extend knowledge by conducting or supporting research of the health, safety environmental effects of the products, processes and waste materials.
- To work with others to resolve problems created by past handling and disposal of hazardous substances.
- To participate with government and other in creating responsible laws, regulations and standards to safeguard community, work place and environment.
- To promote the principles and practices of responsible care by sharing experience and offering assistance to others who produce, handly use, transport or dispose-off chemicals.

Among the measures to prevent acute and chronic poisoning and environment damage by pesticides that should urgently be taken by developing countries are:

- Good agricultural practice and integrated pest control;
- Manpower development in chemical safety—including training in clinical, occupational, analytical, experimental, predictive and regulatory toxicology;
- Risk assessment toxicological surveillance programmes;
- Reliable statistics system on mortality and morbidity data related to pesticide poisoning;
- Monitoring analyses of pesticide residues in staple food, in the environment, and in human biological samples;
- Restricted use of highly toxic and persistent pesticides;
- Multi-level courses on safe use of pesticides;
- Certified operators, periodically, trained, and responsible for the acquisition and safe use of pesticides;
- Enforcement of the legislation;
- Intensive effort to reduce illiteracy among rural workers; and
- Establishment of an Interdisciplinary National Committee on Pesticides, acting as an advisory body to the Ministries of Health, Agriculture, Labour and Environment.[26]

Hospital Waste Management

Prof. K.J. Nath in his article Hospital wastes have always been considered as potentially hazardous. The major identified hazard was that of infection, because over millennia, communicable diseases had been the most common use of morbidity and mortality in the community and majority of persons receiving treatment in the hospitals were suffering from communicable diseases. Until the second half of the present century, there was due emphasis on safe collection, storage and disposal at site to minimize, if not eliminate, the health hazard associated with hospital waste. The advent of antibiotics led to complacency regarding infection control and safe disposal of hospital waste. This has resulted in increased risk of infection in health care setting both to the seekers and providers of health care. The rising prevalence of HBV and HIV infection in the community and among health care providers has led to an increasing awareness about the risks associated with this lackadaisical practice and the need to evolve and implement strategies for safe and sustainable methods of disposal of waste material generated at different sites in health care delivery system.

It is estimated that inpatients in India generate between 0.5 to 1 Kg of solid waste per person/day. Over 75% of hospital waste is non-hazardous. There is no well established system of segregating hazardous from non-hazardous waste in majority of the hospitals. This mixing of the various components results in increased quantity of hazardous wastes that require safe disposal. Very often the hospital wastes are dumped alongwith the municipal wastes. Sometimes the hospitals are provided with incinerators, but very often these are inappropriate in design, improperly operated or remain out of order.

CRITICAL ASSESSMENT AND SUGGESTIONS TO IMPROVE THE PROGRAMMES

The situation pertaining to environmental sanitation is horrifying at the global, regional and national levels. It has been admitted by various agencies responsible for it at all levels. Attainment of the global target of the UN Second Development Decade had not been feasible in most countries of the region. The Regional Director of the WHO in his Annual Report has warned the member-states:

> "In spite of the continuing efforts of governments and international and bilateral agencies, only the fringe of the problem has been tackled. ..there is an urgent need to mobilize further support from all available sources to solve this difficult problem. Investment in this field will be amply rewarded not only in terms of reduction in the incidence of communicable diseases, but also by substantially contributing towards an improvement in the standard of living."[27]

Dr. Abel Wolman, one of the "father-figures" of environmental health and Professor Emeritus of Sanitary Engineering at the Johns Hopkins School of Engineering, Baltimore, USA says while talking of the world health situation: "It always leads great conferences to pass resolutions to do something about providing water to impoverished people. Resolutions become opiates because they are gratifying substitutes for action."[28] He warns the policy-makers and administrators against complacence and says, "Viewed on a global basis, we have little to be sanguine about. The disease-consequences of poor and insufficient water, of living with human excreta, and of unhygienic personal habits, are disastrous—they have been familiar for so long a time that they no longer excite even the statistician or epidemiologist. People accept their devastation, as they so often abjectly bear their real and spiritual poverty. We speak of the toll of deaths, due to environmental deficiencies in a casual way, even though the figures mount to hundreds of millions. The communicable diseases, often the sequels of poor sanitation are maiming and killing men, women and children—not computer data."[29] It is beyond doubt that a lasting solution to many of the existing and future problems of public health require control on environment. The question arises as how to provide sanitary facilities to hundreds of millions of people still without even minimum sanitary facilities? How to tackle such programme? How to find the resources required for these programme? What should be the administrative set-up to ensure speedy implementation? What are the responsibilities of planners and policy-makers to ensure integrated approach We shall discuss the facts and suggestions to provide good environment for the healthy growth of the people.

(1) Cooperation and Coordination among Allied Programmes

There is a close relationship between the environmental programmes and other programmes. In practice, this relationship is ignored by the planners and administrators of these programmes, e.g., a dam has to be constructed for irrigation and power purposes; its consequences on human health or soil salinity are ignored or underestimated. To remedy such unfortunate situations it is suggested that an 'integrated' approach may be adopted. It presumes an unprecedented, ungrudging cooperation between different services, as well as between various brands of natural scientists on the one hand and of social and human scientists on the other. We have to encourage such integrated approach to have full impact rather than piecemeal goals and approaches. It was mentioned in a WHO document that, "more effective administration requires that planners and managers take account of the full range of implications of their own programme goals and further, that they actively seek to participate as consultants and collaborators in the planning and execution of other community programmes that demonstratively or potentially interact with environmental health."[30]

UNESCO's MAB Programme (Man and the Biosphere Programme) coordinates various disciplines by mobilising applied research efforts allover the world on major man environment resources interactions. It relies on international cooperation among governments and the participation of all specialists. A major UNESCO research programme is closely studying the effects of human interventions in the environment and man himself in all the major socio-economic systems. We can get benefit out of such programmes.[31]

(2) Improve Administrative Capability and Competence

Environmental health programmes are administered by technically qualified people but such people lack administrative capability and capacity, i.e. the ability to achieve results. We have doctors, engineers, town planners, inspectors, nutritionists, geologists who are responsible for improving the environment. Every programme has its administrative component which is the heart and soul of that programme. It is suggested that the persons engaged on these programmes may be given suitable training in administration to enhance their competence.

(3) Deploy more Resources

The Environmental Health Improvement programmes require considerable financial investment. The World Bank and WHO reported to the Mar Del Plata Conference that S 140,000 million would be needed to reach the target of clean water for all by 1990. Today, we need double this amount to cater to increased population. Where will it come from? External aid is limited. So, there is a need to exploit the resources available within each country. It is only a question of proper allocation of resources. Voluntary effort can be encouraged to accelerate the pace of development.

With exploitation of local self-help, money can be generated. It is also a question of political will. This programme must be made an integral part of the community development programme. It should take the form of self-aided programme. The funds allocated should be used to achieve the aim of the policy and care should be taken that the funds are not diverted for other purposes. It was mentioned by Dr. B.H. Dieterich, Director, Division of Environmental Health, WHO that "Development planners confronted with meagre budgets are often forced to keep some projects in abeyance and give priority to others that may bring immediate economic benefit. It is now being increasingly realised that it is not a practicable or economically sound idea to defer environmental health projects. Planners are beginning to look at environmental health projects in the context of the ultimate socioeconomic objectives of the development process."[32]

(4) Research to Meet the Requirements of Different Geographical Areas

There are many potential health hazards. We know much about some of these hazards and little about many of them. We must encourage research in the experimental laboratory and epidemiology to pin-point the areas of ignorance. Secondly, national institutes should carry out research to develop models for adapting measures to reduce costs. They may also find simple disinfection devices suited to rural needs. We may not adopt costly western models to supply safe water and sewerage disposal, e.g., the British Development Agency, Oxford has made a latrine which turns the human exereta into organic manure producing some 6,000,000 tons a year. In the Republic of Korea, human excreta is being exploited to produce methane gas. There is need to change the attitudes of experts so that they can design the machinery and equipment suitable and feasible in our country.

(5) Local Participation

Public Health administration is manned by and meant for human beings. It is therefore necessary to associate the people with the progranunes of water supply and rural sanitary latrines. Sociologists, behavioural scientists and public relation experts should be associated with programmes to make the local involvement more effective.

Social mobilisation, People's participation and health and sanitation education are essential inputs into water supply and sanitation programmes. These help to make sure that the proposed activities fit into the targeted population's habits and socio-cultural environment where they do not suggest changes, it intends to ensure that the proposed water supply and sanitation technologies and activities are appropriate to men, women and children.

(6) Strong Political Will and Determination

It has been mentioned that the programmes of environmental health are deferred because of the lack of resources or the apathy on the part of the politicians. This assumption is totally wrong and baseless. "The major cause for delinquent action lies in the motivation of governments. Do they really mean what their resolutions say-militantly enough to go into action? Is only lip service the main response of Presidents, Prime Ministers, kings and ministers? The task for the future is difficult but possible. People should not be consigned to premature death simply because we are less than courageous and diligent. The pace must be accelerated."[33]

(7) Effective Maintenance

It is not only important to build the infrastructure for the environmental sanitation programmes but also to see that these projects function efficiently and regularly. We must ensure their competent construction, efficient and fool-proof operation and maintenance of completed supplies and effective surveillance on quality of drinking water. The maintenance is very poor in the developing countries. Even in the planned cities like Chandigarh, the headquarters of three governments—we are shocked to find germs, mosquitoes and flies coming in the tap water. Besides, the dirt is scattered in the whole of the city. Thus, there is a need to maintain the services once provided to the people through efficient and economical administration, involving the people.

(8) Guidance and Assistance from Bilateral and Multilateral Agencies

The capacity of the developing countries to solve the problem pertaining to environmental sanitation programmes are limited. International and bilateral agencies should be encouraged to increase their direct technical assistance to member-countries in the following ways:

(a) In making assessment studies;
(b) In the establishment of information systems and programme formulation, implementation and evaluation;
(c) In identifying and helping to meet specific needs for multilateral or bilateral assistance by way of expertise, equipment, materials and soft loans;
(d) In setting up research and training centers and collaborating laboratories;
(e) In assisting training programmes, including programmes for the production of manuals and training guides;
(f) In establishing health criteria and codes of practice; and
(g) In the local production of materials.

In addition to providing assistance itself, WHO should act in a coordinating capacity in respect of assistance received from these and other sources.[34]

(9) Civic Consciousness

Environmental sanitation cannot be achieved by the effort of the

Government alone. It requires the active support and cooperation of the people It was indicated to the writer by the authorities responsible for water supply that 25 per cent of the resources are being wasted because the people do not care to use the services only when in need. Most of the public and private taps remain working without any utility. Besides. the people lack civic consciousness and they do not cooperate in the maintenance of hygienic conditions. One is shocked to see the beautiful city of Chandigarh with heaps of debris all around. The difficult task of improving environmental sanitation is possible only if the people develop civic consciousness.

(10) Environmental Education

Dr. T. Sundaran in his Article, "From Literacy to Health" in *Kurukshetra* (Oct. 1992), suggests Health education and personal hygiene are necessary components of all such plans. Such education inputs may relate to:

(a) washing hands before collecting and carrying water, and pouring out water from a storage container without touching it or using a clean long handled dipper to take the water out;
(b) making sure that the water container, the cups and mugs used for drawing water are clean and that the water is kept covered at all times; and
(c) washing hands after defecation, before preparing and eating food, cutting of nails and other such basic measures.

Special care to ensure implementation of these measures in hotels and other public eating places is more difficult but essential to really checking diseases like typhoid.

The Stockholm Conference held in 1972 drew the urgency of tackling environmental problems through various efforts. One recommendation of this conference called for development of 'environmental education' as one of the most important steps to attack world's environmental crisis. The conference pleaded that "new environmental education must be broad-based and strongly related to the basic principles outlined in the United Nations Declaration on the New International Economic Order."

Environmental education has been defined as an educational process dealing with men's relationship with his natural and man-made surroundings, and encompass the relation of population, health, pollution, technology, urban and rural planning, housing, proper nutrition to the total human environment. The scope of environmental education is vast, touching every aspect of man and environment. The purpose of environmental education is to provide knowledge to the people so that they can adjust with the environment and enjoy decent environment. The goals of environmental education as discussed in the Inter-Governmental Conference on Environmental Education, organised by the UNESCO in cooperation with UNEP, at Tbilisi (USSR), from October 14-26, 1977, are mentioned below:

(a) To foster clear awareness of and concern about economic, social, political and ecological interdependence in urban and rural areas;
(b) To provide every person with opportunity to acquire the knowledge, value, attitudes, commitment and skills needed to protect and improve the environment; and
(c) To create new patterns of individuals, groups and society as a whole towards the environment.

The Secretary-General of the UN in his report on Population, Resources and Environment sums up the benefits of environmental improvement programmes. He mentions four social and economic benefits that would result from government action for environmental betterment in the poor countries besides the improvements in the people's health from control of infectious diseases.

(a) Employment of large number of poor people in public works projects;
(b) Reduction of food requirements and costs by lessening the mal-absorption caused by intestinal parasites. This might ultimately save $ 2,000 million per annum in India alone. This annual saving would be equal to the entire capital cost of needed water supply improvements in the whole of rural India;
(c) Increases in potential economic productivity through improved health of adults; and
(d) Greater receptivity of children at the early ages by improvements in health."[35]

(11) Appropriate Technology

A.S. Bal, A.N. Khan and P.R. Sarode in their Article, "Technological Options for Rural Sanitation" in *Kurukshetra* (October 1992), rightly suggest that high incidence of excreta related diseases in the developing countries warrants that the sanitation programmes be designed with the primary objective of bringing about improvement in public health. This objective can be achieved through alternate sanitation technologies which are simpler and cheaper as also socially acceptable. An inter-disciplinary sanitation programme could prove to be more successful not only from the sanitation point of view but also from the point of view of problems faced by the local bodies by way of poor financial returns from provision of sewerage facilities in the low income areas. Selection of appropriate sanitation technology for a given community and its proper operation and maintenance after installation is ensured only when socio-cultural aspects are considered along with economic, financial, ecological and technical features in the planning process. The task of providing water and sanitation to the unserved population is so immense that it would be almost impossible to accomplish it without the development and application of low-cost technologies. Low-cost technologies are generally applied at the peripheral level, where construction, operation, maintenance and surveillance may vary greatly from one location to another, affected by the level of community motivation and participation.

Non-sewerage onsite sanitation facilities may be all that are needed when water supplies are limited, but if improvements result in greater water usage then eventually the need will escalate for sewers and offside disposal. In this case it can create a need for concentrated population to be controlled by treatment.

(12) Holistic Approach

Ninnta Deshpande, an eminent Gandhian has stressed the need to adopt holistic approach to sanitation, it is necessary to approach the problem in a holistic manner by linking sanitation with religion, culture, health, agriculture, environment and production of energy. The basic attitude that needs to be formed is to link it with Bhakti. It has to be stressed that cleanliness is godliness and unless cleanliness becomes a part of our lives, we cannot be true devotees of God. Construction of toilets, their proper use, maintenance and clean habits should form part of the psyche. The wrong notion that night soil is not to be touched has to go. Cleaning should become a part of daily practice. The linkage of cleanliness with health is also very important. It has to be impressed upon the minds of the people that this programme is essential for keeping good health and protecting the family and village from various diseases. With charts, slides, films, songs, cultural shows, this knowledge can be imparted. Imaginative and innovative methods have to be adopted to make people aware of health.

CONCLUSION

Dr. Zbigniew Bankowski,[36] spells out the code of ethics to protect the environment. It would be unrealistic, however, to suppose that the damage that has been done, and still continues to be done, can be arrested and undone in the short-term. Rather, long-term global policies must be envisaged and, if they are to be successful, they will require changes in our perceptions of man in nature. If our global physical environment is not to be further degraded, we must change our conceptual environment, our ways of thinking and behaving. Perhaps the worst environmental pollution is pollution of the mind, and the greatest need is for well thought out principles of environmental ethics.

All spheres of human conduct private and public, are subject to ethical principles or rules. When governments or other corporate bodies despoil the environment in the name of development or political dominance or national security, when government adopt *laissez faire* policies that permit the exploitation of nature for narrow, short-term gains, they contravene the basic ethical principle of the greatest good for the greatest number of people.

Sh. M. Akhtar, Chief WESS/ICO UNICEF, New Delhi in his Article, "Strategies for rural sanitation (UNICEF Experience)" suggested the following based upon UNICEF experience to ensure fruitful application of strategies for safer water supply and sanitation. (*Kurukshetra*, October 1992).

1. If sanitation has to be a 'way of life' it should be treated as a package of facilities/services and not identified with latrines. All the low-cost sanitary facilities, both at domestic and community level, such as latrine, soak pit, garbage pit, smokeless chulha, bathing cubicle, drainage improvement, ground water sources and other community-based facilities should form a part of the package. A distinction may have to be made among 7 components of sanitation. These are: (i) Handling of drinking water; (ii) Disposal of waste water, (iii) Disposal of human excreta; (iv) Garbage disposal; (v) Home sanitation and food hygiene; (vi) Personal hygiene; and (vii) Sanitation in the community. This should be supported by a strong IEC back up to create awareness with regard to various sanitary practices including personal hygiene. It is necessary to modify the guidelines both at the Government of India and State Government levels to reflect the package deal and how to achieve the same.
2. In order that sanitation becomes a "peoples' movement", it is essential that their active involvement and participation receive due importance. In this regard subsidy can play only a limited role. Alternate financing mechanisms have to be developed to facilitate greater adaptability.
3. The low-cost sanitary facilities should have different technological options to suit different geohydrological; conditions and also the varying socio-economic segments of the population. Such technologies should be affordable, acceptable and replicable. Identification and use of alternate materials should be a continuous process so as to keep the cost escalation under check.
4. Demand generation for sanitary facilities should get a high priority in Rural Sanitation Programme. For this purpose, a comprehensive and systematic communication strategy has to be developed and all possible methods and channels should be used to motivate people. In this regard inter-personal communication through village level motivators seems to be quite promising. Willing village level functionaries like Anganwadi workers, DWCRA group organisers. Traditional

Birth Attendants, primary school teachers, Youth Club/Mahila Mandal, office-bearers, etc. could be the core group of motivators. The panchayat members can also play an active role in this regard.

5. The demand generation strategy should be backed up by an efficient delivery system which need not be a part of the subsidy-oriented programme. At present, even if a person wants to have his/her own latrine in rural areas, it is not easy to find the required pan/trap/pit cover, etc. as adequate infrastructure has not developed as yet. Only in an area where government programme is under implementation, things are more readily available. It is, therefore, necessary to create alternate delivery channels/mechanism to have improved sanitation coverage.
6. Private initiative is a must to make the sanitation programme a success. The government-supported activity could at least be a stimulant. The results of the 44th Round on Sanitation Coverage is a pointer to this assumption. While figures from the government sources show a 3 percent coverage, the NSS survey reveals that more than one-tenth of the households were using latrines. The difference could be accounted for by the spread effect of the government programme. It is high time that a clear cut policy on how to encourage private initiative outside the subsidy-oriented approach is laid down. The policy should keep a flexible approach and suggest alternate social marketing strategies to promote sanitation through private initiative. Involvement of industrial houses/public sector units including the manufacturers of sanitary goods could form a part of it.
7. NGOs can play a very crucial role in promoting rural sanitation. They can very effectively be used to encourage private initiative because of their rapport with the community and can serve as an efficient channel for information dissemination, awareness creation and motivation. Only those NGOs who have the required capacity to take up activities at a district level or at least for a group of blocks should be encouraged. The Government should come out with separate guidelines for involving NGO's in the Rural Sanitation Programme. The State Government should be well aware of such guidelines.

Dr. Martin Kaplan[37] has desired to look positively and is hopeful of solutions by mankind. He stated, "hazards to human health arising from environment factors are many and varied. We know much about some and little about many of them. We must therefore depend on future research both by the experimental laboratory and by epidemiology to clarify many of our areas of ignorance. The development of surveillance and monitoring mechanisms for changes in health status correlated with environmental components should provide the warnings necessary to avoid serious harm to present and future generations of the human race.

In reviewing all these environmental effects and their possible Dangers, we should not however reach too gloomy a conclusion. A comforting finding, which may be extended to many other aspects, is the recent discovery that fish caught in the last century and preserved in museums have been found to have similar mercury levels as those found in fish today. And after all, the human race with its great adaptability has survived the innumerable disasters and environmental hazards it has encountered for several million years. Modern life and times represent for man merely a new set of problems replacing old ones, and there is no reason to doubt that man's ingenuity and intelligence will prevail as far as environment problems are concerned.

Notes and References

1. T.N. Chaturvedi, Editorial, in *IJPA*, July-Sept., 1989.
2. Hiroshi Nakajima, "A Wounded Planet", in *World Health*, January-February, 1990, p. 3.
3. Dr Wilfried Kreisel, "Environmental Health in the 1990s.' in *World Health*, January-February, 1990, p. 5.
4. WHO: SEARO, Declaration on Health Development in the South-East Asia Region in the 21st Century, New Delhi, 1997, pp. 17-18.
5. WHO, *World Health*, May, 1972, p. 28.
6. U. Thant quoted in Clellan, M.C. and S. Grant (ed.), Protecting our Environments (New York, 1970), p. 206.
7. WHO, *World Health*, May, 1972, p. 29.
8. Edwards S Roggers, Human Ecology and Health Environment, Administrator. New York, 1960.
9. WHO, Samuel Halter, "Man and his Environment," in *World Health*, July 1975, p. 18.
10. GOI, Planning Commission, Draft Five Year Plan (1978-83), p. 117.
11. WHO, World Health Paper, 59, p. 12.
12. Karnataka towards Equity, Quality, and Integrity in Health, Final Report, Government of Karnataka, April, 2001, p. 52.
13. *Ibid.*, p. 56.
14. Nikolas P. Napulbow, Water For All: A human right, in *World Health*, July-Aug., 1992. p. 3.
15. Karnatka towards Equity, Quality, and Integrity in Health, Final Report, Government of Karnataka, April, 2001, p. 52.
16. Barbara Ward, "The Key to Health" in *World Health*, January 1977, p. 3.
17. UNICEF, Assignment Children, 34, April-June 1976, p. II.
18. A Newsletter of Building Materials and Technology, Promotion Council, India, p. 13.
19. WHO, *World Health*, January 1979, p. 3.
20. UN, 1970, Report on the World Social Situation, New York, 1971, pp. 167-68.
21. *World Health*, July-August 1992, p. 7.
22. A Newsletter of Building Materials and Technology, Promotion Council, India, p. 22.
23. Purshotam Khanna and Bindo Koshy, "When City Growth Exceeds Supply" in *World Health*, July-August, 1992. p. II.
24. The Work of WHO in the South East Asia Region, Report of the Regional Director, 1 July, 2006, WHO, pp. 47-48

25. *Ibid.*, pp. 48-49.
26. Waldemar F. Ahmedia, The Dangers and the Precaution in *World Health*, Aug.-Sept. 1984, p. 12.
27. WHO, SEARO: Annual Report of the Regional Director, 1976-77, pp. xii-xiii.
28. WHO, *World Health*, January 1977, p. 17.
29. *Ibid.*
30. WHO, Public Health Papers, 59, p. 116.
31. Batisse Michel, "Man and Biosphere" in *World Health*, June 1978, p. 4.
32. WHO, *World Health*, May 1972, p. 29.
33. WHO, *World Health*, January 1977, p. 17.
34. WHO, SEA/RC27/p. 41.
35. UN. ST/ESAJSERA/S7, New York, 1975, p. 101.
36. Zbigniew Bankowski, "A Code of Ethics" in *World Health*, January-February, 1990. p. 18.
37. Dr. Martin Kaplan, "Environmental Hazards for Human Health" in *World Health*, May, 1972, p. II.

2

Health Education: Nature and Scope

For thousands of years, disease and death have been accepted with resignation as normal ingredients of daily life—aspects of a tragic destiny, which strikes some and spares others without rhyme or reason. Today this resignation is unacceptable. We are aware that the dangers that threaten our health are often caused by imperfections in our social structures or in our own behaviour. We can afford to scoff at some of these threats, now that a correct application of new discoveries in medicine enables us to reduce them to reasonable proportions.

The task of education is to apprise people of their responsibilities, since diseases and accidents are so often linked with ignorance, carelessness, and inadequate precautions on the part of national authorities.

—*Etienne Berthet*

AIMS OF HEALTH EDUCATION

The most important aim of Health Education is to alter behaviour, which may have directly or indirectly influenced occurrence of spread of diseases in a given cultural setting. A culturally relevant health education programme can be planned only after understanding the behaviour in all its manifestations. One of the best definitions of Health Education was offered by Wood in 1926: "Health Education is the sum of experiences which favourably influences habits, attitudes and knowledge relating to individual, community, and racial health."[1]

Different authorities have differently viewed the aims of health education. According to one source:[2]

"The aim of health education is to help people achieve health by their own actions and efforts. Health education begins therefore with the interest of people in improving their condition of living, and aims at developing a sense of responsibility for their own health betterment as individuals and as members of families, communities or government."[3]

Another source[4] highlights that, "Health education aims at promoting the greater possible fulfilment of inherited powers of the body and the mind and the happy adjustment of individual to society. It is the educational approach to health problem and as such is concerned with practical measures for the promotion of health and the control and treatment of diseases."

Studies made in different countries of the world have shown that fluctuations in the toll of disease and death depend even more on the level of education than on the social and economic conditions in which people live. Ignorance can be just as much a killer as poverty, and these two often go hand in hand.[5]

An excellent examples of the success of health education can be cited from Egypt. Esmut Mansour in his article, "Egypt Tackles Polio", rightly suggests the role of health education in polio eradication. To quote:

In fact, women in Egypt represent a considerable proportion of all private and public physicians and health service administrators. As in may other countries, the nursing staff are predominantly women and are therefore engaged in the front-line battle to eradicate polio. The nurse's role here is much broader than the one she plays during clinic hours, and her value to her community and its welfare should not be underestimated.

Not only does she routinely give the polio vaccine, but she is the primary mechanism for dispensing health care information to each child's carers, thus increasing their awareness about the dangers of disease, the importance of vaccination, and any possible side-effects of the vaccine. Therefore, she acts as the first defence line against the disease, and her understanding of the early effects of polio and her ability to recognize the disease is essential.

Egyptian society is particularly blessed by a culture and history that produces strong family ties. So ultimately the success of our programme to eradicate polio must also credit the mothers who have listened to the information provided at the official level of health care and who have been convinced that the health of their children is worth all the expense and effort they make.

Egypt's Expanded Programme on Immunization is one of the most effective in the world. Reaching our goal of eradicating polio will be a worthy tribute to the hard work contributed by all of us—women and men together—to protect out children.[6]

MEANING OF HEALTH EDUCATION

"A term composed of two concepts, the first one denoting the content (health), and the second is the process (education)"[7]

James McCormick,[8] defines health education:

"The purpose of health education is not, as it is often seem to be the transmission of knowledge, but altered behaviour."

The Health Education Steering Committee of Association of School of Public Health[9] (1966) defines health education as:

"A process, which effects changes in the health practices of people and on the knowledge and attitudes related to such changes."

Sanjay Salooja in an article, "Knowledge to Action" suggests the following top 7 "E"s to Motivate and Influence an Audience

Speak with "E"s. Be a speaker of influence—not control or guild. With the privilege of the platform comes the awesome responsibility of educationing, motivating and influencing your audience to feel/think/act differently.

1. Educate—provide your audience with extensive information on your topic. This will empower audience to feel competent and knowledgeable. Support your points with stories. Adults delineate their thoughts visually.
2. Entertain—give them the facts laced with a good dose of humour. Adults learn better when they are lightening up! Here's the place for some magic tricks, handwriting analysis or a song.
3. Experience—get the audience involved. When they interact, they "get it" better and retain it longer. Group exercise, simple questions and answers, role plays.
4. Enthusiasm—vary your tone of voice, smile often, show passion for your subject matter. Make your body language reflect your comments.
5. Example—be the speaker/person who motivates the audience to admire and respect you. You have succeeded when people say "I want to be like him/her."
6. Encourage—be supportive to your audience—believe in them. Say "I did it . . . and so can you."
7. Excellence—hold yourself accountable for excellence. And then help your audience to be accountable and live up to its potential. Speakers need to give audience what they need, not what they want.

Hiroshi Nakajima in his article editorial "The State of the World's Health" in *World Health,* March-April, 1995, stresses the need of the health education to control lifestyle and other diseases. To quote:

> Our future depends to a large extent on being adequately informed. The World Health Report 1995 is a response of this more and more acutely felt need. Reliable health information is demanded not only by health professionals, politicians and business people who need it to meet the various responsibilities of their jobs, but by individuals and families in every walk of life. Their questions extend from universal concerns about what is happening in the world to very particular ones such as how to avoid diabetes, or how to look after a sick child, or how to ensure the safety of a blood transfusion. As the world's health authority, WHO is uniquely well placed to gather and publicize whatever information is available on such questions.[10]

Top 7 Insights to Effective Health Education

1. The most important objective of any Health worker is credibility and being knowledgeable about health education, i.e. speak to your audience as if you were having a conversation to have an impact.
2. Divert the audience's attention in the first few minutes with a question, starting comment, inspiring story, or funny experience about health education. This will help you connect immediately with everyone and reduce the tension. Stay away from jokes!
3. Feel confident and have faith as faith be gets faith.
4. Shift your focus from one to the other so that all persons remain attentive.
5. Use visual aids to increase audience retention of message. But NEVER become a master of ceremonies to overheads. Use case studies about health education.
6. Personal benefits from acquiring excellent speaking skills and knowledge of health education include: more self-confidence, becoming more persuasive and evolving into a magnetic or dynamic speaker.
7. Keep the people involved in the process of lecture—
   "Health education is not the same thing as health information. Correct information is certainly a basic part of health education; but health education must also address the other factors that effect health behaviour such as availability of resources, effectiveness of community leadership, social support from family members and levels of self-help skills. Health education, therefore, uses a variety of methods to help people understand their own situations and choose actions that will improve their health. Health education is incomplete unless it encourages

> involvement and choice by the people themselves. Merely telling people to follow good health behaviour is not health education."[11]

Baric, while describing relationship between behavioural sciences and health education maintains that health education can be defined in many ways based on the interest of the definers. He feels that whatever number of definitions one could find in the past are too general or cover all activities relating to health in its broadest sense of physical, mental and social well-being or have been operation definitions based on-the-job of health educators.[12]

The concept of health education defined by Wood in 1925 is one of the best-known and still applicable one. It withstood many pedagogical changes; and it also appears sounder today than when it was written. He defines health education—

> "represents the sum of experiences which favourably influence habits, attitudes; and knowledge relating to individual, community, and racial health."[13]

Unfortunately, the experts and development planners have failed to improve the lives of the people as they do not understand properly the science to communicate effectively with each other or with the people they are trying to help. Most of the people in authority today, who are guiding the people in this field, have not realized the urgency of such education and the benefit it can generate; consequently governments have not taken any substantial steps in this direction.

Health education does not mean merely removal of ignorance. On the contrary, it involves three important things:

(i) It provides a person with appropriate knowledge to enjoy decent health and also the knowledge about the occurrence and spread of disease thus enabling him to adopt relevant preventive measures;

(ii) It creates in him an interest for the health of other members of his family as well as of those living in his surrounding; and

(iii) It creates in him a desire to support health education programmes in his area.

Besides, Health Education should make the people understand the benefits that they can derive from modern medicine. K.S. Sanjive, Professor of Medicine has said:

> "It will not be an exaggeration to say that the paramount step in the effort to take modern medicine to every corner of the country and every citizen is health education. Health education in its widest sense

of getting every one to understand what modern medicine can do to diminish disease and death and to be properly motivated to utilize this knowledge in their daily lives, requires the simple quality of sincerity more than highly specialized techniques."[14]

Neglect of health education is one of the main reasons why scientific medicine is not taking root in the country and people are steeped in ignorance and superstition.

ESSENTIALS OF HEALTH EDUCATION

Health education would be possible only if the health educator and the receiver are in constant dialogue with each other. It is not wholly correct that the purpose of health education is to manipulate the receiver. What might be more appropriate is a circular diagram in which the parties to the "Communication Contract" as it is sometimes called, function dually as senders and receivers.

CHART 2.1

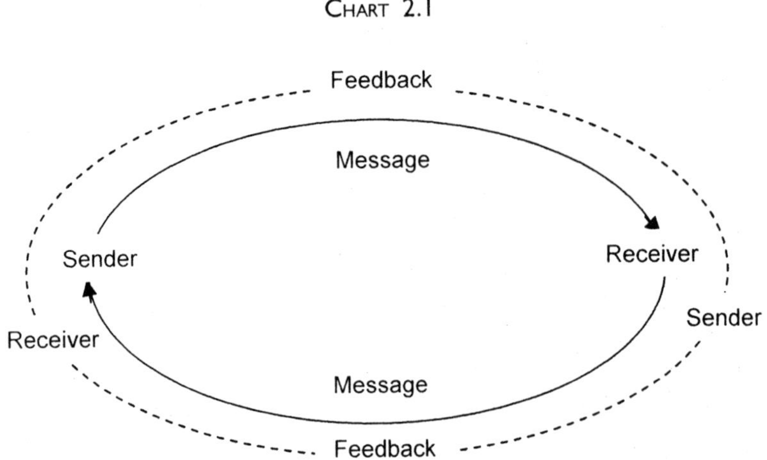

This model would avoid the possibilities of misinterpretation. We know that even well planned campaigns can end in failures if there is no proper monitoring or feedback to make sure that the wrong effect is not being created by the communicator, however innocently.

In a democratic society, the dynamic power, which impels governments to action, is the voice and enlightenment of the people. People can only pressurize their executive or legislative machinery to undertake suitable health measures when they themselves are aware of the means of warding off disease and promotion of positive health. This knowledge (Health Education) is therefore a pre-condition and prerequisite to creating the demand for health and setting the pace of implementation of environmental sanitation and the total health policy.[15]

According to the World Health Organisation Expert Committee, health education serves three main general purposes.[16]

1. To make Health a Valued Community Asset

The value assigned to health by a particular organisation, the level of general education, the concern of the community for its members, the number and ability of its health workers, and financial resources of the people. High educational level of the community is important to enhance the value of health in a given culture. It also encourages people to join hands to find out many ways to solve public health problems faced by them. It is recognized that the needs for education in health matters is intimately linked with other social, cultural, educational and economic problems, which have direct or indirect influence on determining health status of the people. A number of rural studies, mostly in developing countries report that the first concern of the family is agriculture, housing, irrigation or "mere subsistence" but not health. Health Education, therefore, has a significant role to play to help people to come together and to achieve health through their own actions and efforts. It aims at developing a sense of individual as well as collective responsibility in the community for its own health betterment on which its intellectual, physical, mental, social and economic development depends.

2. To help individuals to become competent in and to perform those activities which they must undertake as individuals or in small groups, in order to realize fully the state of health as defined in the Constitution of the World Health Organisation.

In any community, many activities directed to achieve health development are initially launched by the government; but in the long-run, these activities need to be carried out by the individuals, families and community. In the health programmes such as childcare, feeding practices, food hygiene, first-aid, and many such programmes designed to educate the public about the health hazards caused primarily by the changing lifestyle of the individual; education of public is needed.

Health practices and values attached to health behaviour have roots in the social system of a given society or a group. These practices conflict with the improved or modern practices based on scientific findings. In such situation health education has a greater role to play to synthesize the old and new practices without modernizing the values attached to old practices by the community.

3. To Promote the Development and Proper use of Health Services

No matter how best health service delivery system exists and health services are offered to the people; their full utilization by the latter depends on their awareness of availability of services; their judgment of the value of the services; the distance between the health centre and the community; their confidence in effectiveness of services; attitude of health personnel towards people, etc. In other words, the utilization of health services depends on predisposing, enabling and reinforcing factors. Here health education is necessary to prepare people to make adequate use of such services so that they can avoid economic loss incurred by wrong or inadequate use of services, which are often expensive.

PRINCIPLES OF HEALTH EDUCATION

Some of the most important principles underlying the practice of health education are:

1. Planning for health education should be an integral part of all health planning.
2. Since learning is a change in individual's ideas and practices, and since health education aims at changing people's ideas and practices, effective health education planning should be based upon the theories and principle of human learning.
3. People tend to accept change more readily when a change is directly relevant to their aspirations, needs and fulfilment of words, quick returns, personal goals. Therefore, health education should be in line with people's goals, needs, and interests.
4. Group norms and influences are the basic principles of individual behaviour, which also includes health. If a health norm is to change, it is desirable that such changes are compatible with group norms. Health education can succeed in changing individual health behaviour if it addresses itself to group's standards and norms.
5. An internalized change is a stable change. An individual learns better through his own action and effort. Health education, therefore, should aim at creating such a situation so that individual takes initiative for the change.
6. Belief in the dignity of man—Health education is based upon the conviction that individual has the right and ability to make his own decisions; and democratic change should always aim at stimulating the individual to decide his action by his own efforts.
7. Start where the people are if education efforts are not consonant with the level of understanding and needs of the people, people will not easily and promptly assimilate the ideas of change. Health education, therefore, aims to start where people are; and build from this base the necessary ingredients for better healthy life.
8. Plan with the people—Health education ideally is a catalytic process. It does not aim to force a change by manipulating forces without the involvement of the people. Therefore, involvement of the people is the most crucial factor in effective health education. Planning for health education is done with the people, and by the people.
9. Self-help—The concept of self-help for better health is one of the

basic principles in health education. The objective of health education is not to provide temporarily a solution of people's problems but to develop the ability among them to identify problems, find solutions and practice it. Health education, therefore ultimately aims at developing the potentiality of self-help in a community.[17]

CONTROL OVER DETERMINATION OF HEALTH EDUCATION

Health Education is the combination of planned social action and planned learning experiences designed to enable people to gain control over the determinants of health and of health behaviour and the social conditions that affect their health status and the health status of others.[18]

Further development based on human ecology has been spelt out by WHO expert Committee—"In recent years, however, a better understanding has developed of the processes that have a positive or negative influences on the harmonious functioning of a person, both as an individual and as a social being. This has prompted study of the role society plays in influencing the individual's health behaviour. It is now recognized that a community's values and norms play a vital part in defining the general approach of people to illness and health as well as to treatment and prevention, and that the process of socialization is one of the most important mechanisms in transmitting certain values and norms from one generation to the next. This has resulted in the development of social intervention models of health education, in which the emphasis is placed in influencing social, instead of individual, factors associated with health and illness."[19]

Health education is a 'process', which needs effective planning and implementation with appropriate consideration of ultimate goals and the best means for achieving them physical, mental and social health.

The World Health Organisation expert committee on health education of the public (1954) has defined:

> "Health Education like general education is concerned with changes in knowledge, feelings and behaviour of people. In its most usual forms it concentrates on developing such health practices as are believed to "bring about the best state of possible well-being."

The International Union of Health Education (1988) defined:

> "Health Education is the combination of planned social action and planned learning experiences designed to enable people to gain control over the determinants of health, health behaviour and social conditions that affect their health status and health status of others."[20]

HEALTH EDUCATION FOR QUALITY OF LIFE

1. The value placed on health by people depends mainly on social and cultural factors such as the needs, problems, social organisations, the standard of general education and the economic resources of the people for individual, family and community betterment.

To enhance the importance of health in one's culture, education encourages people to come together to find ways of tackling the general problems of their community. The immediate problem concerning the community may not directly be related to health. This active participation being responsible for their own health is enhanced by insisting the people to find solution to the problems of immediate interest.

2. To help individuals to become competent in and carry on those health activities for themselves, as individuals or in small groups, in order to realize fully the state of health.

Health is not a commodity, which can be bought by individuals for their improvement. Individuals have to accept the scientific knowledge and health practices and act accordingly. Therefore, health education, aims to encourage the individual, family and community to take responsibility for their own health.

3. To promote the development and proper use of health services.

The usefulness of any health service depends on the peoples' utilization of the services provided by the health agency. It depends upon the confidence of the people in the health personnel and the attitudes, which health workers have towards the people. By Educating the people one can avoid the economic loss incurred by wrong or inadequate use of services.

Health education begins with the people and leads them for broadly understanding the activities for better health. It translates the findings of the laboratory into language and activities understood and accepted by people. Health education is more showing and doing than mere telling.

When health education is skillfully done, people continue with pride on what they themselves have accomplished.

Health education should produce a cooperative relationship between the people and health personnel. Many workers in health profession are engaged in doing things to and for the people. They should understand and be able to apply the principles of the educational process in their contacts with people, as well as in their working relationships with others. Health education is a basic function of all health workers and all the personnel of allied health organisations and agencies.

Health education is an essential component of any programme to improve the health of a community, and it has a major role in promoting:

(a) good health practices—for example, sanitation, clean drinking water, good hygiene, breast feeding, infant weaning, and oral rehydration;

(b) the use of preventive services—for example, immunization, screening, antenatal and child health clinics;

(c) the correct use of medications and the pursuit of rehabilitation regimens—for example, in tuberculosis and leprosy respectively;

(d) the recognition of early symptoms of disease and promoting early referral; and

(e) community support for primary health care and government control measures.

Despite the potential benefits of health education, existing schemes are often inadequate and ineffective. The key decisions that form the basis for any planning are decisions over what the desired change should be, where the health education should take place, who should carry it out, and how it should be done.[21]

The following remarks of a working group on communications in family planning,[22] which summarizes the value of the mass approach in family planning, are of value in health education planning as well "Mass communications cannot replace fact-to-face approaches. Each has its definite and well-defined objectives. Mass communications can inform, help to create a favourable social climate, counter hostile propaganda, dispel rumours and clarify doubts and misunderstandings. They may motivate a relatively small section of the public to adopt contraceptive practices. But, for the large majority of the people, a sustained programme of education, persuasion and motivation, obviously in a fact-to-face situation, is necessary."[23]

However, education for health and training are both crucial to the successful implementation of a water supply and sanitation project, because they promote, on the one hand, favourable attitudes towards, and community participation in, the project, and on the other hand, provide the participants with a wide range of knowledge and skills contributing to a better standard of hygiene and health.

The Decade programme in the Philippines is moving towards its objectives, and there are many factors, which have contributed to its success so far. These include community participation, a primary health care approach, and increased emphasis on education for health; the financial help received on an international as well as a bilateral basis, and the technical support lent by WHO; the close cooperation between the various bodies concerned with carrying out the work, and with training administrators and primary-level workers. Finally, mention must be made of the importance of relying on appropriate technology and effective control measures carried out by the field staff in bringing the Programme's activities to a successful conclusion.[24]

PROCESS OF HEALTH EDUCATION

Understanding Behaviour

The knowledge of the people's behaviour is essential before planning for health education. Understanding Behaviour is basic to influence through health education. Behaviour includes the following:

(a) Knowledge;
(b) Beliefs;
(c) Attitudes; and
(d) Values.

(a) Knowledge

Knowledge about health can be gained through personal experience or through teachers, elders, friends, reading material that is why, there has been a constant demand to include health education as subject so that students can get correct knowledge about health.

Knowledge is attained either through experience or reading books or the information provided by parents, teachers, elders. If we have some health problems and we have the knowledge for that, that in future we try to avoid this.

(b) Beliefs

Beliefs dominate our life as they pass on from generation to generation. People accept the belief since these have been handed down from their old traditions. Some of these may be good for health while others may be harmful. It is the duty of health educators to change these beliefs slowly keeping in view their sensitivity. If the people are too much attached to these beliefs, health educators may ignore them as co-operation of people may not be solicited.

(c) Attitudes

Attitudes are based upon our small experience or may be based upon the experience of others. Health educators must change the attitudes, which have taken roots wrongly and are harmful for health. It requires strenuous efforts on the part of health workers.

(d) Values

People in a community share some values, which they consider as important. What status we accord to women differ from community to community. The behaviour, beliefs, values when put together constitute culture, e.g. eating habits, marriage, etc. differ from community to community.

Thus, there is a need to understand beliefs, behaviours, values of people or a community before introducing any health education, which can cause natural change or a planned change. Planned change is better, as the impact of health education would be lasting.

Health educators can use health education successfully by:

- Talking to the people and listening to their problems;
- Thinking of the behaviour or action that could cause, cure, and prevent these problems.
- Finding reasons for people's behaviour (beliefs, friends' ideas, lack of money, and others).
- Helping people to see the reasons for their actions and health problems.
- Asking people to give their own ideas for solving the problems.
- Helping people to look at their ideas so that they could see which were the most useful and the simplest to put into practice.
- Encouraging people to choose the idea best suited to their circumstances.[25]

World Health Organisation defines Health Education as:

Health education does not replace other health services, but it is needed to promote the proper use of these services. One example of this is immunization: scientists have made many vaccines to prevent diseases, but this achievement is of no value unless people go to receive the immunization. Similarly, incinerators for burning refuse are useless unless people will make the effort to put the refuse inside the incinerators.

Health education encourages behaviour that promotes health, prevents illness, cures disease, and facilitates rehabilitation. The needs and interests of individuals, families, groups, organisations, and communities are at the heart of health education programmes. Thus, there are many opportunities for practicing health education.[26]

Health Education is a part and parcel of every health activity and the health professional who ignores health education cannot be successful in any health programme.

Function of Health Education Programme

No health education programme can function in isolation. A health education programme has to be an integral part of various other development programmes. Functionally, a health education programme should aim at bringing about the following changes as shown in Chart 2.2.

A Change in Knowledge

The most important need which health education programme can serve is to provide appropriate knowledge about health and diseases to the people. This knowledge should be provided in such a way that the recipients do not find it hard to accept it. How to provide this knowledge in an acceptable way? This is the first challenge faced by a health educator. Meaningful responses are relatively easier to learn than the meaningless ones. The health educator can do a lot better by making his demands on

CHART 2.2

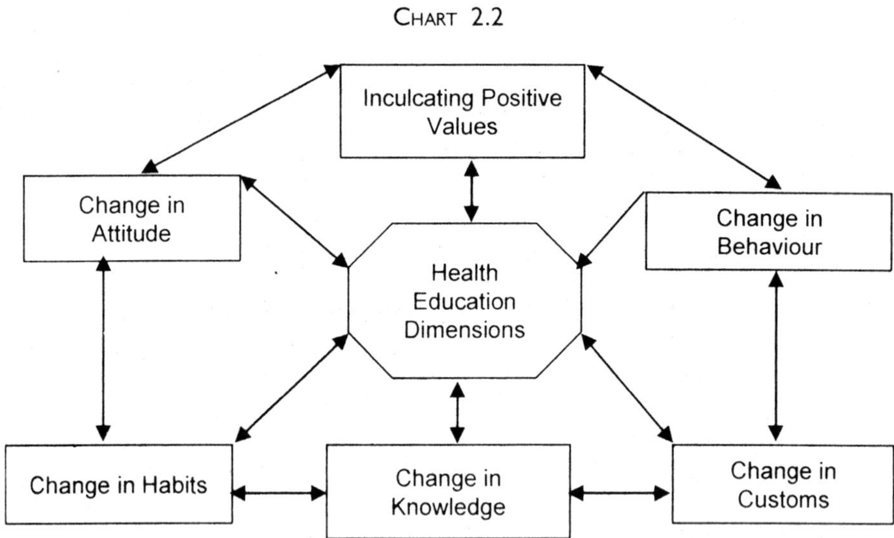

the response of receivers, which are meaningful. For instance, the health educator who gives a big lecture to the mother on the value of practicing family planning without indicating its benefits to her as an individual would be showing inadequate understanding of this principle, for she has to look into her own benefits first. Vigorous efforts would be required to proliferate suggestions that are realistic and meaningful.[27]

Education for Family Health (An Example)

Although the basic conditions of organisation of services for family health are necessary, the attainment of true family health depends upon the education both of members of families (nearly every member of the general public is a member of a family) and of health workers of all categories. (See Table 2.1). This education and training will be effective only when behaviour is altered and decisions are made with new knowledge and different attitudes as the family member understands more of family dynamics and relationships, and as the health worker sees beyond the individual into the family. This is manifestly easier said than done. For instance, the idea that the family itself is the greatest potential contributor to family health is not new, but the incorporation of education for family members at different ages as integral parts of health and educational services is far from being realized in practice. The education of health workers in family health, getting them to see the family as a group of inter-related persons, would also be a radical departure from almost every type of traditional training.

Thus, medical and health training for primary health care would once again be shared between community and hospital, the "normal" family and its dynamics would be understood as a background to the "abnormal" just as "physiology" and "anatomy" can be integrated with "pathology." Teaching and learning would then be related to the social context of the region in which the teaching organisation was situated, and the hospital would act as an institution within society rather than the centre of society as it seems to appear to so many medical teachers.

In all health care there is a large element of education yet generally speaking health workers are relatively ineffective as educators. The reasons for this are complex; one is because most of their training is still directed to the alleviation of symptoms or of episodes of illness or disability, and does not lead or compel them to think through the symptoms of illness to its prevention in the future or to consider the long-term prevention of disease by changing patterns of individual or family behaviour. No one pretends it is easy to change such set patterns of human behaviour but it is regrettable that most training schemes for health workers do not even make the student aware of the problem, let alone give them any grasp of the techniques by which changes can be accomplished.

The delivery of health care will vary from one society to another and, as it does, so too will the roles of the various categories of health workers. Yet ultimately the effectiveness of all health workers depends upon their awareness of their own role in society and their attitude towards and understanding of the society in which they work. Understanding of society in its turn begins with understanding of family, so that an awareness of family dynamics and family health should form an integral part of the training and later of the practice of every health worker whatever their role or category. (Appendices 2 and 3 for National Health Policy, 2002 and 1983).

The organisation of primary care service to provide family health care with the family as a health unit would require an educational set-up very different from that, which obtains today. Our submission is that at whatever level of development it could be applied, beginning with maternal and child health and family planning and progressing to a full primary care health team, such a set-up would give a better return for expenditure, lay a better foundation for health and provide a scheme for continuous development of family care and family health. The primary problem is to change the outlook, attitude and education of the health workers themselves.[28]

A Change in Attitude

A change in attitude is possible only when the new knowledge that is offered is acceptable to the recipients. Its utility should also be well known to them. Normally, provision of appropriate knowledge should lead to formation of positive attitudes not only towards a person's own health but also towards the health of other members of the community.[29]

Ann Goerdt in an article, "Disability Prevention and rehabilitation", observes that Reduction of handicaps requires a great effort on the part of all sectors to promote changes in beliefs and attitudes which limits the activities of people with disabilities.[30]

Health educators should see to it that they put an abrupt end to that type of health education, which was concerned with telling people how to

TABLE 2.1

Areas of Family Functioning

Biological	*Psychological*	*Socio-cultural*	*Economic*	*Educational*
(i) Reproduction of the species	(i) Emotional Security of members	(i) The transfer of values relating to behaviour, tradition, language and mores	(i) Acquisition of resources to fulfil other functions	(i) Inculcation of skills, attitudes and knowledge relating to other functions
(ii) Rearing of children	(ii) Sense of identity for members	(ii) Socialization of children	(ii) Distribution of resources, expenditure, saving	(ii) Preparation for adult life
(iii) Nutrition of family members	(iii) Maturation of personality	(iii) The formulation of norms of behaviour for all stages in development and adult life	(iii) Economic buffering of members of family	(iii) Fulfilment of adult role
(iv) Protection of health of family members at all ages	(iv) Psychological protection			
(v) Recreation for family and its members	(v) Ability to make relationships outside the family			

Source: WHO: *World Health*, August-September 1975.

act. They should instead put all the emphasis on understanding all those social forces, anywhere in the world, that cause people to act as they do.

Recently there has been a rediscovery of the contribution that lay people can make to health care. Lay self-care is a fact. It has been a fact ever since people were born. Today however it is realized that, far from reflecting mistrust in the health services or disappointment with their effectiveness, lay self-care offers a real potential for improving health status and decreasing health costs. Such care, however, must be applied intelligently and this is why health education is essential for ensuring appropriate self-care.

In the area of educational technology, heath education needs to develop the educational technology most appropriate to promote individual and community involvement and self-reliance.

Health education needs to provide the individual with knowledge about alternative types of behaviour and their outcomes, so that she or he can be in a position to make choices and accept their consequences. We must not forget that it is at the level of the individual and the family that values are formed. It is in the home that the child first learns how to behave. Of course, individuals and families are affected by the society in which they live, but they also influence that society. In the final analysis the choice is theirs.

But education and information can themselves be powerful tools for influencing society as a whole. They must be used as a permanent operational arm of strategies for mobilizing not only popular support but also the political support of decision-makers. The methods used must have social relevance. They must encourage people to become more self-reliant. They must develop in individuals and communities a will to lead a healthy life.

Next, health education needs to strengthen its multisectoral approach, and to increase the coordination of health education efforts through appropriate technology.[31]

A Change in Behaviour

Once positive attitudes are formed, these must reflect in the behaviour of the recipients. They should not only become mindful of their past behaviour but should also avoid doing things which can in any way influence occurrence or spread of diseases.[32]

A central point in the definition of McCormick is that health education is directed to change the behaviour of an individual so as to adopt advocated health practices. The change in the behaviour of an individual depends on individual decision (in the case of adult) in response to a number of factors; and knowledge, and awareness of risk of health hazard is one. Elaborating more of altered behaviour, the individual has to conform to the prevailing norms of the group and society in which he lives. Accepted norms by the family and society have equal influence in changing the behaviour as that of knowledge of risk. Behaviour of an individual has to be seen in the context of existing values and norms, which have greater influence; thus the efforts to change a behaviour needs to be gradual and slow. Behaviour is not arbitrary. It is the outward manifestation of values, which are deep-rooted and which can only be changed by an alteration in the individual's perception of him/her. For example, to stop smoking, the individual must perceive himself as a non-smoker and he must begin to dislike himself as a smoker and ultimately finds it intolerable to continue. McCormick believes that 'a form to non-directive counselling is much more like to facilitate behavioral change than didactic advice'.[33]

Abdulmoneim Aly in an Article: "Health Education through Religion", Achieving Health for all requires much more than just setting up a health centre in every high standard of medical care within easy reach of everyone.

A key element in the primary health care approach to Health for all is health education, which seeks to bring about a change in behaviour patterns by making essential health information available to all people in a simple, direct and effective manner. It is hoped that people will thus be motivated to evaluate their habits and practices, and will modify them according to the requirements of health protection and promotion.

Behavioural change, however, is too complex a process to be initiated simply by providing a set of facts. The motivation to break a habit must be much stronger than the force of habits or the pleasure derived from a certain practice. The spiritual dimension can be highly influential in this process of behavioural change.[34]

A Change in Habit

The change in the behaviour of the recipients must lead to habit formation. A habit can be formed only when the behaviour becomes repetitive. If proper habits are formed, not only the individual's concerned but the whole community will be benefited. Habit formation, however, is a slow process and it has been well said, that 'habits die hard'.

The persuasive communication or health educator should be interested both in the long-range effects of his messages and in their initial effects. As a matter of fact, he should be interested in turning the learned responses into habitual ones. What are the other principles that guide the establishment of a response? First, the probability of response will increase with the increase in the number of rewarded repetitions. As long as the stimulus with reinforcement following each correct response is not adequately repeated, it will not become a habitual response. Many messages are short-lived because of lack of reinforcement and are likely to become extinct. Second, in order to establish habit patterns, it would be necessary to have a shorter interval between response and reward. Third, habit formation is easier when stimuli are presented in isolation. A nutrition message when unaccompanied by another message such as sanitation message facilitates habit formation. Fourthly, timely increase in reinforcement will further strengthen habit formation. Fifth, receiver's original level of motivation will also influence her habit formation. The mother having a better level of motivation from the beginning will find habit formation much easier. Sixth, providing timely information about receiver performance, would lead to further improvement in performance. Providing selective information to a mother on the positive aspects of her performance will also improve her performance. Thus, communication of health ideas can yield the desired result if the above principles are followed religiously.

A Change in Customs

Acquisition of positive attitudes leading to appropriate habit formation must sooner or later, evolve into customs. Only when a substantial number of people in a given cultural setting start behaving in a customary manner, one can say that behaviour has become a part of their customs.

Don Palmer in his article, "Social Health: A True Story, Culture and Tradition as Medicine" in *The Daily Tribune,* dated 26th January 2000, rightly stresses the need of health education. Modern urban life, devoid of the goodness of social health, can be particularly tough for young indigenous inhabitants of developed countries. Some kill themselves, while many more drift into drugs, alcohol and crime. Now a prison programme is helping in rehabilitation of aboriginal offenders by reintroducing them to their cultural traditions.

Contents

It needs to be re-emphasized that health education is a slow process and that it proceeds gradually a part of the process may get established without any problem but additional efforts may be required to complete the whole process. This process may be directed towards the following important programmes: (See Chart 2.3)

(a) Personal hygiene;
(b) Knowledge of modern medicine, i.e. use of health services;
(c) Nutrition;
(d) Mental health;
(e) Prevention of communicable diseases;
(f) Care of children;
(g) Environmental sanitation;
(h) Human physiology;
(i) Lifestyle diseases; and
(j) Education about Alcohol and Drugs.

Health education must be imparted keeping in mind latest developments in the field of health. Life is changing fast and the individuals must be educated in the new technology—its role and

CHART 2.3

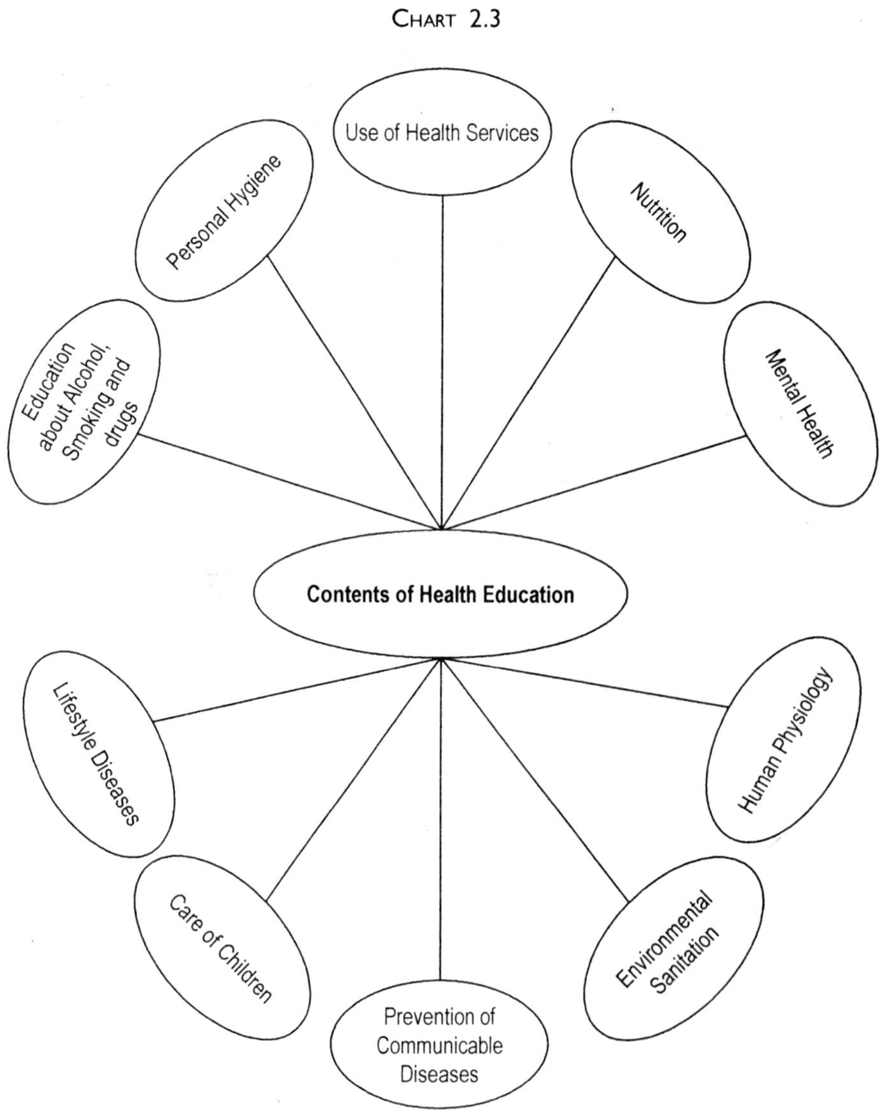

limitations. Mr. V. Tatochenko, a member of the WHO Expert Panel on Maternal and Child Health in his article on "Education for Health" said, "Rapid changes in lifestyles and the evolution of views on health and disease call for new departures in health education. A quick glance of health education material of even one generation ago will show how fast it tends to get out of date. Medical facts, it has been estimated, get outdated within a decade or so. Effective health education, therefore, requires a continuous stream of knowledge, development of the people's ability to absorb it, and decisions taken on the basis of a constantly changing body of information.[35]

Let us give some studies to support our thesis:

Children become volunteers to change Asia's biggest slum. Using children as volunteer health educators is one of the methods being employed in an extensive programme taking place in Dharavi, an area of Bombay that is Asia's largest slum.

Four hundred thousand people live in one square mile, and 50,000 of them are the target of a primary health care project directed by Professor Gopa Kothari of the Lok Manya Tilak Municipal Medical College and General Hospital.

The aim is to improve the health and nutritional status of all the people, particularly children under five and women aged from 15 to 45.

The project began in 1981, with an extensive survey of behaviour and beliefs. The results were used to develop health education activities and a community-based health care programme with three main components—medical, welfare, and social activities.

Three doctors, three medical social workers, a nurse, and 14 community health workers from the staff, with the active participation of local residents.

Training programmes were designed for health workers, traditional birth attendants, child volunteers, and other groups, Immunization, oral rehydration therapy, good nutrition, and personal and community hygiene were major elements in the training, with the young volunteers, aged from eight to 14, carrying the messages home to mothers and grandmothers, as well as to other children.

Opening a dialogue with community leaders helped to bring informal health committees into being, and adult literacy schemes were launched, as well as ideas on how to generate income by selling vegetables or making articles for sale.

Competitions were also held for different groups.

Educational aids such as posters, flannelgraphs and slide shows were prepared locally, and used in-group meetings and at exhibitions.

Experience has shown that the most successful health education activities have been the training programme, demonstrations of oral rehydration therapy, the production of flannelgraphs, and the establishment of a printing unit to produce posters. Cookery demonstrations and the provision of small feeding centres have also been successful.

Evaluation shows that, since the programme began, breast-feeding has increased from 60 per cent to 90 per cent, and immunization rates have increased to 100 per cent, except for measles, which has risen to 60 per cent from a low base. A 68 per cent improvement in personal hygiene has been noted.

"Well-planned communication makes an individual health-conscious, provides him with knowledge on health matters, and promotes the requisite desire and motivation to avail of health services and stay healthy," says Dr. Kothari. "It also encourages measures at both the individual and community level to prevent sickness."

Rural Water Schemes Need Women if they are to Achieve Success

"As the International Drinking Water Supply and Sanitation Decade was nearing its end, enough evidence has accumulated to show that community involvement and responsibility are essential if rural supply and sanitation programmes are to be successfully introduced and sustained."

Reports over the decade have clearly established the need for safe water supplies and sanitation, with million of preventable deaths each year. The vast majority of rural populations do not have access to such supplies, nor adequate facilities for disposing of excreta. And knowledge of basic hygiene practices is low.

Hygiene education programmes must become an integral part of all community partnership programmes and must be planned, designed and initiated before, during and from five to ten years after the construction of facilities. The primary purpose is to create a desire in the community to use facilities, and to keep them functioning.

Community preparation and hygiene education constitute a support programme which appears to be vital to the development of effective community management, and to the success of the community management, and to the success of the community partnership approach advocated by WHO.

In order to create a strong enough demand, materials used to convey messages about the benefits of safe water, adequate sanitation and hygienic practices must be realistic, believable, and acceptable to the target population. This is why village groups should be organized, and particularly groups of women, since this tends to ensure that the information conveyed is sensitive to the socio-cultural characteristics of the people.

Educational materials based entirely on the 'germ theory concept' are not always acceptable to rural people, nor are they always particularly effective, because it is hard to give a meaning to invisible organisms. To suggest that people are drinking water, which contains the fasces of their friends and neighbours can be considerably more effective.

Religious beliefs, superstitions and taboos all contain some positive elements, which can be used. In Papua New Guinea, for example, most people do not mind drinking from surface water sources (even though they may be contaminated), but are careful to avoid sources, which enemies might use to poison them.

Many religious and supernatural beliefs are concerned with water quality, sanitation, and proper hygienic practices, and can be used as a means of communicating positive messages. When developing educational materials, this type of information should always be considered.

Whether people feel the need to maintain and repair the systems, and maintain acceptable levels of sanitation and hygiene because of fear of 'germs' or fear of 'enemy poisons' is irrelevant, as long as they use, manage, and maintain their programmes effectively.

A planned programme is the basis of the community partnership approach, with a national plan being established, and refined according to the circumstances of local communities.

National specialists, such as sociologists, anthropologists, health educators and community development personnel should be seconded to work with women's groups, and other organized groups in the project area. The aim should be to identify the most effective methods of implementing a programme through mass media techniques. Education and preparation should come before any facilities are constructed at community level.

After educational materials have been developed, and an educational programme has begun in a project area, the materials should be refined to fit community requirements. Women and community leaders should be recruited and trained to organize, promote, and implement the programme.

Community hygiene education sessions should take place at least once a quarter, and no less than once every six months.

Village caretakers should be trained in the operation, maintenance and repair of water supply and sanitation facilities, and latrine construction. They should work with women's groups and project personnel to advise on latrine construction in villages.

The health and hygiene curricula of rural primary and secondary schools should be reviewed by the expert group, who should develop teaching materials. They should also develop practical exercises to involve students in building latrine slabs, making shallow wells, and installing hand pumps. The curriculum should include practical training in the operation, maintenance and repair of community facilities.

This schools programme should be launched not later than a year after the introduction of a community hygiene programme.

But it is women who hold the key to success, since they are responsible for most water collection and use. They should be asked to advise on the acceptability of hygiene education materials, technologies, the location of facilities, and so on. Women should be trained by national project staff to promote programmes, construct systems, and operate them.

Only when a community has been prepared, and hygiene education programmes successfully run, should facilities be constructed.

The link between community water supply, sanitation, and health education is well established. With the promotion of the community partnership approach, even closer collaboration between these two fields will be necessary of design and implement successfully programmes which will enhance the quality of life, and the maintenance of life, in the rural populations of the world.[36]

Methods of Health Education

Health education are set-up to promote positive health. A good health education must establish environmental linkages—points of interactions with the environment. These can be classified into four categories: enabling, functional, normative and diffused. The enabling linkage ensures and protects the organisational authority to operate, its access to resources and its power to achieve results. Functional linkage is to link the programme with the task environment. Normative linkages try to modify the behaviour of the people into the existing value system of the society. Diffused linkages imply reaching the clients through public relation (health education).

Sociologists have categorized diffusion process, which leads to a widespread acceptance of the programme into five critical stages: awareness (the individuals first introduction to a new idea or practice), interest (the stage at which he actively seeks further information and background data), trail (a limited phase of experiment), and finally acceptance or adoption. These processes have been occurring for centuries. The need of the present day health administration is to accelerate adoption of the health programmes and to control diffusion process in a short span of time to achieve effective implementation of health programmes.

Changes in knowledge, attitudes, behaviour, habits and customs can be brought about by 'personal' as well as 'impersonal' methods of health education. These methods have certain advantages and disadvantages. While personal methods involve face-to-face interaction, the impersonal methods do not require such a close personal contact. Personal methods are indeed more convincing and generally more successful. However, the success of personal methods greatly depends on the establishment of a good rapport between the health educator and his recipients. The impersonal methods are relatively simpler and even less time-consuming. The radio, the newspapers, the posters, and the pamphlets, etc. can all play an important role in imparting health education. Experience with personal and impersonal methods of health education have revealed that if both the methods are used simultaneously one can obtain better results than simply using one or the other method. The most important aspect in the adoption of the programme is the use of interpersonal relationships. Alastair Metheson, Deputy Director of UNICEF's division remarks on the basis of his research that:

> "To get people to act in ways that conform to new values almost always requires that mass communications need to be reinforced by personal influence."[37]

Thus, we see that communication, i.e. dissemination of information is only an important element in health education. The adoption or acceptance may not take place simply by communicating health information. A study conducted by United States Public Health Services has revealed that, "Unfortunately knowledge alone does not motivate a person to act in accordance with it. He may well know the correct answers to questions without really believing and accepting such information as the basis for his own action."

Dr. Gisela Gastrin, a Finnish physician mentions in his article, "How Education Helps", "People can be motivated to adjust their outlook towards health and disease, but before this can happen their negative attitudes have to be countered with factual information. . . . Education needs to be a part of a comprehensive programme in which responsibilities involving the health authorities and others are clearly delineated and resources allocated."[38]

For effective health education, people's involvement is essential. Eric R. Ram[39] in his article, "Information is Power" in *World Health* rightly says that making people aware of their rights and responsibilities helps them to determine their own health priorities and take part in solving their own health problems, a step so essential in the process of empowerment of the people. We have to employ all credible channels of communication, including the traditional methods of story telling and drama, in order to reach all people. Films, radio and television whenever available can be useful, but we have to recognize their limitations; they are useful in creating awareness among people in their communities, but to bring about a real change in health practices, people have to decide for themselves and take responsibility for their own health.

It was mentioned by Dr. E. Berthat in his article, "A New Role for Teachers" that besides information and motivation, action is indispensable. He said that "information and motivation are not enough; it remains for governments to ensure that a good health infrastructure is available to all the people. Health education has to convince the men and women who are responsible for taking decisions that health is a basic raw-material for their country's eventual social and economic development."[40]

A health educator, as a persuasive communicator can make the best possible use of the personal methods of health education. But he has to see that the messages, which he is delivering, get mentally registered with his recipients. Actually, he can present his message and then wait until he gets the requisite response from his recipients. D.F. Skinner has distinguished between two types of approaches to the learning situation, as 'operant behaviour' and 'respondent behaviour'. The two situations have also been described as involving instrumental learning and conditional learning. In 'instrumental learning situation', which involves 'operant behaviour', the health educator will present his message and then wait for the receiver to make a correct response. When the receiver makes this response, the health educator will attempt to fix the response by the appropriate award or reinforcement. On the other hand, in 'conditioned learning situation' which involves 'respondent behaviour', the health educator presents his message in such a way that he elicits the response that he wants from his recipients and thus the stimulus that originally served to elicit the response becomes the reinforcing or rewarding element in conditioning. Undoubtedly, conditioning is much more efficient than instrumental learning. It is, however, necessary for the health educator to be aware of both kinds of situations since the condition for using 'respondent behaviour' may not be present in the persuasive situation. The health educator has to be aware that the recipients of his messages differ in the ways in which they learn a given response. They may give different responses essentially in the same situation because of certain specific reasons.[41]

COMMUNICATION IN HEALTH EDUCATION

1. "Health Education, like general education is concerned with changes in knowledge, feeling and behaviour of people." This definition implies that health education has knowledge, attitude and behaviour components.
2. "Health Education is translation of what is known about health into desirable individual, family and community behaviour patterns by means of educational process." This Statement implies that health education aims at individual, family and community behaviour and their interaction patterns.
3. "Health Education is a process . . . leading to programme planning, utilizing available resources, modifying health behaviour, breaking down barriers of ignorance, prejudice and misconceptions after the intelligent and thoughtful consideration of relevant health knowledge . . ." This statement means that health education is a process involving a series of steps and efforts by people and is not a single procedure.
4. Health education provides situations in which people educate themselves. This statement means that learning takes place through the efforts of learner and that the health educator provides the circumstances in which this learning takes place.

The principal objective of Health Education is to help people to achieve health by their own action and efforts. Its general purposes are:

1. To make health a valued community asset,
2. To help individuals to become competent in and to carry out the activities, and
3. To promote the development and proper use of health services.[42]

CONCLUSION AND RECOMMENDATIONS

Without evaluating the impact of health education programmes on the bulk of the people, one cannot possibly identify positive as well as negative aspects of the programme. An objective evaluation of the health education programme alone can help one improve the guidelines for future action. 'Cost-benefit' analysis should be an integral part of this evaluation, so that one may assess how available resources have been utilized. Through objective evaluation; one may also be able to curtail mass production of ritualistic health education material as produced by various health education bureaus. The amount thus saved can be effectively utilized for a more purposeful and meaningful health education programme.

Health education is the most difficult task as habits, usages and customs are deeply entrenched. But health administration would fail in its purpose if it could not produce social change through health education.

That is why it has been said that "it is easier to destroy mountains than to change our customs."[43] Professional training helps the health experts to deal with the health changes effectively. Their pharmacopoeia in both fields must be strong in order to translate the findings of biological investigations into social application. So over and above each technical act; there is a corresponding education function which doubles the value of the act, increases its efficiency and endows it with real human and social value.[44] G. Borkar in his book, "Health in Independent India" writes that all progress in public health depends ultimately on the willing assent and cooperation of the people and their active participation in measures intended for individual and community health protection, considering how much of illness is the result of ignorance of simple hygienic laws or indifference to their application. In practice, no single measure is productive of greater returns to outlay than health education.[45] Thus, health education can influence the lives of people for many generations. WHO conducted an interview of a Mongolian Feldsher. He stated that "conducting continuous health education is my first duty, prevention is our basic principle. Every effort is made to raise the health knowledge of the people. Child Care, correct feeding and vaccinations are among the most important topics for health education."[46]

In order to improve the functioning of the administration of health education at the Union and State levels in India, the following facts and suggestions may be taken into consideration:[47]

1. Effective Role for Hospitals in Health Education as Patients are Amendable to their Advice

Hospitals within the country are not serving as agencies of health education. Health education can be imparted to mothers when they come to hospitals with their babies. During their stay in the hospital, mothers can be taught how to care for their children during sickness and how to feed them correctly. The mental field is also full of promise. Hospital physicians can do much in this direction by their own attitude to patients, give them simple instructions and, above all, treat them as persons rather than cases.

2. Modernize Health Education Institutes

Those very institutions responsible for imparting health education courses are lacking in standards for sanitary facilities. It is difficult to see how the concepts of sanitation can be effectively imparted among trainees, under such conditions. The curricula and contents of health education need careful planning. The educational methods for health education used in a country or community should be regularly evaluated and revised in line with socio-economic development. Health education should be oriented to health consciousness and not disease consciousness.

3. Constant Research and Evaluation

There is the necessity of research in behavioural sciences for the improvement of health education. Dr. B.S. Sehgal, Director, CHEB, New Delhi, said, "It was essential to conduct research on the behavioural sciences, in order to build up a body of knowledge for meeting the challenges posed by the health programmes."[48]

4. Special Attention to Training of Trainers

Training for trainers needs re-orientation and re-examination. We should supplement classroom-based academically-oriented training strategy in health education with the actual practice based on models of social change. The emphasis should be on learning by doing and not by listening alone. To quote a UNICEF/WHO study:

> "Efforts in health education have often been limited to giving information dogmatically, as if this alone would bring about a transformation. Inevitably, the outcome has been disappointing. The pattern of existing resources—economic, human and cultural—has been forgotten and this too has contributed to health education's failure."[49]

5. Creation of Women's Club as in Democratic Republic of Korea (DRK)

Women can be effectively approached only by women workers. The experiment of mother's club has been sufficiently rewarding and useful in the People's Democratic Republic of Korea as agencies of socio-economic development. The process of social and economic development is a process of human development for people is the target as well as essential variable in development. Communication being a two-way process provides for participation at whatever stage of enlightenment the individuals composing a society find themselves. Mother clubs if established in India in right earnest can be the key factors in both the communication and development process since they can be the instruments for getting facts to the people upon which decisions can be based.[50]

6. Understanding Local Social-cultural Issues

Before launching any programme of health education, the health educator must assess the local problems and possess the knowledge about the beliefs, conceptions and misconceptions, which the people have formed about diseases, their causation and cure. This is possible provided the multi-disciplinary studies of rural communities are encouraged. Such studies would throw light about the cultural background of the people. He can arrange his programmes accordingly and this will save him from antagonism and hospitality.

7. Create Good Relations with Mass Media

There is less coordination between health education and the means of mass media communication, which need strengthening on positive lines. It needs to be recognized that most of our health education programmes and activities are so ritualistic in nature that they rarely correspond to the realities of the situation. In most situations the health educator's knowledge of the cultural content of health education programme is often so deficient that they find it hard to deliver the health education messages in a culturally acceptable manner. It needs to be stressed that the cultural aspect of health education programme is of the greatest importance in the Indian situation. Anthropological and sociological studies in the area of health education are so few in our country that health educators find it extremely hard to understand the many changing aspects of the communities they deal with. There is, thus, an urgent need to study the social and cultural context of health and disease, and to design health services in such a way as will gain the acceptance and support of the people involved. The social scientists can help the health educator in the following ways:

(1) to understand the role of socio-cultural factors in health, including people's beliefs about etiology, diagnosis and therapy of prevalent diseases;
(2) to understand the food culture including people's belief regarding consumption or rejection of various foods on socio-cultural consideration;
(3) to understand people's attitudes towards acceptance or rejection of health education programmes; and
(4) to help them plan and develop culturally relevant health education programmes.

South-East Regional Office of WHO has also expressed its dissatisfaction over the lack of importance to health education in its report "Health Situation in the South-East Asian Region, 1994-97."

Despite these achievements, health education and promotion practices are faced with major constraints—the low priority accorded to health education at the policy level, high illiteracy levels, inadequate resources, poor social status of women, and limited capacity for health promotion research are but only a few examples. To overcome such constraints, new thinking and innovative approaches are required. As we move into the 21st century, the challenges for health promotion go beyond the wider articulation of the concept of health promotion, to building infrastructure and achieving adequate levels of resources, both technical and financial, in order to respond effectively to the increasing demands for health promotion in the Region. "Settings for Health" represent the organisational base of the infrastructure required for health promotion.

Partnerships, which effectively respond to the health needs of specific population groups, such as workers, women and school children, need to be more vigorously pursued. Healthy public policies need to be developed to ensure supportive environments for individual and community health action, and to protect people from lifestyle-related problems such as those due to tobacco and alcohol. Documentation and dissemination of health promotion outcomes are also critical to the legitimization of the cause of health promotion in the Region.

New health challenges mean that new and diverse networks need to be created to achieve intersectoral collaboration. Such networks should provide mutual assistance within and among countries, and facilitate the exchange of information about which strategies have proved effective. All countries need to develop the appropriate political, legal, educational, social and economic environments required to support health promotion. In this venture of health education, mass-media if properly used can help solve the problems.

Health promoters and educators need to be convinced that the mass-media can operate in the public interest and should play a critical role in social affairs, including health issues. The health concerns or readers, listeners and viewers are very much the concerns of the print and broadcast journalists. The basis of the relationship between the health and media sectors should therefore be one of partnership, not one of user-helper.

Health and media are not naturally inclined to work in unison. Historically, medical scientists trained in the methodical and meticulous search for knowledge have been somewhat skeptical of any effort at popularizing their work. Some doctors even view the media with suspicion and ambivalence. Media people, on the other hand, need to have their source material in language understandable to the layman; they have motive to dwell on technical details, and often loose patience with lengthy scientific papers.

Yet media and health in a close partnership have much to contribute to the public's welfare. Without the involvement of the media, the health sector cannot hope to inform the public on health issues or to help stimulate a community's involvement, which is critical to the success of any health effort. Without the technical input of the health sector, the media cannot fulfil their obligations to serve the interest of the public and these public interests certainly include health.

The complexity of the media, with their obsession for meeting dead lines and their own technical constraints, is little appreciated or understood by health professionals. Those in health who work in partnership with the media need to acquire a rudimentary knowledge of how media works—not in order to become media specialists but to be more empathetic in their dealings with the journalists and broadcasters. This in turn will call over a good hard look at the core curriculum of the training of health promoters and educators.

Whether the health professionals can play their rightful role in battling successfully against lifestyle-related illness—including AIDS and whether health education and promotion practitioners will enter the 21st century adequately prepared of the communication challenges, will depend on the actions that health authorities take now.[51]

In the new millennium, we need to harness all the resource especially the mass media in a planned manner. This would require active collaboration between media and health specialists. Jack Ling[52] in his article, "Health and the Media" has rightly stressed that the health sector should focus on making technical subjects digestible and understandable to the layman. In particular, the health professionals should identify existing, credible channels of communication, including traditional ones, in order to reach the public. The media offers the public health community more than just access to air-time and newspaper space; they are also a source of communications expertise that is needed to ensure the success of large-scale health promotion campaigns and transmit technical information about health to a mass audience.

What is more useful is the follow-up of media-transmitted message that can be effected by village health workers. For instance, primary health care workers can be an effective channel of communication by delivering in person the same messages that have been delivered to a target audience in print or over the radio, thus increasing the overall impact of the educational drive.

A dialogue has to be initiated between decision-makers in media and in public health. The object of that dialogue should be to heighten awareness among the media personnel about the important responsibility they hold for the health and well-being of their people, and equally to alert health professionals to their own responsibility for ensuring that their health initiatives reach all people. Without this whole-hearted backing form the media in conveying health messages to the greatest number of people, we risk having only Health for Some and not Health for All.

However, the success of health education would depend in the long-run upon the shoulders of the providers of health care to the people. They should be motivated to do this job as a part of their medical duties. S.S. Sooch in his Article, "Revamping Health Care" in *The Daily Tribune*, (26 January 2000) rightly remarks that there is a general feeling that most of the health care providers in the government-run hospitals are indifferent, apathetic and insensitive and a few even outrightly arrogant in their behaviour. A sense of compassion and human touch is simply missing. A series of crash courses should be arranged to expose the entire staff to the art of public relations.

Health Education is vital to provide health to all in 21st century. This is the cheapest and most effective tool of health care. The success of Primary Heath Care in 21st century depends upon the identification of community needs through community needs assessment surveys and later on providing health education to the community so that they can solve their problems themselves.[53]

Notes and References

1. John J. Hanlon, Principles of Public Health Administration, St. Louis, 1960, p. 402.
2. WHO: *Technical Report Series*, No. 89, p. 4.

3. S.L. Goel, Health Care Policies and Programmes, Deep & Deep Publications, New Delhi, Vol. 2, p. 6.
4. WHO: *Technical Report Series*, No. 156, p. 3.
5. WHO: Etienne Berthet, A new role for teacher, *World Health*, May 1979, p. 23.
6. WHO, Esmat Mansour, "Towards a World without Polio", January-February 1995, p. 27.
7. Adopted from: Behavioural Sciences, Medicine and Health Education by Leo Baric in (Ed.) *Behavioural Sciences in Medicine and Diseases*, The Health Education Council, London, 1972.
8. McCormick, James: The Doctor-Father Figure or Plumber, Croom Helm, London, 1977.
9. A report prepared for the 1965 Annual Meeting of the Association of Schools of Public Health, Health Education Monographs, No. 21, 1966.
10. WHO: Hiroshi Nakajima, "The State of the World's Health", *World Health*, March-April, 1995, p. 3.
11. World Health Organisation (1988), Education for Health—A Manual on Health Education in Primary Health Care, Geneva.
12. Baric Leo, (1972): Behavioural Sciences in Health and Disease (Ed.), The Health Education Council, London.
13. Wood, T.D., and C.L. Brownell (1925), Source Book in Health and Physical Education, Macmillan Company, New York.
14. K.S. Sanjive, Planning India's Health, Orient Longman, New Delhi, 1971, p. 94.
15. S.L. Goel, Health Care Policies and Programmes, Deep & Deep Publications, New Delhi, Vol. 2, pp. 7-8.
16. World Health Organisation (1954): WHO: *Technical Series Report*, No. 89, Expert Committee on Health Education of the Public, Geneva.
17. A.B. Hiramani, Health Education—An Indian perspective, Delhi, B.R. Publishing Corporation, 1996, pp. 47-48.
18. H.S. Dhillon and Dennis D. Tolsma, 1991 meeting global health challenges—A position paper on health education, XIV World Conference on Health Education, Helsinki, Finland, June 16-21, 1991.
19. WHO, 1963, New Approaches to Health Education in Primary "Health Care", *Technical Report Series*, 690, WHO, Geneva.
20. V.D. Sarangapani, Health Education: Concept and Scope, in K. Mahadevan (Ed.), Health Education for Quality of Life, Delhi, B.R. Publishing Corporation, 2002.
21. *Ibid.*
22. Economic Commission for Asia and the Far East, Communication in family planning, Bangkok, (Asia Population Studies Series, No. 3).
23. K. Mahadevan (Ed.), Health Education for quality of life, Delhi, B.R. Publishing Corporation, 2002.
24. WHO: Pablo R. Imperio, Primary Health Care, *World Health*, 1986, p. 9.
25. WHO: Education for Health: A manual on Health Education in Primary Health Care, Geneva, 1988, p. 22.
26. *Ibid.*, p. 23.
27. WHO: S.L. Goel, Health Care Policies and Programmes, Deep & Deep, New Delhi, Vol. 2, pp. 8-9.
28. WHO: F.J.W. Miller, The Target, *World Health*, August-September 1975, p. 15.
29. WHO: S.L. Goel, Health Care Policies and Programmes, Deep & Deep, New Delhi, Vol. 2, pp. 9-10.
30. WHO: September-October 1995, p 4.
31. WHO: Dr. Halfdan Mahler, Health For All—Everyone's Concern, *World Health*, April-May 1983, pp. 2-4.

32. WHO: S.L. Goel, Health Care Policies and Programmes, Deep & Deep, New Delhi, Vol. 2, p. 10.
33. McCormick, James, The Doctor-Father Figure or Plumber, Croon Helm, London, 1977.
34. WHO: Abdulmoneim Aly, Health Education through Religion, *World Health*, July 1989, p. 27.
35. WHO, *World Health*, Feb-March 1979, p. 24.
36. WHO: June 1988 (Booklet inside), Education for Health, pp. 8-12.
37. UNICEF, *UNICEF News*, "Communication": A Tool for Development", Issue 84/1975/12, p. 18.
38. WHO, *World Health*, Nov. 1975, p. 14.
39. *World Health*, Jan-Feb. 1989, p. 9.
40. *World Health*, May 1979, p. 25.
41. WHO: S.L. Goel, Health Care Policies and Programmes, Deep & Deep, New Delhi, Vol. 2, pp. 12-15.
42. K. Kaliy appraisal, Communication in Health Education: Perspective on methods in K. Madhawan, *op. cit.*, pp. 312-13.
43. Bosnian proverb.
44. WHO: *Technical Report Series*, 1954.
45. Borkar, Health in Independent India, p. 217.
46. WHO, *World Health*, April 1977, p. 20.
47. Based on personal discussion and interview.
48. WHO, SEARO: SEA/RC 23, p. 88.
49. UNICEF, Health and Basic Services, Keys to Development, *op. cit.*, p. 46.
50. For further details refer to author's article, "Role of Communication in Family Planning: Setting up of Mother's Club in PEN", Family Planning Association of India, Haryana, Branch, May, 1977.
51. Jack C.S. Ling, "The Media its Role," in *World Health*, January-Feb. 1989, p. 25.
52. *Ibid.*, March 1986, p. 18.
53. S.L. Goel, Health Care Policies and Programmes, Deep & Deep Publications, New Delhi, Vol. 2, pp. 23-29.

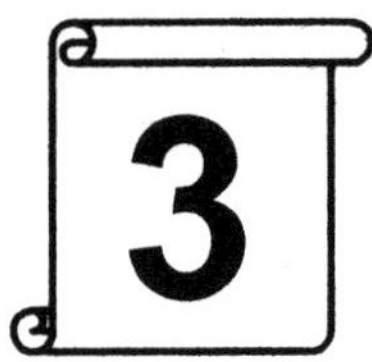

Population Policy and Family Planning

> The ultimate goal of the world's population policy must be to achieve an equilibrium based on low birth and low death rates that can be sustained throughout a distant future for the world and its several parts.
>
> —*F.W Notestein*

> The programme of family welfare and family planning is in the interest of peace and humanity in order to improve the quality of life for families in developing countries particularly in rural areas and in urban disadvantaged poor.
>
> —*Tokyo Declaration of Parliamentarians issued in March, 1978*

ADMINISTRATION OF FAMILY PLANNING PROGRAMME

The growth rate in population absorbs the national income and lowers the standard of living. The world population conference indicated in the population plan of action that population growth and population policy must be viewed not in isolation, but in the context of development. It was mentioned by the Secretary-General that "Current and potential world-wide population trends evidently cannot continue for as long as even one century without causing serious dislocations and crises in many areas.[1]

Myrdal in his book "Asian Drama" gave a stem warning to the world in regard to population explosion when he said, "Demographers are of the view that if fertility does not decrease, a time will come when mortality will lose its relative independence of levels of living and begin to rise again."[2]

Alexander Kessler[3] in his article, "Family Planning and the role of WHO" in *World Health*, May-June 1994 stated that the success of family planning programmes has led to a considerable decrease in average family size in developing countries, yet actual numbers continue to increase. This poses enormous challenges in terms of providing food water, energy and services, let alone improving the quality of life. Far more emphasis must be placed on the importance of family planning services. (See Appendix 5 for National Population Policy, 2000)

Family planning and health are intimately related. Family planning can promote women's health through the prevention of unwanted pregnancies, limiting number of births, and proper spacing, timing of births and foetal health. Family planning also promotes the health of the child through the reduction of child mortality, and promotion of the child development. Maryellen Fullam stresses the importance of family planning as instrument for the promotion of health. He says:

"Uncontrolled fertility directly threatens the health of mothers and infants and may undermine the health of other family members. Today, no health programme can be considered complete unless it offers ready access to the appropriate family planning measures for all potential parents."[4]

Rapid population growth leads to social and psychological tensions, and breakdown of a distribution system. Civil amenities such as water and power supply, housing, transport and social utilities like schooling, educational, health and medical services fall much short of demand in spite of their constant expansion. Besides, it leads to political and social corruption and accentuates economic disparities.

The experiences and lessons gained from Indian Planning suggests that effective population control, designed to restore the balance between vital rates by reducing the level of fertility, has a positive influence on the process of economic development and modernization. An eminent scholar has rightly mentioned that "A reduction in fertility would make the process of modernization more rapid and more certain. It would accelerate the growth of income, provide more rapidly the possibility of productive employment of all adults who need jobs, make the attainment of universal education easier and it would have the obvious and immediate effect of providing the women of low income countries some relief from constant pregnancy, prostitution and infant care."[5]

Thus, we can say that the problem of growing population has reached such menacing proportions that it has become a real threat to the socio-economic stability of the country. The excessive growth in population does not affect the stability of the national economy alone, it disturbs the stability of the entire body politic. It poses a colossal threat to our social structure. In our fight against poverty, disease, hunger, malnutrition and unemployment, checking the rapid growth of population is as important as raising production in the farms and factories and provision of social services. Population control is one of the chief issues which the country has to resolve and accord top priority in its march towards social and economic development. The programme of family planning is of vital importance for our country. It is a positive and constructive approach to the betterment of the quality of life of the community. Thus, it is evident to the key to India's economic future based on social justice lies in the immediate and effective implementation of a nation-wide population programme.

MEANING

Family Planning Programme makes a planned and scientific approach to the issues and problems of family life and attempts to solve them to make the family life happier, harmonious and fruitful. Family planning was thought of as a public health problem. It was stated in the First Five Year Plan:

It is apparent that population at a level consistent with the requirement of national economy should be established. This can be secured only by the realisation of the need for family limitation on a wide scale by the people. The main appeal for planning is based on considerations of health and welfare of the family. Family limitation or spacing of the children is necessary and desirable in order to secure better health of the mothers, and better care and upbringing of children. The measures described to this end should, therefore, form part of the public health programme. A distinction must be made between population control and family planning. Population control is influenced and determined by a government policy motivated by socio-economic considerations. Family planning, on the other hand, is a responsibility of the family. Who has given various definitions of family planning.

An Expert Committee (1991) of the WHO defined family planning as: "a way of thinking and living that is adopted voluntarily upon the basis of knowledge, attitudes and responsible decisions by individuals and couples, in order to promote the health and welfare of the family group and thus contribute effectively to the social development of the country."[6]

Mr. Ramakrishna Mukherjee has defined family planning in broader and narrower context. In broader context, he says that:

(i) It is not matter of mere biological arrangement between a man and a woman, albeit in the "social" setting of a family.
(ii) It is not exclusively a "cultural" issue: culture defined as an aggregate of what a person or group of persons desires and detests in every-day-life, the aggregate being formed, from the past upto date in the course of socialisation and, thus, provides the person or the group with a matrix of perception of life itself.
(iii) It is a matter of systematic understanding of the human kind with reference to the world as a whole and not merely one of its sectors: The Third World.

In the narrower sense, he says, that family planning is, regarded as a managerial issues particularly relevant to the Third World. It involves the following measures:

(a) Propogation of appropriate slogans for a "small family";
(b) Running family planning centres for sterlisation; and
(c) Distribution of contraceptives and education of the people to use them for their own good.

Another Expert Committee (1971)[7] defined and described family planning as follows: "Family Planning refers to practices that help individuals or couples to attain certain objectives:

(a) to avoid unwanted births;
(b) to bring about wanted births;
(c) to regulate the intervals between pregnancies;
(d) to control the time at which births occur in relation to the age of the parents; and
(e) to determine the number of children in the family."[8]

Dr. H. Mahler, ex-Director General of WHO has rightly said in *World Health* June, 1984) that in all societies, the family in one form or another is the Central nucleus for people, for their lives, their loves, their dreams and their health. So the people must be helped to understand that it is in their own interest to plan their families. And when they want to plan their family, appropriate information and services must be available in a context that provides confidence and security. Clearly what most parents want are healthy children who will grow upto become healthy adults. Today, it is possible for families through the use of technically and culturally appropriate contraceptive means to choose the timing and spacing of their children, and thus to complement other traditionally accepted means of child spacing such as breast-feeding. And quite apart from the positive health effects of family planning, the ability of couples to control their own fertility has opened the way for women to achieve the full and equitable participation in social and economic development that is their due.

In *World Health* June 1984), it is correctly stated that healthy families do not just happen, they are planned. The birth of a healthy wanted child is a joyous occasion. A child has chance of being born healthy, of surviving the first few years of life and growing well are enchanced if parents plan their children, so that they are born not before the mother is 18 or after she is 35-at least 2 years apart. Family Planning improves the health of women by helping them avoid high-risk pregnancies.

A WHO Expert Committee (1970)8 has stated that family planning includes in its purview: (1) the proper spacing and limitation of births, (2) advice on sterility, (3) education for parenthood including pre-natal and post-natal care, (4) sex education, (5) screening for pathological conditions related to the reproductive system (e.g. cervical cancer), (6) genetic counseling; (7) pre-marital consultation and examination, (8) carrying out pregnancy tests, (9) marriage counselling, (10) the preparation of couples for the arrival of their first child, (11) providing services for unmarried mothers. (12) teaching home economics and nutrition, and (13) providing adoption services. These activities vary from country to country according to national objectives and policies with regard to family planning. This is the modem concept of family planning.

STATUS IN INDIA

Population of the country has multiplied by more than four times during the century. It became 84.6 crore in the 1991 census and is 1,027 million as on March 1, 2001 (531 million males and 496 million females from 361 million at the time of independence. The India's population now is thrice that of USA (For details see Table 5.1). According to United Nations Fund Population Activities (UNFPA) estimates, world population is currently increasing at the rate of about 80 million per year. India alone is contributing to a fifth of the total increase in world population, every year. This is excessive as can also be seen from the fact that India has only 2.4% of the world land area, while its population constitutes 16% of the present world population. The already unusually large pressure of population on land in India, coupled with still continuing large annual increase indicates that the population situation in India is already critical.

TABLE 3.1

Decadal Variations in Population Growth in India, 1901-2001

Census year*	Total population in million	Average annual exponential growth rate	Progressive growth rate over 1901 in per cent
1901	238.4	—	—
1911	252	10.5	6 5.8
1921	251.3	-0.03	5.4
1931	279.0	1.04	17.0
1941	318.7	1.33	33.7
1951	381.1	1.25	51.5
1961	439.2	1.96	84.3
1971	5482	2.20	129.9
1981	683.3	2.22	186.6
1991	846.3	2.14	255.0
2001	1027.0	1.93	330.6

* Including Assam and Jammu and Kashmir. The 1981 Census was not held in Assam and the 1991 Census was not held in Jammu and Kashmir due to disturbances The 1981 and 1991 census data include estimated figures for these two states.

Source: Census of India, 1981, General Population Tables, Series 1, India, Part II-A (I), pp. 35-50, 536-37; Census of India, 1991, Final Population Totals: Brief Analysis of Primary census-Abstract, Series 1, India, Part 2 of 1992, p 86; Census of India, 2001, Provisional Population Totals, Series 1, India, Paper 1 of 2001, p. 34.

Such large and still increasing population has big implications for availability and incidence of unemployment in the society. The pressure of population is also very relevant for the state of environment. The high levels of population on land, in air and in water in large parts of the country indicate that the carrying capacity of land and environment is being exceeded.[9]

NATIONAL POPULATION POLICY

India adopted a comprehensive and holistic National Population Policy (NPP) 2000 with clearly articulated objectives, strategic themes and operational strategies. The Policy enumerates certain socio-demographic goals to be achieved by 2010, which will lead to achieving population stabilization by 2045. The Policy also prescribes an Action Plan for implementing the strategic themes listed in the Policy.

The National Population Policy, 2000 has identified the immediate objectives as meeting the unmet needs for contraception, health care infrastructure and trained health personnel and to provide integrated service delivery, with the following interventions: (i) Strengthen community health centres, primary health centres and sub-centres; (ii) Augment skills of health personnel and health care providers; (iii) Bring about convergence in the implementation of related social sector programme so that the Family Welfare Programme becomes a peoples' programme; (iv) Integrate package of essential services at village and household level through mobile clinics and counselling services; and (v) Explore the possibility of accrediting private medical practitioners and revive the system of licensed medical practitioners, who could provide specified clinical services.

S.P. Singh in his Article, "Problems of Population and Sustainable Development in India" in *PA*, January-March 2003, observed that, With a population of about one billion, India has achieved many dubious distinctions. Now India is a country with largest number of unemployed youth, handicapped people, beggars, slum-dweller and illiterates in the world. The population of illiterates in India is larger than the total population of any country in the world except for People's Republic of China. Every third illiterate in the world is an Indian. It is irony that in all these areas India, come what may, will lead the world for many more years to come. It is pity indeed that in near future we will be able to achieve a few more dubious demographic distinction.

GENSIS AND GROWTH

Policy-making and Planning for family

Welfare Family planning as an official programme was adopted in India in 1952. Before this, the Family Planning Association of India was formed in 1949 in Bombay. On 11 April 1951 the Advisory Panel on Health Programmes appointed a sub-committee on Family Planning. The sub-committee strongly recommended that family planning should be recognised as an official programme to protect the health and welfare of mothers and children and to aid the national economy by reducing the birth rate concurrently with the death rate in order to stabilise the population. During the first of Five Year Plans (1951-61) the programme was taken up in a modest way with a clinical approach. During the Second Plan period, 549 urban and 1,100 rural clinics were set-up.

The programme was reorganized in the Third Plan after the publication of the 1961 census result which showed a higher growth rate than anticipated. It was towards the middle of the Third Plan that the emphasis was shifted from the clinical approach to the more vigorous extension educational approach for motivating the people for acceptance of the small family norm and for provision of services.

A full-fledged Department of Family Planning was created in the Ministry of Health and Family Welfare. During the three annual plans (1966-69), the programme which was described as the 'kingpin' of the plan was made time-bound and target-oriented with vastly increased funds. In the Fourth Plan, the programme was accorded the highest priority. More emphasis was given to training, research, publicity, organisation, supplies and evaluation. Medical Termination of Pregnancy Act, 1971, was passed which came into force from 1 April 1972. With this Act, State Governments were empowered to constitute relevant boards to certify the registered doctors who were willing to perform the operations causing termination of pregnancy. Though the MTP Act is mainly a health measure, it also supplements the family welfare programme because a large percentage of women undergoing medical termination of pregnancy readily accept family planning measures to avoid future conceptions.

The experiences gained within the country and outside had amply established that health of women in the reproductive age group and of small children (up to 5 years of age), is of crucial importance for effectively tackling the problem of the growth of population. This perception has led to change in the approach from Family Planning to Family Welfare. Since the Seventh Plan implemented during 1984-89, the FW programmes have evolved with the focus on the health needs of the women in the reproductive age group and of children below the age of 5 years on one hand and on the other hand, to provide contraceptives and spacing services to the desirous people. Thus, the family welfare programme has objectives of stabilising population of the country early and to ensure good reproductive and child health status of the existing population. These objectives are pursued by addressing contraception issues, maternal health issues, child survival issues and by encouraging citizens through IEC to use these services.

Various programmes have led to very substantial improvement in health indicators. The achievements with regard to some prominent health and population indicators is depicted in the Table 3.2

TABLE 3.2

Achievements of the National Family Welfare Programme

Indicator	*Past Level*	*Current Level*
Crude Birth Rate	41.7 (1951-61)	25.4 (2001)
Crude Death Rate	22.8 (1951-61)	8.4 (2001)
Infant Mortality Rate	146 (1951-61)	66 (2001)
Maternal Morality Rate	437 (1992-93)	4.07 (1998)
life Expectancy at Birth (years) Est. Male-	37.1 (1951)	63.87 (2001)
Female	36.1 (1951)	66.9 (2001)
Effective Couple Protection Rate	10.4 (1970-71)	48.2 (1998-99)
Total Fertility Rate	6 (1951)	3.2 (1999)

(Relevant year in parentheses).
Universal Immunisation was started in 1985-86.

The Approach Paper to the Ninth Plan brought out by the Planning Commission has shown the inadequacy of the investment made for family welfare. This is a severe handicap, particularly when it is noted that in almost all respects, the health care system needs up-gradation and it needs to reach out to many more people for the national goals to be achieved. While there is a steady improvement due to economic development, spread of education/literacy and empowerment of citizens, substantial problems in regard to education/literacy, particularly among the weak performing states and in regard to empowerment particularly of women, remain. It has been now renamed as Reproductive and Child Health (RCH).

Containing population growth was one of the six major objectives of the Eighth Plan Recognizing the fact that reduction in infant and child mortality is an essential pre-requisite for acceptance of small family norm, Government of India has attempted to integrate MCH and Family Planning as part of Family Welfare services at all levels, NDC approved modified Gadgil Mukherjee Formula which for the first time gave equal weigtage to performance in MCH Sector (IMR reduction) and FP sector (CBR reduction) as a part basis for computing central assistance to non-special category States. This initiative ensured that the inter-linkages between Family Welfare Programme and Development was kept in focus in State Plans.

In order to give a new thrust and dynamism to the ongoing Family Welfare Programme the National Development Council set-up a Sub-committee on population to consider the problem of population stabilisation and come up with recommendations to improve performance. The report of the sub-committee was considered and the recommendations were endorsed by the NDC in its meeting in September 1993. The NDC Committee on Population had recommended that Family Welfare Programme should take cognizance of the area specific socio-economic, demographic and health care availability differentials and allow requisite flexibility in programme planning and implementation. For this purpose the NDC Committee recommended that there should be:

(a) Decentralised area specific planning based on the need assessment.
(b) Emphasis on improved access and quality of services to women and children.
(c) Providing special assistance to poorly performing states/ districts to minimise the inter and intra-state differences in performance.
(d) Creation of district level database on quality and coverage and impact indicators for monitoring the programme.

ORGANISATION

The apex body at the centre is a cabinet committee which is presided over by the Union Minister of Health and Family Welfare. It includes Ministers of States for Finance, Human Resource Development, Home Affairs, It also includes a member from the Department of Electronics and Scientific and Industrial Research. This body has the overall responsibility for the formulation of national policies on the family planning and for reviewing the progress in their implementation.

To Co-ordinate the family planning activities among the different States, the Central Family Planning Council has been set-up as an advisory body for policy-making. It includes Health Ministers from all the States and is presided over by the Union Minister of Health and Family Welfare, Vice-President in Union Minister of State. The Union Deputy Minister in the Ministry of Health. Other members are from the Planning Commission, representatives of the Union Territories, representatives of major voluntary organisations, labour organisations, selected members of Parliament, Eminent individuals in their personal capacity and officials from the various ministries It has representatives from a wider section of interests in family planning, including those that are directly charged with the implementation of the programme.

The Department of Family Welfare (earlier Family Planning) within the ministry is responsible for the implementation of policies. The Secretary to the Government of India in the Ministry of Health and Family Planning is overall in incharge of the Department of Family Welfare. An Additional Secretary assists the Secretary and provides overall direction to programme implementation. He is known as Additional Secretary and Commissioner for Family Welfare. There is a Joint-Secretary who supervises the working of the Technical Wing of the Department which provides technical guidance to the various programme activities, i.e. Sterilisation, IUD, Post-Partum, M.C.H., Training, Mass Education, besides Evaluation and

Research. -The Additional Secretary's duties include policy formulation, programme planning, supervising the programme implementation and co-ordination of activities of the department with other related ministries and departments of the Government of India.

There are two wings of the department: (A) Administrative Wing (the Secretariat), and (B) Technical Wing with many divisions. On the secretariat side, there is: (i) Policy Division, (ii) an Aided Programme Division, (iii) an organised sector, (iv) Voluntary Organisations Division, and (v) a Plan Budget Division.

(i) The Policy Division looks after formulation of policies concerning family welfare.
(ii) The Aided Programme Division looks after the activities of organisations which receive extra government assistance and aims at improving upon the scope and quantum of medical and health care services.
(iii) The Organised Sector Division Co-ordinates Departmental Policies and Measures affecting the family planning activities of public bodies and private organisations which are collectively called institutions in the organised Sector.
(iv) The Voluntary Organisations Division assigns programmes to voluntary agencies and aims at assessing the efficiency and effectiveness of these agencies.
(v) A Plan Budget Division looks after the finances of the Programme.

On the technical side, the following divisions are functioning. The functions are clear from the names of the divisions:

(i) Programme Appraisal, Co-ordination and Training and Sterilisation (including Research) Division.
(ii) Technical Operation Division.
(iii) Maternal and Child Health Division.
(iv) Evaluation and Intelligence Division.
(v) Mass Education and Media (including population education) Division.
(vi) Nirodh Marketing Division.
(vii) Transport Division.
(viii) Projects Division (Area Projects).

Organisation at State Level

In order to co-ordinate the family welfare activities between the State Governments and the Central Government, the Directorate of Health and Family Welfare for each State gives adequate support to the State Health and Family Welfare Departments. Organisation at District and block levels- At the district level there is a Distt. Family Planning Bureau while at block level Family Planning has been integrated with health services. Besides, the Primary Health Care complex is responsible at the village level.

SERVICES

The National Family Welfare Programme provides the following contraceptive services:

- Sterilization as a terminal method.
- Intra-Uterine Devices (IUD) for the spacing births.
- Daily Oral Contraceptive Pill for spacing births.
- Condoms for spacing births.

Emergency Contraceptives Pill (E-Pills)

Department of Family Welfare introduced procurement of Emergency Contraceptive Pills (E-pills) in National Family Welfare Programme during 2002-2003. This contraceptive is used within 72 hours of un-protected Sex. Following quantities of E-pills were procured during 2002-03 and 2003-04 for distribution to states. No procurement has been made during 2004-05 and 2005-06 however, procurement of 10.00 lakh packs is proposed during 2006-07.

The acceptance level of the various methods of contraception during the last two years has been as given in Table 3.3

TABLE 3.3

Acceptance of Various Services from 1995-96 to 2005-06 and 2006-07

	1995-96	*1996-97*	*1997-98*	*1998-99*	*2002-03*	*Compare of two years*		*% change from 2005-06*
						2005-06	*2006-07*	
Sterilisation	4422319	3870226	4127065	1283402	473100	1.53	1/35	(-)11.8
IUDs	6857882	5680671	6085744	263463	6108000	2.76	2.44	(-)11.6
Oral Pills	5090850	5250179	6249222	5081306	16537000	6.93	7.74	11.7
Condom	172974291	17214327	16730468	12984061	8243000	18.03	17.91	(-)0.7

Source: Annual Report, Ministry of Health and Family Welfare from 1995-96 to 2006-2007.

Prevention of Unwanted Pregnancy

The data from National Family Health Survey has shown that awareness regarding contraception is nearly universal, But there is an unmet for contraception, The Family Welfare Programmes will gear itself to meet the unmet need during the Ninth Plan period. Vasectomy is safer than tubectomy and efforts will be made to increase acceptance of vasectomy, so that there is substantial reduction in the morbidity associated with terminal methods of contraception. Quality of contraceptive care will be improved. Couples will be provided with balanced information on all available methods of contraception and the advantage and disadvantage of each of these methods so that they choose the method best suited to their needs. Such a balanced presentation and counselling will in the long-run not only improve acceptance of contraceptive care, but also improve continuation rates of temporary methods of contraception. The quality of services will be improved through appropriate training of service providers at all levels.

MTP Services

Over two decades have elapsed after the enactment of legislation for Medical Termination of Pregnancy (MTP) Act. Over the last two decades the Government of India has taken steps to provide trained manpower and equipment at secondary and primary health care level for safe legal abortion services.

It is obvious that after the initial rise, the reported number of MTPs has remained below 0.6 million for the last 15 years. In 2001, it was 7,66,762. In spite of efforts to improve the availability of, and access to, induced abortions services in the primary health care set-up, safe abortion services are not available to majority of rural population in India. Even today majority of the estimated 7.6 million induced abortions are not carried out in settings recognised for legal abortion and about 8.9% maternal deaths in India are due to septic abortion.

Efforts to improve access to family planning services to reduce the number of unwanted pregnancies and cater to the request for induced abortion will continue to receive intensified attention during the Ninth Plan. In addition, efforts will be made to improve access to safe abortion services by training physicians in MTP and recognising and strengthening institutions which are capable of providing safe abortion services for the first trimester. IEC efforts through appropriate channels of communications to improve awareness among women about availability of safe abortion services at affordable cost through appropriate channels of communication will be intensified. Provision for first trimester abortion will be coupled with appropriate contraceptive care so that these women do not incur the risk of yet another unwanted pregnancy and induced abortion.

RESEARCH AND DEVELOPMENT

The ICMR is the nodal research agency for funding basic, clinical and operational research in contraception and MCH. In addition to ICMR, CSIR, DBT and DST are some of the major agencies funding research pertaining to Family Welfare Programme. The National Committee for Research in Human Reproduction assists the Department of Family Welfare in drawing up priority areas of research and ensuring that there is no unnecessary duplication of research activities. Some of the major institutions carrying out research in this area include the Institute for Research in Reproduction, Bombay, National Institute of Nutrition, Hyderabad, National Institute of Health and Family Welfare, New Delhi, Central Drug Research Institute, Lucknow and the Central Council for Research in Ayurveda and Siddha, Delhi. A network of 18 Population Research Centres conduct studies on different aspects of Family Welfare Programme and undertake demographic surveys."

Bask and Clinical Research

Development and testing of new contraceptives include contraceptives which are considered to be effective in Indian Systems Medicine.

- Research on methods for male fertility regulation,
- Clinical trials on newer non-surgical methods of MTP, and
- Post-marketing surveillance of Centchroman.

Operational Research

- Studies on the ongoing demographic transition and its consequences.
- Studies on continuation rates and use of effectiveness of contraceptives.
- Research on operationalising integrated delivery of RCH services nutrition, education, women and child development, rural development and family welfare' services at village level.

MONITORING OF FAMILY WELFARE SERVICES

Monitoring and evaluation form an essential component of FW programme. Indicators used for monitoring and evaluation include process indicators and impact indicators. Process indicators are used to monitor the progress of implementation of the programme through monthly progress reports as compared to the annual targets/expected Level of Achievements (ELAs).

Training

Training to medical and paramedical health professional is imparted in various training institutes, centres and school. Basic training is imparted in ANM training schools, LHV training schools and MPW M) training schools and selected Health and Family Welfare Training Centres. In-service training is imparted in National Institutes; State Regional Health and Family Welfare Training Centres, HFWTC's and by District Training Teams.

CRITICAL APPRAISAL

To quote S.P. Singh again, What has happened elsewhere can happen in India too provided there is a massive campaign to educate eligible couples, particularly in villages, about the benefits of limiting the size of the family. This point has of course been emphasized innumerable times and at different places but it has never been sincerely implemented. Rural people, steeped in ignorance and obsolete religious relief, still do not know the harm that big family size brings to them and consider every child as a gift of God. This notion must be altered if family planning is to succeed. However, the education campaign must always be backed by easy availability of modem contraceptive measures hat can enable people to plan their families. One of the reasons why family planning measures have not yielded the desired results is that it as not been honestly implemented. The unmet need for family planning as been reported to be quite high. According to the National Family Health Survey 2, the current unmet need for family planning is 16 per cent and it is higher in rural areas than in urban areas.

Inspite of the existence of infrastructure and availability of technology to control the growth of population, we have not been achieving the desired results. K.B. Sahay in his article, "Population: Time for Tough Measures", in *The Daily Tribune* (January 28, 2000) has rightly portrayed the present population scene, which present a depressing picture. To quote him: "It is very well known that we are adding at least about 1.5 crore "additional" children every year to our population. Thus, the reality is that hardly 10 percent of the "additional" children accruing every year in India are getting (even) enrolment in primary schools and the rest 1.35 crore per year are being left to grow up without any school education. Thus, we need to open at least 60,000 new primary schools per year to meet the constitutional requirement whereas we have been opening only 6000 new primary schools per year. Thus, our "educational rate" is, in fact, declining about 1.4 per cent per year. It is feasible now for the country to open 60,000 new primary schools per year and provide free and compulsory primary education to all the children as required in the constitution without first controlling our population growth? And, again, it is possible to empower women without even primary school education?"

It might be recalled that in 1970 Dr. Norman Borlaug, in his speech that he gave on the occasion of receiving the Nobel Prize cautioned that whatever was being done by way of increasing food production would give us a breathing time of not more than 30 years which should be used to tame the population monster. We have now come to the end of that grace period but our population is still increasing by about 1.6 crore per year. Also, according to a recent study report, "Population, Food Production and Nutrition in India", published by UNFPA, India (Oct.1999), "there is an urgent need to reduce population growth so that the demand for foodgrains can be reduced and effectively met."

The question arises as to what is the major problem? It may be mentioned that the main problem in the less developed world including India is that of inadequate and inefficient administration which directly or indirectly impinge on the implementation of family planning programmes. The success of family planning programmes can ensured only through innovative, impartial, honest and efficient administration. There is a need that Family Planning Administration must be modernized, i.e. recreated, renewed and revitalized to achieve the predesigned changes and output. This needs a different trend and magnitude of Administrative Management, culture and capability especially in a challenging area of Family Planning. Let us analyse some of the problems in detail which affect the functioning of family planning programme:

I. Ineffective Environmental Linkages

It is understood that the implication of family planning programme is a quite complex process in which medical, cultural, psychological, social, economic, administrative and even political factors are involved and intermingled. The existing family planning organisations are operating like other government departments and thus their performance is not adequate. A good organisation must respond to and react to the changes in the environment and establish environmental linkages, linkages are points of interactions with the environment. They can be classified into four categories: (a) enabling, (b) functional, (c) diffused, and (d) normative linkages.

(a) Enabling Linkage

It ensures and protects the organisational authority to operate its access to resource and its power to achieve results. One of the most important factors—which impinges on the programmes from its formulation to execution is political and its impingement on both the programme and its executors occur at al levels (national, regional, provincial, district) and at the programme input levels (financial allocations, personnel, material resources). The impact of policies and the political processes on the programme is both positive and negative and this insight provides the directions and options available to ensure greater success in programme implementations. Since political constraints are neither permanent nor inseparable there is urgency in adopting measures designed to optimise the positive contributions of political support as well as minimise and mitigate the harmful effects of partisan interferences. To make Family Planning Programme effective and stronger there is a need of more visible political commitment and commitment for demographic rather than health or welfare reasons.

For Family Planning administrators to operate successfully in this political environment they must acquire not only a deeper insight of the 'political games' as well as the 'political skills' needed to serve and thrive in that environment. An important asset is the capability of programme leaders to seek and maintain support from key political elites both at the national and local levels.

The Family Planning Workers at all levels must keep in touch with political elite to generate favourable public opinion. In this context, there is a great need at the local level where the family planning programmes are being implemented. Here, they must involve the members of Panchayat and other local leaders so that they can help the family planning workers in developing momentum.

(b) Functional Linkare

It is to link the programme with the task environment, i.e. university, research institutes, hospitals, etc. The Family Planning workers must analyse the agencies interested in the developmental activities and then get their support and guidance in their work. Such agencies are existing from national to local levels. For examples, at the grass-root level, we have teaching institutions, extension offices of many development departments. The need is to develop effective linkages in order to get the benefit of their existing structures and mechanisms. Let us discuss some of them.

(i) Collaboration with rile Elites

In this connection, it is suggested that there should be effective collaboration between the universities and the family planning programme as the universities can be a sources of strength to the programme from the policy formulation to evaluation. To quote K.P. Bahadur:

> "The involvement of intellectuals in the programme has distinct advantages. This was done in Turkey with excellent results. They have the ability and the social position to carry its message to the lower classes and to convince those who are hovering on the fringe of doubt."[10]

At the moment there is a dichotomy between the social scientists and the medical specialists which must fade away as early as possible. In South Korea, one of the reasons ascribed for the success of the programme is the association of the university with the family planning programme.

(ii) Collaboration with the Hospital

The success of family planning programme depends to a great extent on the way the programme can operated through the health services network in the country. The hospital provides a good platform from the educational and motivational point of view. About 200 million people approach the hospitals every year in the country and there the people are most amenable to advice upon any aspect of their personal behaviour including family planning. Maternity wards are special places for such work. Moreover, the hospital is the best place for family planning as it can provide all the services to deal with after effects.

Conventional contraceptives are not being used by the people in India because it requires high motivation and good standard of living, e.g., the sale of Nirodh has touched 50 million mark in India while in USA with half the population, sale is about 6000 million per year, in Japan with of fifth of India's population, the sale is 250 million per year. Therefore, the country should rely on sterilization, IUD, etc. Both of these require supervision of a high order. Hence, we must streamline the administration of the hospitals so that the hospital staff can also take up Family Planning Programme work with more earnestness and seriousness.

(iii) Co-ordination with Voluntary Agencies

Voluntary agencies can play an effective role in mobilizing the public opinion in support of the programme. The Family Planning Association of India and its branches in the States are rendering useful service. In this connection, it may be suggested that to revolutionise the programme, FPAI may take initiative in setting up the "Women's Club" in every village South Korea. At present, the 'Mother's Club' having a membership of, 20-40 women in each of 19,000 villages has become a multi-purpose basic organ for the nation-wide 'New community movement' since 1971, in Korea. It is significant to note that the family planning programme became integrated into a broader community movement by the Mother's Club at the village level.[11] This experiment has been a great success in South Korea. We can bring these members in the communication network with the help of a four-step strategy mentioned below:

(a) Provide the opinion leaders with the information necessary for a full understanding of the reasons for family planning including its relationships to national and particularly local development,
(b) Invite their suggestions for local activities,
(c) Involve them in the purview of radio and television programmes, and
(d) Invite them to open discussion about family planning in the community whether formally or informally.[12]

Mrs. Helvi Sipila has also stressed that the associations of women organisations will surely help in checking the menace of population explosion.[13] A study of the inter-relationship of the status of women and family planning was conducted in accordance with economic and social council resolution.[14] The report affirmed:

(a) The right to decide freely and responsibly on the number and spacing of their children is a fundamental right of individuals which facilitates the exercise of other human rights especially by women.
(b) Adequate information, education and services enabling

individuals to exercise this right are essential prerequisites for ensuring their complete integration in social and economic development at all levels.

(c) Family Planning which should constitute an integrated and essential part of development plan and programme in countries suffering from over-population can only succeed in concert with other measures which also improve the status of women.[15]

It can be said that the best contraceptive in the world is the involvement and the overall improvement of the status of women. Meher C. Nanavatty in his Article, "Organising Communities" has rightly stated that the process of Community Organisation, which is necessary for shouldering this work, has to be generated in developing community education for population control. The development of the nucleus of local leadership, involving the community in the study of the needs and requirements of the programme, the association of existing groups and their leader in the promotion of the programme, the effective use of educational and audio-visual aids with emphasis on creating the climate of change for and acceptance of programme. Their inclusion needs to be ensured by the non-official Organisations which would take upon themselves the responsibility of promoting community education for population control.[16]

(c) Diffused Linkage

"Life enlighten movement" means to reach the clients through mass-media. Organized family planning programme requires a high level of user participation. Any successful family planning effort must be understood and accepted by the people and be based on public trust and confidence. It cannot be solely dictated or legislated. Family planning is such a multifaceted personal and intimate subject that its practice can only occur on an individual, voluntary basis.[17]

The art of developing common understanding among people is vital to bring about change of attitudes and behaviour. Sociologists have classified the diffusion process which leads to a widespread acceptance of the programme into five stages:

- Awareness (the individual's first introduction to a new idea or practice).
- Interest (the stage at which he actually seeks further information and background data).
- Evaluation (the stage of assessment on theoretical grounds).
- Trial (a limited phase of experiment), and finally acceptance or adoption.

Naturally, the duration of the process depends upon personality factors which differs with individuals. Mass-media helps in creating awareness, in providing stimulation and motivation and in giving ready access to information. But at the specific stage of evaluation, trial and adoption, inter-personal, face to face, communication counts for much more and the inability of the mass-media to maintain a two-way dialogue with regular feedback restricts their utility.[18] Therefore, no medium of communication is as effective as one human being talking to another. The UNESCO has rightly stated:

The process of social and economic development is a process of human development for people are the targets as well as the essential variable in development. Communication being a two-way process, provides for participation at whatever stage of enlightenment of the individuals composing a society find themselves. Change agents are key factors in both the communication development processes since they are instruments for getting facts to the people upon which decisions can be based.[19]

The function is to be performed mostly by the field workers. At present, the field workers are not fully equipped to do this interpersonal communication resulting into much mis-informed criticism of the programme. For example, on the personal discussion of the writer with a group of rickshaw-pullers, it was revealed that they were not undergoing family planning operations as they thought that they would not be able to ply their rickshaws afterwards. Similarly, in a discussion with educated people one finds that the adoption of family planning programme would lead to many social and psychological maladjustments. It was found in a survey that multi-purpose workers felt a need for more training to develop skills and techniques to contact, communicate and persuade their clients in their own particular setting and identity of personality. Even the Haryana Government has admitted that training of the workers in the field needs re-orientation and pre-service training of multi-purpose workers is absolutely necessary.[20]

The ultimate test of establishing diffused linkage can be ascertained from the following:

(a) Awareness of the needs and problems of population control;
(b) Knowledge of schemes in operation, their objectives, service, eligibility criteria, agencies and functionaries for the delivery of services;
(c) Community's conviction about the efficacy and usefulness of the services;
(d) Community's clear understanding of its participation and contribution; and
(e) Active involvement of the people, their leaders, institutions, organisations.

(d) Normative Linkage

There has been little attempt to incorporate the family planning behaviour into the existing value system of the society. Social values act as a hindrance to ready adoption. For example, if people talk about birth control behaviour naturally related to sex, it is traditionally regarded as impolite. Besides, the demand for sons to carry on the family line has been predominant in the Indian society. Not only social values but also religious values often act as a hindrance.[21] Therefore, the mass-media and communication officers and family planning workers must dispel all these false impressions and taboos after a careful survey and research in demography. Mass-media and communication officers may intensify their efforts by organising public meetings of different groups-labourers, farmers, workers, union leaders and extensive use of various media like, cinema, exhibition, radio, TV, etc. may be made. At present, the full use of mass-media is not being made in the real sense inspite of the availability of the arrangements. More attention is to be paid to uneducated rural people and economically depressed classes. Family planning and fertility control behaviour of the client group especially eligible women have been affected by their socio-economic background.

It is found that the higher educated women tend to have a small number of children and the use of contraceptives and induced abortion is more prevalent among them. The socio-economic status as well as the urban-rural diffusion of client groups are clearly pronounced in their family planning behaviour. The Government of India, Ministry of Health, has also admitted that "high fertility rates have been identified as more a function of poverty than of anything else." Therefore, more attention must be paid to groups living under conditions of poverty.

2. Limited Financial Resources and Absence of Cost Consciousness Among Family Planning Personnel.

The most important aspect about the finances for the Family Planning Welfare is its effective utilisation, i.e. to ensure optimization. This can be ascertained from the physical results achieved. V.M. Dandekar in his Article, "Population Front of India's Economic Development" in *Economic and Political Weekly*, April 23, 1988 has analysed the Family Planning Programmes. He states that the expenditure on family planning increased from Rs. 12.14 per eligible couple in 1980-81 to Rs. 37.7 in 1985-86. There is a great variation in States, the expenditure per eligible couple varied from Rs. 59.59 in Kerala to Rs. 23.47 in Bihar. The cost per birth averted has increased from Rs. 285.63 in 1980-81 to Rs. 590.87 in 1985-86. Study the Deptt. of Family Welfare also found this. Expenditure on Family Welfare per eligible couple is the highest in Punjab.

This analysis clearly indicates that the resources allocated to Family Planning are not being fully utilized. Though, there are no two opinions regarding the urgency of averting birth. To quote Mr. V.M. Dandekar, "Whatever the cost, the Family Planning Programme must be pursued steadily. But, it must perform."

"It has been a matter for concern that there are considerable shortfalls in expenditure and disturbing increase in the cost per acceptor. . . .

Although expenditure has been mounting since the beginning of the Fourth Five Year Plan, Physical Performance has not been keeping pace with it. Capital expenditure on construction activities and vehicles has grown since 1969-70, but the number of equivalent sterilizations has been going down."[22]

3. Not Enough Use of Modem Management Techniques

In a developing country, such as ours, there is a great urgency to control population growth in the shortest time possible before it becomes too late. It is felt that the scope of experimentation is a costly and slow process. As such, we need to apply the new management technique to accelerate the process of population control. Family Planning functions are so pervasive, diverse and vast, in terms of the range of functions, the number of functionaries, and the areas of operation, that it would be risky to fail to appreciate the need for rationalization of the processes of management.

To quote Dr. Chi-Yuen Wu of the UNDP:

> "To create administrative capabilities, commensurate with requirements, developing countries must be able among other things, to use modem management techniques more effectively than in the case of the industrially advanced countries."

Family Planning and Population Programme involve large, complete and inter-related activities which net to be managed consistently to include the desired social change. Though there are a large number of these techniques like PERT/CPM, Operational Research, Organisational Development, Cost-Benefit Analysis, Management Information System; Work Study, Method Study, Performance Budgeting, etc. which can be used profitably to optimise the family planning activities. But, the management techniques suitable for industrial and commercial enterprises may not help in their pure forms. There is a need to modify and develop these techniques to make them applicable to family planning activities. We generally forget it and the result is frustration.

4. Less Emphasis on Relevant Research

Mr. Prodipto Roy in his Article, "The Uses of a Rapid Survey and Feedback to Accurately Assess Demographic Trends" has emphasized the need of co-ordination between researchers and policy-makers, planners and decision-makers. He states that the dialogue between the research workers, decision-makers and action workers must be maintained. The latter must feel free to ask foolish but sometimes difficult research question and the research machinery must be geared to answer these questions. A continual feeding of problems from high political places or low action places to simple or complex research design and execution must maintain a steady cycling and recycling. It is only when this level of research capability is built flexible, fast and with the capacity to save the entire range of problems that arise, will the population problem be put on an intelligent footing so that the policy can be based squarely on scientific facts.[23]

The researches so far conducted have not devoted sufficient attention to fields of organistional structure and functioning of family planning program and modem methods of administrative management. Evaluation machinery needs strengthening at all levels. Independent evaluation may be undertaken to ensure that qualitative aspects of the programme have not been ignored by the states.

Research is not an end in itself, it is only a means to an end. There has been a lack of co-operation and co-ordination among the institutions engaged in teaching and research. This resulted in disjointed, isolated and rank duplication of scientific research in the institutions engaged in population/Family Planning Research resulting in waste of scarce resources. Thus, there is a need that energetic steps may be taken to enlarge the scope of collaboration to avoid repetitive research. Besides, over the years, for a variety of reasons, the medical and family planning programme in the country could not follow the path of problem-oriented research in priority areas. The Sixth Draft Plan (1978-83) was also critical of the research policy pursued so far. It was stated that medical research in the past had by and large failed to lay emphasis on problems of immediate practical importance. The Estimate Committee in its 102 Report pointed out that it is unfortunate that resources, time and talent of the medical community of the country have not been meaningfully utilized over the years according to well thought out prioritity.[24]

5. Lack of Area Development Profiles and Programmes

The policy of the Family Planning Programme Organisation in terms of targets are made only for the state or country as a whole. No attempt has been made so far to prepare action plans for each sub-centre/primary health centre or urban centre in terms of money, equipment, personnel, time, physical targets, etc. Such action programme if designed would help in effective implementation and monitoring. Here, we can make use of the new techniques of management-PERT/CPM for proper programme planning and resource deployment.

It is understood that planning covers not only the determination of programme objectives and overall targets but also the detailed specification of activities and projects as well as resources allocation for the achievement of specific project targets during a given period of time. In the case of most Asian countries, planning of FP programmes covers only the official statement of programme objectives in terms of national demographic goals and the determination of the overall targets of FP acceptance. There is no such management planning that is conducive to programme implementation through the provision of guidelines for managers and administrators of FP programmes at every level regarding specific actions to be undertaken in terms of what to do (specification of activity design), how much to do (individual activity targets and budgeting), what is required (standard of performance), how to secure the desired performance (monitoring), how to co-operate (organisation)., etc. In most Asian countries, FP programmes are conceptually specified into primary functional categories such as: (1) contraceptive services and supplies (FP delivery), (2) information, education and communication; (IEC) for mass education, (3) training of FP personnels, (4) research and: training, (5) administration, etc. According to information revealed in the plan documents of programmes, however, the elaboration of these: activities into further specific sub-functional categories is not made and thus managerial strategies for achieving the programme targets are hardly demonstrated. The lack of specification of FP programmes in the planning stage does not help in guiding adequately the administrators' role in management planning, monitoring and evaluation.

6. Lack of Team Work in Family Planning

Besides Planning and Training, we may keep in mind that team-work among different categories of personnel engaged in family planning activities is of vital significance.

Most of the Family Planning workers are working in isolation i.e, their activities are not co-ordinated properly resulting into lower output of services. According to Antonia Ordonex-Plaja: "Team work requires, among other things, that the members have an image of their team-mates, which coincides as precisely as possible with reality. In addition, each member must have a self- image which adjusts to reality as much as possible and thus coincides with the image the other members have of him."[25]

The team work would develop common practices and shared practices. This would also raise the morale of the personnel working at the grass-root level.

Another important area is of Organisational Communication which can bind and keep united all the Family Planning workers. Effective communication in the Family Planning organisation is very important because:

(i) Unless employees know the organisational objectives, they cannot associate them with their own;

(ii) It is essential to the management of change in the organisation. Without facts, understanding, and acceptance, efforts to change are doomed to failure, without well directed communication, are is not a chance; and

(ill) Without a communication, sharing of ideas with others will take place.

Let us now mention some other problems:

1. No reliable criteria for evaluation of the impact of family planning programme.

2. Inadequate Management Information System to Monitor Family Planning Programmes to ensure effective policy-making, implementation and evaluation.
3. Lack of dedicated and committed leadership.
4. Inadequacy of personnel planning and development.
5. Lack of effective public responsibility and accountability.
6. Lack of adequate administrative machinery for implementation.
7. Increasing women's status through women empowerment.

CONCLUSION

Joung Wahang has identified some potential areas where administrative reforms and improvements can help in increasing operational efficiency, i.e.

(a) To get F.P. methods (including instruments and services) identified and defined;
(b) To get sufficient amount and reliable quality of F.P. instruments and services available to the clients;
(c) To get F.P. instruments and services available to clients in the most appropriate places;
(d) To get F.P. instruments and services available to clients at the most reasonable price and costs; and
(e) To get F.P. instruments and services available without any psychological embarrassment and disturbance to the privacy of clients.

We should not be pessimistic. We should hope that the present momentum built-up since the Sixth Plan would continue. We should not hesitate to bring about innovative changes to make the programme realistic. We cannot afford to allow the programme to go slow as the programme is a source of strength to all other schemes of socio-economic development, whatever may be their immediate goal. Prime Minister Indira Gandhi, has rightly said on September 30, 1983, at New York while receiving the United Nations Population Award.

The enabling objectives during the Ninth Plan period, therefore will be to reduce population growth rate by:

(a) meeting all the felt needs for contraception, and
(b) reducing the infant and maternal morbidity and mortality so that their is a reduction in the desired level of fertility.

The strategies during the Ninth Plan will—

(a) To assess the needs for reproductive and child health at PHC level and undertake area specific micro-planning, and

(b) To provide need-based, demand-driven high quality, integrated reproductive and child health care.

The programmes will be directed towards:

(a) Bridging the gaps in essential infrastructure and manpower through a flexible approach and improving operational efficiency through investment in social; behaviour and operational research.
(b) Providing additional assistance to poorly performing districts identified on the basis of the 1991 census to fill existing gaps in infrastructure and manpower.
(c) Ensuring uninterrupted supply of essential drugs, vaccines and contraceptives, adequate in quantity and appropriate in quality.
(d) Promoting male participation in the Planned Parenthood movement and increasing the level of acceptance of vasectomy.

Efforts will be intensified to enhance the quality and coverage of family welfare services through:

(a) Increasing participation of general medical practitioners working in voluntary, private, joint sectors and the active cooperation of practitioners of ISM and H.
(b) Involvement of the Panchayat Raj Institutions for ensuring inter-sectoral coordination and community participation in planning, monitoring and management.
(c) Involvement of the industries, organised and unorganized sectors, agriculture workers and labour representatives.

It is said that prosperity is a good contraceptive. But the effects of development submerged unless we bring about a low birth rate. Family Planning is an input for development, an indispensable exercise in human capital formation. Education, better capacity for producing and earning a higher rise in per capita income are possible only when population growth is curbed.

Government of India has enunciated the new Population Policy in February, 2000, Commenting on the New Population Policy Business Standard Editorial, "Sense on Population" dated February 17, 2000 commenting on the New Population Policy Business Standard Editorial, "Sense on Population" dated Feb. 17, 2000, remarked, The new national population policy, 2000, however may have a greater chance of acceptance it incorporates some of the lessons learnt from recent successes in curbing population growth. While the earlier attempts merely emphasized physical targets and ignored the vital aspects of health and education, especially that of the girl child, which are vitally linked to birth rates, the latest policy seeks to squarely address these issues. Besides, it also makes the right kind of noises about investment in social infrastructure as an essential prerequisite for promoting small family norms.

Success of the new policy will depend largely on the way it is implemented by the laggard states and the pace of socio-economic development (including in the field of health and education) that accompanies it. Measures like freezing the number of seats in the Lok Sabha at the current level are essentially facilitators, dispelling states fears that population control will reduce their quota of MPs. There has to be an adequate political will to achieve the twin, variably inseparable, objectives of reducing family size and improving the quality of life. However, The Tribune Editorial "Gaps in Population Policy" dated February 17, 2000 suggested the gaps in new policy and stressed the need to make up these gaps. Increasing population packs a greater destructive power than what Pakistan can cause by hurling a few nuclear bomb blasts. That is because it is concentrated at the bottom of the social and economic pyramid covering three-fourth of the population. The failure to control the exploding numbers is the most damaging of all failures. What the country needed was a radical review of the old policies, alertness to deploy all available instruments and establish enduring contacts with the target segment in rural India. Sadly these are missing in the New National Population Policy unveiled. The document still pins its hopes on a few tired incentives and shapeless promises to rein in population growth. Such sops will be available only after the event — that is, after individuals or couples take themselves out of the reproduction cycle. Actually, the concentration should have been on goading people to enter the charmed circle.

To quote S.P. Singh again, According to the provisional results of the 2001 Census, India's population stood 1,027 million on March 1, 2001, comprising 531 million males and 496 million females. From 361 million at the time of Independence the population reached one billion in 2001, registering an increase of nearly three times. All this had happened when country is not in a position to guarantee adequate nutrition, health- and education to the burgeoning population. At the same time, it is true that all this has happened because of mass poverty in the country. Indifferent government is also partly responsible for the current graphic and health scenario. Every year about 18 million people added to India's population during 1991-2001 as against 16 million during 1981-91 (Table 3.1). In other words, each year India's on Increases by the equivalents of the number of inhabitants of Australia, Mozambique or Saudi Arabia

Notes and References

1. UN: E.F.S. 75, XIII. 4, p. 76.
2. Gunnar Myrdal, "Asian Drama: An Inquiry Into the Poverty of Nation", Vol. III, London, 1968, p. 154.
3. Alexander Kessler, Family Planning and the role of WHO" in *World Health*, May-June, p. 30.

4. Maryellen Fullan, "*People*—A Journal of the International Planned Parenthood Federation", Vol 5, Number 4, 1978, p. 27
5. Ansley, J. Coale, "Population and Economic Development", in Phillip M. Hauser (ed.), The Population Dilemma, p. 69.
6. WHO, (1971) Technical Report Series, No. 483.
7. WHO, (1971), Technical Report Series, No. 473.
8. WHO, Technical Report Series, No. 442.
9. *The Daily Tribune*, January, 28, 2000.
10. KP Baholdur, Population Crisis in India, National, New Delhi, 1977, p. 37.
11. Joung, Whaff, Ph.D., Graduate School of Public Admn., Seoul, National University, Seoul, Korea, Seventh General Assembly and Conference on "Implementation—The Problem of Achieving Results", EROPA, 24-31, October 1973, Tokyo, Japan, pp. 69-106.
12. U.N, F/F/S. 75, XIII, 5, p. 383.
13. Mrs. Hevli Sipila, Assistant Secretary General, "Social Development and Humanities Affairs", UN, June 17, 1975, *Weekly News Letter*, UN Information Centre, New Delhi, Vol. 25, No. 3.
14. UN, 1326, (XLIV).
15. UN, F/C/N/6/5755, Add 13, ECOSOC.
16. Council for Social Development,, New Delhi, 1969.
17. UN, Public Administration Division of the Department of Economics and Social Affairs, "Organisation and Administration of Family Planning Programme", UN: F/E/75, XIII, 5, p. 494.
18. UNESCO, Communication Media, Family Planning and Development, No. I, Paris, 1975.
19. UNESCO, Communication in Support of Population, Family Planning and Development, E/F/S.75, XIII, 5, p. 482.
20. State Family Planning Bureau, Haryana: National Population Conference (6th to 8th December, 1974), Population Statement of Haryana State
21. S.S. Kamalai, and C Parvathemma, "Family Planning and Social Values", *Family Planning News*, March 1970, Vol. XI, No. 3.
22. Fourth Five Year Plan, Mid-Term Appraisal, pp. 223-24.
23. Council for Social Development, Aspects of Population Policy in India, New Delhi, 1969, p. 56.
24. Lok Sabha Secretariate Estimates Committee, 102nd Report (5th Lok Sabha), New Delhi, 1975, pp. 92-94.
25. Antonio Ordonex—Plaja, Teamwork at Ministry level in Teamwork for World Health, (ed.) *op. cit.*, p. 170.

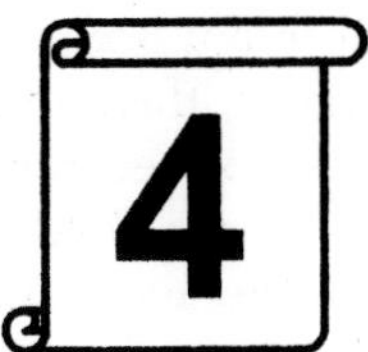

Challenges of Infectious Diseases in Community Health Care

India has been striving to achieve its goals of health, i.e. to prevent various ailments through better immunization, nutrition, environmental improvements and increasing awareness through various educational means. It has also been making provisions for healthcare to its populations by setting of hospitals in rural as well as urban areas. The concept of providing palliative care to those who cannot be cured or where the prevention of ailments was not possible is relatively a new concept. There have been loopholes in all the areas. Similarly, the aspects of proactive promotion of health through yoga, sports, and gyms have been rather sketchy. India today possesses the human power, infrastructure, financial resources and appropriate health care know-how to ensure quality health care for all its citizens. However, several loose ends need to be tied for better management of resources and better outcome for its citizens.

Many of the Ailments are Preventable

India is a victim of double whammy in the field of health care. While lifestyle diseases are invading the health scenario in a big way, infectious diseases have continued to show their ugly head. Environmental degradation combined with weakening public health systems have contributed to the resurgence of Diarrhea, dysentery, acute respiratory infections and asthma. Around 6 lakh children die each year from an ordinary illness like diarrhoea. While diarrhea itself could be largely prevented by universal provision of safe drinking water and sanitary conditions, these deaths can be prevented by timely administration of oral re-hydration solution, which is presently administered in only 27% of cases. Cancer claims over 3 lakhs lives per year and tobacco related cancers contribute to 50% of the overall cancer burden, which means that such deaths might be prevented by tobacco control measures. Estimates of mental health show about 10 million people suffering from serious mental illness, 20-30 million having neuroses and 0.5 to 1 percent of all children having mental retardation. The Infant Mortality Rate in the poorest 20% of the population is 2.5 times higher than that in the richest 20% of the population. In other words, an infant born in a poor family is two and half times more likely to die in infancy, than an infant in a better off family. A child in the 'Low standard of living' economic group is almost four times more likely to die in childhood than a child in the better off 'High standard of living' group. A girl is 1.5 times more likely to die before reaching her fifth birthday, compared to a boy! The female to male ratios for children are rapidly declining, from 945 girls per 1000 boys in 1991, to just 927 girls per 1000 boys in 2001. This decline highlights an alarming trend of discrimination against girl children, which starts well before birth (in the form of sex selective abortions), and continues into childhood and adolescence (in the form of worse treatment to girls). Dalit Women are one and a half times more likely to suffer the consequences of chronic malnutrition (stunted height) as compared to women from other castes. The delivery of a mother, from the poorest quintile of the population is over six times less likely to be attended by a medically trained person than the delivery of a well off mother, from the richest quintile of the population. An adivasi mother is half as likely to be delivered by a medically trained person. Thus preventive health and public health spending are closely related.

Only five other countries in the world are worse off than India regarding public health spending (Burundi, Myanmar, Pakistan, Sudan, and Cambodia). The W.H.O. standard for expenditure on public health is 5% of the GDP. The average spending today by Less Developed Countries is 2.8 % of GDP, but India presently spends only 0.9% of its GDP on public health, which is merely one-third of the less developed countries' average. The consequence of this dismally low allocation, which stands at the lowest levels in the last two decades, (in contrast to 1.3% of GDP achieved in 1985), is deteriorating quality of public health services. Over 2 crores of Indians are pushed below the poverty line every year because of the catastrophic effect of out of pocket spending on health care. Irrational medical procedures are on the rise. According to just one study in a community in Chennai, 45% of all deliveries were performed by Cesarean operations, whereas the WHO has recommended that not more than 10-15% of deliveries would require Cesarean operations.

Cigarette smoking in public places

One million Indians die every year from tobacco-related diseases. Cigarette smoking is the primary cause of lung cancer, chronic obstructive pulmonary diseases (COPD), coronary artery disease and a major risk factor for coronary heart disease. It is also the primary cause of chronic bronchitis and emphysema. "Passive smoking also called environmental smoke exposure is the phenomenon where non-smokers involuntarily inhale the smoke of nearby smokers. Wives, children and friends of smokers are a highly risk -prone group. Passive smoking is associated with an overall 23 per cent increase in risk of coronary heart disease (CHD) among men and women who had never smoked. A lot of harm is caused due to the inhaling of the side stream smoke." "Side-stream smoke is the smoke issued from the burning end of a cigarette between puffs. Mainstream smoke, as distinguished from side-stream smoke, is the one that is exhaled by the smoker after inhalation. Side-stream smoke contains three times more nicotine, three times more tar and about 50 times more ammonia. Inhalation of side-stream smoke by a non-smoker is definitely more harmful to him than to the actual smoker as he inhales more toxins."

"Supreme Court directed all states and Union Territories to immediately issue orders banning smoking in public places and public transports, including railways."

"The order banning smoking in public places would include hospitals, health institutes, public offices, public transports including railways, court buildings, educational institutions, libraries and auditoriums, the court said." "How practical is it to regularly pick up people seen smoking on the road or in other public places and take them to court? Does our police force have the time, manpower and infrastructure to concentrate on smoking offenders, unless they institute a separate 'anti-smoking squad'?"

Fluorosis affects drinking water in several areas of the country

Our bones are brittle, our teeth come in color, we seem to age faster and our babies do not have normal childhood—all works out to a different lifestyle. All of this we owe it to Fluoride. We also owe it to several successive central and state administrations, local and other leaders that conveniently forgot about our drinking water problems. We stand corrected! They remind us constantly at every five years or sooner at every election cycle. Our drinking water problem was an election agenda for 4 decades and unfortunately it still is!

Commercialization and Corruption issues in medical education

Medical education is commercialized by opening private colleges and makes a business out of it. Most of these colleges are not in rural places. Some of the medical colleges do not have enough infrastructure—the hospital, number of beds, and most important, the faculty. According to the report, out of 172 medical colleges and 123 dental colleges in the country, 23 medical and 38 dental colleges are in Karnataka alone. There is 30 to 40 per cent of the shortage in teachers in all the health science institutions in the state, resulting in substandard professional education in healthcare. According to the report, commercialization and corruption are two important issues that need to be tackled firmly. Corruption in medical education has raised its head at various levels, and a mechanism should be evolved to root out this cancerous growth, as otherwise it will erode the credibility of the healthcare system in the country. Corruption is visible at every stage, including that of examinations at the undergraduate and postgraduate levels. Starting from joining the medical college—you can buy a seat, you can buy the examiner, the corrupt examination system, you can get question papers. In the viva-voce and practicals, many people have paid and it is still continuing. Can we expect better treatment from the doctors who graduated in these circumstances? What are the steps we need to suggest to the government? There is a need to focus our concept of the health care services on the following observations:

(1) Metros and cities are becoming crowded; there is plenty of contaminated stagnant water, poor sewage system, poor drainage system, and new form of living style in the house without using mosquito nets, lack of adequate public health care facilities.
(2) It is not possible to check outbreak of any febrile illness like Dengue in crowed cities and metro despite of the large number of hospitals.
(3) Present day hospital system dictates maximum bed strength up to 300/350 beds only with more emphasis on ambulatory care, day care treatment, advanced technology with minimal post procedure stay in the hospital, promotion of home care treatment with family, with more emphasis on utility and supportive services unit of hospital system, more emphasis on preventive and rehabilitative care, integration and innovation of various other technology with health care technology and recently new form of medical education system separated from patient care system under single roof with the use of telemedicine, virtual communication technology, more emphasis on use of computers in medical education, more awareness of advanced technology in education with emphasis shifting to research division in education sector.
(4) If we observe our strength in nursing care, which is most important, it is insignificant. The present ratio with doctor is 1 nurse to 4 doctors. But it should be 4 nurses to one doctor.
(5) If we observe the history and geography of epidemics, we can see maximum outbreak of febrile and communicable diseases were seen in cities, metros except nutritional related epidemics in rural areas.

Telemedicine can promote health in the following manner—

(1) The two-way communication of health care in distant medical education, training in new technology, patient referral, and distant medical care, distant follow of care,

(2) Integration of clinical, experimental and research data in a multi-centric study all over the country in a single theme.
(3) Clinical marketing for the top dedicated clinicians and surgeons (who can not be made available in various parts of the country and he has to take care of his own institution).
(4) Feed back information network for clinical, administrative management of one sector, may be government, private, for organisational and policy matters of health care at a distance.
(5) Accreditation for qualifying doctors as present scenario dictates not-only recognized qualification, recognized training, but also utilization of qualification and training and the performance through tele network.
(6) Help lines for rural-based doctors for the management of complicated cases.
(7) Future progress of tele -surgery and satellite surgery in the country.
(8) Increases awareness among the receivers of health care regarding modern treatment and removes the age old taboos from the minds of people

A uniform system of telemedicine should be made by integration of private telemedicine network with government owned like isro-sponsored telemedicine under one national telemedicine council.

Health promotion

Health promotion is "the process of enabling people to increase control over and to improve health." It is not directed against any particular disease, but is intended to strengthen the host through a variety of approaches. Health promotion implies general measures undertaken to improve the health of community at large. Health promotion generally refers to broad measures undertaken in pre-pathogenesis phase, i.e. before the occurrence of disease. Providing safe water supply is not directed towards cholera or jaundice only rather provision of safe water is a general measure and a part of quality of life. Similarly ensuring provision of safe blood transfusion facilities as a health promotion measure is neither directed towards a particular individual or community nor towards a specific disease (HIV/AIDS). Health promotion measures are, because they address the whole society, large scale ventures and hence are very costly.

The well-known interventions in this area are:

(i) health education
(ii) environmental modifications
(iii) nutritional interventions
(iv) lifestyle and behavioral changes

The Ottawa Charter for Health Promotion (WHO, 1986) has led to the development of a series of health promotion initiatives based on settings. The pressures for hospitals to broaden their role from the focus on treating diseases towards health promotion have been felt for a long time.

Hospitals are in a strong position within the health care system to be advocates for health promotion. The hospitals are seen as credible sources of advice and expertise on health issues beyond their responsibilities for sick care services.

The key elements of a health promotion programme should include:

- strong leadership at different levels of the organisation (especially from the Board of Management, Chief Executive Officer, Assistant Chief Executive Officer, Health Promotion Consultant and several champions from corporate and clinical areas);
- incorporation of health promotion into the hospital's vision and strategic role statements, policies, service agreements with divisions, and job descriptions for staff, as well as a specific health promotion policy;
- strategic, operational and evaluation plans for health promotion;
- staff development and education; and
- resources allocated (human, physical facilities and financial).

Delegating health promotion

This approach has been observed in hospitals that have a health promotion unit, have designated health promotion workers, or have established community-oriented visions or departments who 'do health promotion' or 'have a community orientation' for the hospital. A common phenomenon observed in organisations with this orientation is that staff working in these roles, departments or divisions often became limited in the impact they can have on re-orientation of the broader hospital, as health promotion was often seen as 'their job'. Hospitals in the United States are increasingly positioning themselves as the leading provider of health promotion services within the community. Traditionalists argue that hospitals should maintain their long-established role as centers for acute care, relegating the responsibility for public health education to other community agencies. Progressive hospital leaders, however, are establishing integrated health care systems as a strategy for long-term survival.

In today's health-conscious environment, physicians continue to be perceived as the primary source of useful and reliable health information, but few people are satisfied with the information they receive from their physicians. Most people associate hospitals with physicians and transfer this perceived reliability and credibility to hospital-based activities. In many communities the hospital is identified as a centre for health. It seems likely, therefore, that people would want hospitals to take a leading role in health promotion.

Patient Education

One of the earliest health promotion initiatives within a hospital was the establishment of formal programmes for patient education. Many social factors led to the increased interest inpatient education observed in the late 1960s and 1970s including: the increased prevalence of chronic diseases requiring long-term and continuous management, often self-administered; a growing social concern about containing costs, the utilization of health services, and quality care; the consumer movement, public demand for influence in medical care decisions, and frustration with the complexities of the health care delivery system; documented evidence that patient education helps attain treatment goals; legislation related to informed consent; and malpractice issues. In response to these factors and others, supportive documents, mandates and guidelines have evolved to further entrench patient and family education as an integral component of quality care and professional practice in hospitals.

Many studies have demonstrated the benefits that patients realize from a planned and coordinated approach to patient education. Reductions in length in stay, reductions in complications, and reductions in admissions and readmissions to hospital are the benefits to patients most widely documented in research on patient education.

Clinical rehabilitation programmes that incorporate exercise therapy and health education enhance the continuity of care and treatment of people moving from the inpatient unit to the outpatient unit or home treatment. Following the treatment and stabilization of an illness, a rehabilitation programme is designed to return the person to a level of health equal to or greater than the level before the illness. The goal of clinical rehabilitation programmes is to improve stamina and strength, return people to their homes and activities of daily living, and at the same time prevent recurrence of the illness or injury.

Clinical rehabilitation programmes typically provided by hospitals include: cardiac rehabilitation and pulmonary rehabilitation; exercise therapy to rehabilitate mental health patients and those suffering from substance abuse and eating disorders; and sports medicine. Self-directed, home rehabilitation programmes are prudent alternatives to structured hospital-based programmes. Typically, the guide for the home programme is provided on discharge from the hospital. Rehabilitation professionals carefully educate people in exercise and lifestyle modification. Home programmes require frequent follow-up to evaluate progress, encourage adherence, and provide support.

Community and Corporate Wellness

Wellness programmes are designed to educate and motivate individuals to reduce their risk of preventable diseases. By adopting healthy lifestyle practices, the individual decreases the risk of premature death and disability, and the costs associated with medical care. The enhanced community relations and direct revenue resulting from providing health promotion services can justify entry into the wellness arena for many hospitals. Hospital-based programmes are typically directed at three audiences: apparently well groups or individuals within the community, employees of local businesses and industries (and their dependants), and the health professionals and other staff employed by the hospital. The programmes encompass a broad spectrum of activities and services, and are planned to address the health-related needs and interests of the target population.

It is a truism to say that education and counseling are most effective provided as near as possible to the time when need arises. In a study by Wallace (1988) patients expressed a consistent preference for preparation (including booklets) prior to hospitalization rather than after admission. With the use of individualized care plans and the encouragement of active participation of patients in their care, there ought to be a continual monitoring of educational need and organisation of appropriately timed response. Much of this response may take place on a one-to-one basis in association with other ongoing activities. In addition, there may be needs which could usefully, and cost effectively, be met through group methods.

A model of health promotion

Tannahill has developed an elegant model in which health promotion is viewed as a number of different combinations of prevention, health protection and health education (Downie, Fyfe and Tannahill, 1992). The model however, differs in its concern to emphasize and explicate the contribution made by education; its structure represents a development of the familiar health field concept.

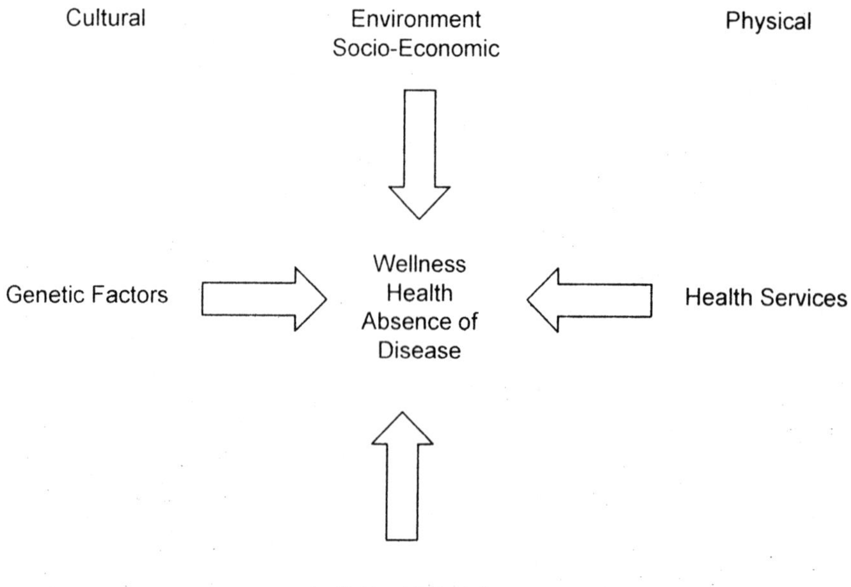

The health field concept

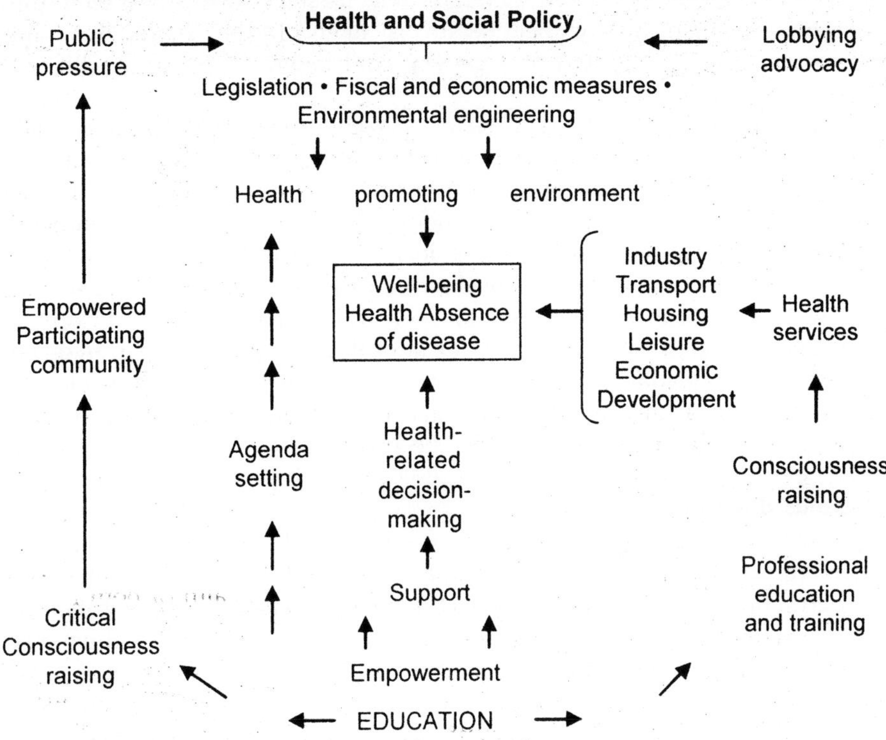

The contribution of health education to health promotion

The Alma Ata and Ottawa declarations insist that neither people nor health should be seen in isolation. Each is nested in systems that profoundly affect behavior and health. Health promotion must take this ecological fact into account. Such an ecological view represents a move away from the educationist tendency of biomedical science and some applications of health education in the service of centralized, categorical, and vertical programs, to a broader systems view. This view recognizes the interaction of lifestyle and environment when health is being considered. In this view, the individual and the context are of equal account. It legitimates both a lifestyle and a systems approach to health promotion.

An ecological model of health promotion says that health is the product of the individual's continuous interaction and interdependence with his or her ecosphere—this is, the family, the community, the culture, the societal structure, and the physical environment. Characteristic modes of interacting over time constitute a lifestyle, as distinct from discrete acts or behavior. The determinants of a lifestyle must be seen as a combination of intrapersonal and external environmental forces, continuously interacting. In some instances, health promotion programs need to emphasize the individual or behavioral side, in others, the environmental side needs emphasis as the point of intervention. If the individual has a sense of harmony with, or a degree of mastery over, the everyday environment, then his or her health is likely to be good. But with oppression, poverty, limited opportunity, and lack of mastery, health will suffer.

Health, in the Ottawa Charter, is still given the original WHO definition of a state of complete physical, mental, and social well-being, to reach which "an individual or group must be able to identify and to realize aspirations, to satisfy needs, and to change or cope with the environment" (WHO, 1986). Of special importance is inclusion of yoga in the management of illnesses. Sufficient evidence need to be collected on this aspect so that a scientific basis can be provided to yoga training in hospitals. Hospitals should be projected as role models for adopting HP practices e.g. hygiene, environmental cleanliness, food hygiene, safe water supply, provision of healthy food, clear air. People's religious sentiments may also be respected by providing prayer facilities within the premise.

Infectious diseases

When in 1967, US Surgeon General William Stewart made a statement that "...the time has come to close the book on infectious diseases", little did he realize that in the next 30 years or so more than 30 organisms would be newly discovered (Fauci, 2001). Some of them like HIV/AIDS have given more pain and misery than the pandemic of Spanish flu in first quarter of 20th century. With the emergence of new infections and re-emergence of known diseases, the books on infectious diseases might never be closed. Emerging disease is a term used to include diseases of infectious origin, new or whose incidence in humans has increased within the recent past or threatens to increase in the near future or those which are re-emerging after a period of quiescence. These new organism emerge from the dynamic interaction between the classical epidemiological triad of agent, host, and the environment.

A large number of factors are thought to be playing a role in this, with varying degrees of contribution in emergence of each infection. Examples of some of selected factors are microbial adaptation and change, human susceptibility to infection, climate and weather, changing ecosystems, human demographics and behaviour, economic development and land use, international travel and commerce, technology and industry, breakdown of public health measures, poverty and social inequality, war, and famine and intent to harm (Committee on Emerging Microbial Threats to Health in 21stCentury 2003).

In an analysis of emerging infectious diseases between 1940 and 2004, it has been observed that a majority (about 60%) are caused by zoonotic pathogens and vector borne diseases are responsible for 23% of them. The predicted emerging disease hotspots due to zoonotic diseases and vector borne pathogens are more concentrated in lower latitude developing countries (Jones et al 2008). It is also feared that in all probabilities the next flu pandemic too would raise its head from Asia. Multiple factors mentioned above are perhaps present and interacting with one another at the same time and at the same place. Main factors believed to drive the increased incidence, geographic range or both of emerging and re-emerging pathogens have been identified by conducting a systematic review of emerging diseases literature. Changes in land use or agricultural practices and changes in human demographics and society are the most common drivers. Followed by poor population health (e.g. HIV, malnutrition); hospital and medical procedures; pathogen evolution (e.g. antimicrobial drug resistance, increased virulence); contaminating food sources or water supplies; international travel; failure of public health system; international trade and climate change (Woolhouse and Gowtage-Sequeria Sonya, 2005).

A five pronged strategy has been suggested for countries of the South East Asia region, i.e. epidemic preparedness and rapid response; vibrant public health infrastructure; effective risk communication; appropriate research and its utilization; and passionate advocacy for political commitment and partnership building (WHO South-East Asia Regional Office, 2005).

Amongst the South East Asian countries, India is the big brother. It should be able to provide leadership in the region and assist other countries in their fight against the emerging infections. I would focus on the health research component of the strategy. In India, the research domains in emerging infectious diseases are in various stages of development, i.e. basic and fundamental, applied and strategic, translational and operational. Some of our infrastructural facilities are comparable to the best in the world. We also have a large pool of talented scientists. But we have not always clicked as an orchestra to produce symphonies. India has had its share of emerging infections (Vibrio cholerae 0139, plague, Gp–B rota virus, HIV/AIDS, Nipah virus, chikungunya fever, Chandipura encephalitis, H5N1 influenza, etc.) laced with successes and controversies. The Indian Council of Medical Research (ICMR) is the apex organisation for health research within the country, and it has played a very significant role in research on these organisms.

Over the past two decades, explosive epidemics of unidentified and re-emerging diseases have given the world a few close calls. Some have affected international trade and tourism. Others have led to the mass slaughter of poultry and farm animals. Some have overwhelmed a country's health services and diverted resources from elsewhere. Almost all have caused fear and panic. The appearance of pneumonic plague in Surat in India in 1994 led thousands to flee to other areas—at the risk of spreading the epidemic elsewhere. The outbreak highlighted the need for good disease intelligence systems. Early identification of the cause followed by a rapid response can prevent a small outbreak from becoming a major epidemic.

During 1997, the vast majority of countries had at least one infectious disease outbreak. Several had as many as eight. Some of the diseases involved—cholera, plague, typhoid, and meningitis—were old foes. Others —like the new variant Creutzfeldt-Jakob disease, a bird influenza affecting humans for the first time and a virus carried by pigs—were less familiar. If a global disease surveillance system had not been in place the outcome could have been disastrous. Ultimately national surveillance systems need to be strong enough, not only to provide constant alert and rapid response to outbreaks of endemic diseases, but also ready to respond to a sudden unexpected outbreak of a known or unknown disease. The emergence of the HIV/AIDS pandemic in the 1980s is a devastating example of what can happen when the world is looking the other way. Reporting systems are the intelligence network that underpins disease control and prevention. Without this framework in place it is impossible to track where disease is occurring, measure progress in disease control targets, monitor antimicrobial drug resistance, or provide an early warning system for outbreaks and the emergence of new diseases. Surveillance data is also needed to assess where resources should go for maximum cost-effectiveness.

At a global level, WHO has established an epidemic intelligence team, who monitor and verify reports of outbreaks anywhere in the world and provide a response team, where needed. WHO has also developed a global alert system which prioritizes surveillance for diseases such as influenza (FluNet), rabies (RABNET), HIV/AIDS, Creutzfeldt-Jakob disease and related diseases. In 1997, FluNet picked up reports of a new form of human influenza transmitted from birds. This virus had killed a three-year-old boy in Hong Kong. The incident sparked off fears of a new pandemic which—unless contained—could spread to other continents and kill millions. In the 1918 influenza pandemic 20-40 million people died in one year—more than the total deaths during the First World War. It could happen again. Six months later another outbreak caused 17 cases and five deaths. Through a rapid outbreak response—which sampled over 1,800 animals and birds—the virus was traced to live poultry. The authorities responded by establishing an intensified surveillance network and by destroying all live poultry stocks. By the end of 1997, only 18 cases had been confirmed. The virus did not appear to have been transmitted person-to-person and the threat of a pandemic receded. In 1999, the new system detected and reacted to yet another new type of animal influenza in humans. Every year FluNet gathers surveillance data from around the world on the various strains of flu virus that affect humans. Twice a year, recommendations are made to manufacturers on the content of the next year's influenza vaccine so that effective vaccines are available each year.

In 1996, Africa experienced the world's largest recorded epidemic of meningitis involving over 187 000 cases and 20,000 deaths. At the time, vaccine stocks were exhausted and countries were late in recognizing the outbreak. To make matters worse, the wealthier countries started buying up vaccine—in excess of real needs. Countries with vaccine stocks were using it sometimes in an unplanned way and with unsafe injection equipment. In response WHO established an interagency group to monitor the incidence of meningitis and coordinate the emergency supply and fair distribution of meningitis vaccine for countries in greatest need and ensure that it was used safely. The group estimates vaccine needs, and oversees the purchase and distribution of an emergency stock of high-quality vaccine and injection equipment. Countries get rapid access to the emergency stock of vaccine at a preferential price.

Early warning systems and prompt intervention to contain an outbreak can be highly cost-effective as well as saving lives. In Peru, an epidemic of cholera in 1991 cost an estimated $770 million in lost trade and tourism—almost one-fifth of normal export earnings. Three years later the epidemic of plague in India resulted in losses totalling $1.7 billion. Hotel bookings fell by 20%-60% and one airline lost $1 million a week. Elsewhere, the mass slaughter and destruction of cattle, pigs and poultry in the United Kingdom, Malaysia and Hong Kong SAR respectively, have caused heavy economic losses.

India is a hotspot for emerging infectious diseases (EIDs)

A study by an international team of scientists which recently published its findings in the journal Nature has warned about the old infections and new emerging infections. Of special concern are zoonoses (diseases that travel from animals to humans) such as bird flu, incidences of which have risen worldwide. Researchers from the Zoological Society of London (ZSL), the US-based University of Georgia and Columbia University's Earth Institute analysed 335 incidents of previous disease emergence, beginning from 1940, and determined that zoonoses are the current and most important threat in causing new diseases to emerge. And most of these, including SARS and the Ebola virus, originated in mammals. "India risks new epidemics as the human population expands into natural wilderness, coming into contact with a diverse range of wildlife that harbor unusual diseases," said Kate Jones, a biodiversity scientist at the Zoological Society of London. She said there was an urgent need to prevent further intrusion into areas of high biodiversity. Other zooneses in India include incidences of Japanese encephalitis in UP, the Surat plague, leptospirosis and more common infections such as rabies and anthrax.

Worldwide, the study found that disease emergences have roughly quadrupled over the past 50 years. Also, more diseases emerged in the 1980s than any other decade—likely due to the HIV/AIDS pandemic, which led to other new diseases in immune-compromised victims. In the 1990s, as per their report, insect-transmitted diseases saw a peak, possibly in reaction to rapid climate changes that started taking hold then. The team also prepared a detailed map highlighting the world's hotspots for emerging infectious diseases. Besides India, China and sub-Saharan Africa are the regions where there is increasing likelihood of EIDs. According to the researchers, about 20% of known emergences are multi-drug-resistant strains of previously known pathogens like tuberculosis.

Diseases are organized into the following 6 exposure categories and listed in typical descending order of risk.

1. Food or waterborne diseases acquired through eating or drinking on the local economy

Hepatitis A—viral disease that interferes with the functioning of the liver; spread through consumption of food or water contaminated with fecal matter, principally in areas of poor sanitation; victims exhibit fever, jaundice, and diarrhea; 15% of victims will experience prolonged symptoms over 6-9 months; vaccine available

Hepatitis E—water-borne viral disease that interferes with the functioning of the liver; most commonly spread through fecal contamination of drinking water; victims exhibit jaundice, fatigue, abdominal pain, and dark colored urine

Typhoid fever—bacterial disease spread through contact with food or water contaminated by fecal matter or sewage; victims exhibit sustained high fevers; left untreated, mortality rates can reach 20%.

2. Vector borne diseases acquired through the bite of an infected arthropod

Malaria—caused by single-cell parasitic protozoa Plasmodium; transmitted to humans via the bite of the female Anopheles mosquito; parasites multiply in the liver attacking red blood cells resulting in cycles of fever, chills, and sweats accompanied by anemia; death due to damage to vital organs and interruption of blood supply to the brain; endemic in 100, mostly tropical, countries with 90% of cases and the majority of 1.5-2.5 million estimated annual deaths occurring in sub-Saharan Africa.

Dengue fever—mosquito-borne (Aedes aegypti) viral disease associated with urban environments; manifests as sudden onset of fever and severe headache; occasionally produces shock and hemorrhage leading to death in 5% of cases.

Yellow fever—mosquito-borne viral disease; severity ranges from influenza-like symptoms to severe hepatitis and hemorrhagic fever; occurs only in tropical South America and sub-Saharan Africa, where most cases are reported; fatality rate is less than 20%.

Japanese Encephalitis—mosquito-borne (Culex tritaeniorhynchus) viral disease associated with rural areas in Asia; acute encephalitis can progress to paralysis, coma, and death; fatality rates 30%.

African Trypanosomiasis—caused by the parasitic protozoa Trypanosoma; transmitted to humans via the bite of bloodsucking Tsetse flies; infection leads to malaise and irregular fevers and, in advanced cases when the parasites invade the central nervous system, coma and death; endemic in 36 countries of sub-Saharan Africa; cattle and wild animals act as reservoir hosts for the parasites.

Cutaneous Leishmaniasis—caused by the parasitic protozoa leishmania; transmitted to humans via the bite of sandflies; results in skin lesions that may become chronic; endemic in 88 countries; 90% of cases occur in Iran, Afghanistan, Syria, Saudi Arabia, Brazil, and Peru; wild and domesticated animals as well as humans can act as reservoirs of infection.

Plague—bacterial disease transmitted by fleas normally associated with rats; person-to-person airborne transmission also possible; recent plague epidemics occurred in areas of Asia, Africa, and South America associated with rural areas or small towns and villages; manifests as fever, headache, and painfully swollen lymph nodes; disease progresses rapidly and without antibiotic treatment leads to pneumonic form with a death rate in excess of 50%.

Crimean-Congo hemorrhagic fever—tick-borne viral disease; infection may also result from exposure to infected animal blood or tissue; geographic distribution includes Africa, Asia, the Middle East, and Eastern Europe; sudden onset of fever, headache, and muscle aches followed by hemorrhaging in the bowels, urine, nose, and gums; mortality rate is approximately 30%.

Rift Valley fever—viral disease affecting domesticated animals and humans; transmission is by mosquito and other biting insects; infection may also occur through handling of infected meat or contact with blood; geographic distribution includes eastern and southern Africa where cattle and sheep are raised; symptoms are generally mild with fever and some liver abnormalities, but the disease may progress to hemorrhagic fever, encephalitis, or ocular disease; fatality rates are low at about 1% of cases.

Chikungunya—mosquito-borne (Aedes aegypti) viral disease associated with urban environments, similar to Dengue Fever; characterized by sudden onset of fever, rash, and severe joint pain usually lasting 3-7 days, some cases result in persistent arthritis.

3. *Water contact diseases acquired through swimming or wading in freshwater lakes, streams, and rivers*

Leptospirosis—bacterial disease that affects animals and humans; infection occurs through contact with water, food, or soil contaminated by animal urine; symptoms include high fever, severe headache, vomiting, jaundice, and diarrhea; untreated, the disease can result in kidney damage, liver failure, meningitis, or respiratory distress; fatality rates are low but left untreated recovery can take months.

Schistosomiasis—caused by parasitic trematode flatworm Schistosoma; fresh water snails act as intermediate host and release larval form of parasite that penetrates the skin of people exposed to contaminated water; worms mature and reproduce in the blood vessels, liver, kidneys, and intestines releasing eggs, which become trapped in tissues triggering an immune response; may manifest as either urinary or intestinal disease resulting in decreased work or learning capacity; mortality, while generally low, may occur in advanced cases usually due to bladder cancer; endemic in 74 developing countries with 80% of infected people living in sub-Saharan Africa; humans act as the reservoir for this parasite.

4. *Aerosolized dust or soil contact disease acquired through inhalation of aerosols contaminated with rodent urine*

Lassa fever—viral disease carried by rats of the genus Mastomys; endemic in portions of West Africa; infection occurs through direct contact with or consumption of food contaminated by rodent urine or fecal matter containing virus particles; fatality rate can reach 50% in epidemic outbreaks.

5. *Respiratory disease acquired through close contact with an infectious person*

Meningococcal meningitis—bacterial disease causing an inflammation of the lining of the brain and spinal cord; one of the most important bacterial pathogens is Neisseria meningitidis because of its potential to cause epidemics; symptoms include stiff neck, high fever, headaches, and vomiting; bacteria are transmitted from person to person by respiratory droplets and facilitated by close and prolonged contact resulting from crowded living conditions, often with a seasonal distribution; death occurs in 5-15% of cases, typically within 24-48 hours of onset of symptoms; highest burden of meningococcal disease occurs in the hyperendemic region of sub-Saharan Africa known as the "Meningitis Belt" which stretches from Senegal east to Ethiopia.

6. *Animal contact disease acquired through direct contact with local animals*

Rabies—viral disease of mammals usually transmitted through the bite of an infected animal, most commonly dogs; virus affects the central nervous system causing brain alteration and death; symptoms initially are non-specific fever and headache progressing to neurological symptoms; death occurs within days of the onset of symptoms. New Infectious Diseases recognized in India since 1973.

Year	*Agent*	*Type*	*Disease*
1973	Rotavirus	Virus	Major cause of Infantile Diarrhoea worldwide
1975	Parvovirus B19	Virus	Aplastic crisis in chronic haemolytic anaemia
1976	Cryptosporidium parvum	Parasite	Acute and chronic diarrhoea
1977	Ebola virus	Virus	Ebola haemorrhagic fever
1977	Legionella pneumophila	Bacterium	Legionnaires' Disease
1977	Hantaan virus	Virus	Haemorrhagic fever with Renal Syndrome (HFRS)
1977	Campylobacter jejuni	Bacterium	Enteric pathoger distributed globally
1980	Human T-Lymphotrompic virus 1(HTLV1)	Virus	T-cell lymphoma leukaemia

1981	Toxin-producing stains of Staphylococcus aureus	Bacterium	Toxic shock syndrome
1982	Escherichia Coli 0157:H7	Bacterium	Haemorrhagic colitis; haemolytic uraemic syndrome
1982	Borelia burgdoferi	Bacterium	Lyme disease
1982	HTLV-2	Virus	Hairy cell leukaemia
1983	Human Immunodeficiency Virus	Virus	Acquired Immuno-deficiency Syndrome (AIDS)
1983	Helicobacter pylori	Bacterium	Peptic Ulcer disease
1985	Enterocytozoon bieneusi	Parasite	Persistent diarrhoea
1986	Cyclospara cayetanensis	Parasite	Persistent diarrhoea
1986	BSE agent?	Non-Conventional Agent	Bovine Spongiform encephalopathy in cattle
1988	Human herpesvirus 6 (HHV-6)	Virus	Exanthum subitum
1988	Hepatitis E virus	Virus	Enterically transmitted non-A, non-B virus
1989	Ehrlichia chaffeensis	Bacterium	Human ehrlichiosis
1989	Hepatitis C virus	Virus	Parentally transmitted non-A,non-B liver hepatitis
1991	Guanarito virus	Virus	Venezuelan haemorrhagic fever
1991	Encephalitozoon hellem	Parasite	Conjunctivitus, disseminated disease
1991	New Species of Babesia	Parasite	Atypical babesiosis
1992	Vibrio Cholerae 0139	Bacterium	New strain associated with epidemic cholera
1992	Bartonella henselae	Bacterium	Cat-scratch disease; bacillary angiomatosis
1993	Sin Nambre virus	Virus	Hantavirus pulmonary syndrome
1993	Encephalitozoon cuniculi	Parasite	Disseminated disease
1994	Sabia virus	Virus	Brazilian haemorrhagic fever
1995	Human herpesvirus 8 (HHV-8)	Virus	Associated with Kaposi's sarcoma in AIDS patients

Global warming and infections

The outbreaks of highly infectious tropical diseases like dengue, chikungunya, encephalitis, etc., in India, is due to global warming and climate change, which are proving to be advantageous to the mosquitoes, to breed and flourish. Warmer weather and high humidity help vectors like mosquitoes, to breed more effectively. Chikungunya and dengue outbreaks have claimed hundreds of lives across India. Environmentalists in India believe that irregular weather and rainfall patterns, induced by global warming, are the main reasons behind the recent outbreaks and environmental management is the only solution to control such outbreaks of infectious diseases. Chikungunya, a disease characterized by high fever, joint pains and severe headache has claimed hundreds of lives and infected nearly 1.3 million people, across the country.

Incidence of malaria and tuberculosis

Why there is large increase of malaria and TB? These could include: (1) deteriorating standards of living, (2) mis-measurement in this standard, and (3) self-reporting bias.

1. *Deteriorating standard of living*: One possibility that comes to mind is that the people who are skeptical of the liberalization are right and life got harder for poor people in the 1990's and it's taken until the middle of the next decade to recover (at least for TB, for malaria we just don't know). However, this would not explain the upward shift in the whole function relating wealth and health, just a movement along the function due to deteriorating income. Further, on the basis of the index of "wealth" there doesn't appear to be deterioration among the poor in either period. Banerjee and Picketty (200_) looked at incomes of the top 1% of tax return filers and find their share of total income increased enormously since 1991. In fact, the change in wealth and the steepness of the function at the low end make the problem seem even worse.

2. *Mismeasurement of standard of living*: What is this measure of wealth anyway? Maybe the problem lies with that. The NFHS asks a battery of questions concerning what the family owns, what the nature of their house is (materials and number of rooms), landholding for rural households and the family's source of light and heating. The measure is simply the weighted average of these ownership patterns based on the first principal component of the variance/covariance matrix of this set of variables. Simple diagnostics for this exercise suggest the index is a reasonable measure of standard of living. For example, having a "kutcha" (bad) house, almost always associated with having a dirt floor, has a large negative weight as does using cow dung as the primary source of cooking fuel. The little jump way at the high end of the index is associated with automobile ownership.

A third criterion of "reasonableness" is how well the index performs relative to conventional measures. In the paper that best advocates the use of this measure. Filmer and Pritchett (2003) show that the error in measurement of conventional measures (relying, for example, on questions like "how much rice did you eat in the last two weeks") is much larger than the error for elements of the index ("do you own a bicycle?").

3. *Self reporting bias*: Some of the observed increase in infectious disease between the first and second rounds could be due to relying on self-reporting of clinical conditions.

Officially reported malaria cases were virtually identical at 2.2 million in the two survey periods and rainfall was similar in the two years as well. As for TB, official statistics show a substantial fall in prevalence from about 550 cases to 510 per 100,000 in the period between the surveys. The latter survey was done during a well-publicized and re-energized TB campaign in 1997 that appears to have had no impact on case detection rates (70, 68 and 72% in 1997-99 respectively).

What can be inferred, however, is that little if any improvement in the functional relationship between infectious diseases since the beginning of the reform era. While levels seem to be hard to compare across surveys, a safer inference applies best to shape and pattern of the functions. The function for malaria clearly gets steeper over the 1990's unless there is systematic reporting bias across income groups between the rounds—that is the cross derivative of bias with respect to time and income—is large. This increase in slope indicates that while people may protect themselves or be more resistant to disease to some extent, the role of public policy to reduce and flatten these curves has not been played well. For TB, the reverse is true for period 1992-98 where there is some flattening of the function even as it increased (as unlikely as that is). The improved shape seems to have persisted through the subsequent period as the function as a whole fell back to its original average level.

Infectious versus chronic problems

It is also the case that chronic conditions (blindness especially—from either cataracts or diabetes) are much more common at older ages. Many more, richer, people live to older ages than do poor. While poor people suffer from every disease more than do the less-poor, the rate of decline is much faster with infectious disease than with chronic conditions. A direct implication is that, ceteris paribus, any reallocation of a fixed budget from infectious to chronic problems will hurt poor people and help the non-poor. Further, unless one of the diseases is actually eradicated, this applies regardless of the overall numbers of people who suffer from each disease within an income group, being based on the marginal impact of spending. That is, this is true even if more poor people suffer from chronic diseases than from infectious. That being the case, the relative gradient argues for more concentration on infectious rather than chronic disease as a matter of policy.

What is shocking is the negligible amount spent by the public sector on traditional (in the Western sense) population based public health interventions such as ensuring safe water (as opposed to simply extending piped water with no attention to health at all), vector control, health education, drainage of swamps and a host of other obviously public responsibilities.

People appear to know when they are seeing "quacks" but prefer them to public providers because they are more reliably available and courteous. Similarly, if poor people received the majority of the benefits from PHC services, this would be another possible justification even if very inefficient.

Given that the evidence appears to show a deterioration of infectious disease control (or, at least, no evidence of improvement), that amounts of money spent on activities with large market failures are so small and that money that is spent does not tend to help the poor much, the experience of the 1990's shows substantial government failure in the health field. This was made worse by the central government in 1997 with the implementation of the Fifth Pay Commission recommendations to increase salaries.

Health is a relatively labor intensive ministry in comparison to many others and the higher salaries raising the wage bill did not help in supporting non-salary inputs such as pesticides, earthworks, drainage installation and maintenance equipment and drugs (for TB, say). Health education is usually expected from "Anganwadi" workers associated with the ICDS program (a central government initiative) but they did not benefit from the pay increase. They are paid nominal contributions and are not on official pay scales.

Auxiliary Nurse Midwifes are on government pay scales but their performance (in terms of attendance, say) has been questionable as they are paid via salary with little or no performance-related incentives. Health is a "state subject" meaning allocation decisions are made by the states but the Pay Commission decision was an unfunded mandate to increase wage bills. Given the difficulty of firing civil servants, this had a direct, if unintended implication of the relative spending priorities of the states toward Health along with other, labor intensive, Ministries. It also shifted the budget towards personnel within the Ministry.

The special case of sanitation services deserves some mention here. The bulk of spending for improved sanitation in rural areas is through the budgets of Ministries of Water and Sanitation or of Rural Development (depending on the state). Here the problem has been less one of low spending, though in many states it is that too, but of extraordinally poor implementation. Usually the problem is that such services are provided without concern for the health impacts of programs. For example, Kerala had a very extensive sanitation campaign of building latrines. It had a separate program for water supply. It was frequently the case that there was no coordination between the two and that the seepage of the new sanitation infrastructure directly contaminated the new water sources.

Malaria is usually a rural problem and, indeed, urban expansion crowding out breeding areas for Anopheles mosquitoes has been the main factor in malaria eradication in richer countries. Curiously, urban malaria seems to have shifted up more than rural between the rounds so that the functions are not very different and, at the same time the gradient in urban incidence appears to have increased noticeably over the period. Even if we remain skeptical about the interpretation of levels across the years, the change in slope is more disturbing. Official statistics could have systematic urban/rural differences (the location of health officials versus private practitioners influences reporting) but it is unclear why survey based data would have this problem. India has been urbanizing unusually slowly for a country whose economy is increasing so the expansion of cities couldn't have reduced malaria overall in the 1990's. If there is, indeed, an increase in malaria within cities, particularly among the poor, there is further reason to continue to fear continued problems with the disease.

However, political pressures seem to bias spending patterns toward curative care. From the politician's perspective, facilities have opening ceremonies in which they can officiate and are easy to observe by their constituents. They also open job opportunities which can be handed out as patronage. The outcome of this expenditure in terms of health status improvements is much harder for constituents to observe and to attribute to the policies that lead to better health. No one may connect the reduction of malaria mosquitoes with public works projects even if it was a major factor. Ironically, it is easier to claim credit politically for private goods rather than truly public goods. Beneficiaries know who they are.

Combating emerging infectious diseases in India

In late 1990s the ICMR stepped up its funding in communicable diseases which also accelerated research inputs for emerging infections diseases. One of the unparralled strengths of the ICMR is the network of institutes devoted to specific infectious diseases, and a chain of regional centres which are strategically located in areas where the chances of new and emerging infections raising their heads are high like in the North-Eastern part of the country, the Andaman Islands, and the like. The Government of India had started an Integrated Disease Surveillance Project (IDSP) in 1997-98. Surveillance forms an important cornerstone for control of emerging infections. The ICMR addressed the needs of the programme by providing inputs in capacity building, strengthening of laboratories, developing diagnostic tests especially the rapid ones, characterization of pathogens, surveillance of drug resistance, etc. In order to facilitate research in the unknown, new and exotic agents with minimal or no risk to the scientists and the environment, a chain of bio-safety level-3 laboratories has been set-up with largest being at the National Institute of Virology's Microbial Containment Complex at Pune. A modern BSL-4 facilities is also under construction in the same complex. A BSL-3 laboratory for aerosol animal experiments has also became operational. A state-of-the-art modern biology laboratory complete with transgenic animal facility has been created as a support to research in enteric infections at Kolkata. The animal experiment facilities in almost all its Institutes have been upgraded to conform to accepted national standards. Obtaining good quality animals for laboratory experiments had become extremely difficult because of some strict regulations. The ICMR stepped in to fill this void and has started to set-up a center for non-human primate breeding and research at Susnavgarh, Maharashtra. A world-class facility for providing biological resources especially the large animals is also expected to come up shortly in Genome Valley, Hyderabad. Microbial repositories for organism of major public health importance have been created, these repositories house large number of strains which are made available to other research organisations, for testing new tools, understating host-parasite interaction, etc. Rapid molecular tools for virus identification have been installed, (like real time polymerase chain reaction [PCR], nucleic acid sequence-based amplification [NASBA] platform, micro-array technology).

Other examples of some major equipments installed include confocal microscopes, sequencers, flow-cytometers, micro-array facilities, high throughput screening equipment, gas chromatography mass-spectroscopy, and DEXAs. Several of ICMR laboratories have been equipped with electron microscopes notably the digital cryo transmission electron microscope at Pune. It was with this frontline tool in rapid diagnosis that SARS virus was picked up, in a urine sample of a suspected person. The first indication that encephalitis outbreak in Andhra Pradesh may be due to Chandipura virus in 2003 also come from electron-microscopy studies. Very useful information about circulating strains, seasonality and other epidemiological factors is emerging from surveillance for influenza, rotavirus, measles, leptospirosis, etc. When chikungunya fever started in India in 2005 and spread to large number of states in 2006, it was an ICMR institute which created a diagnostic test and made it available to all the States. Early warning tools for dengue, Japanese encephalitis, malaria are being better refined using geographic information system (GIS) and remote sensing. A warning to the impending Japanese encephalitis out break was given to Tamil Nadu Government in 2006. As many of the new and emerging infections are viruses, and realizing that there is an acute shortage of training virologist and infrastructure in the country, the ICMR is addressing this issue at two fronts. A Masters course in virology has been started at Pune, and it is planned to create regional centers of excellence in viral diseases in the country.

To mount an effective public health response to a disease outbreak a vibrant public health system with skilled professionals is necessary. Complementing the Government's steps to augment training in epidemiology and public health an Institute of Epidemiology was started in Chennai which offered a two years masters degree in Applied Epidemiology and from July, 2008, a Master of Public Health (MPH) course has also started. Training courses of other support facilities are also organized, i.e. conventional diagnosis, diagnosis using tools of modern biology, rapid response modules, rapid assessment techniques, quality assurance and control and bio-safety measures. For the country of size and population of India, these laudable efforts are not enough. A well coordinated and an integrate approach is essential to tackle the threat of emerging infections. The doors of modern biology have opened almost endless potential, and we must harness them to combat emerging infectious diseases.

The potentials of genomics, proteomics and nano-technology are beginning to be appreciated and need to be further explored in diagnostic, therapeutic and microbial research applications and in drug and vaccine design. A beginning has been made of using gene and protein-based micro-array, it should be expanded to detect pathogens, to monitor drug-resistance, characterize responses to recent infections, and facilitate development of new drugs and vaccines. Laboratories have acquired the ability to sequence microbial genomes in a few days, this period could be further shortened. Studies on host-vector-microbe interactions are few and far in between. They must be promoted to understand the molecular mechanisms that underlie the pathogenesis of infectious diseases and host defences. Geographical information system and satellite imaging should be more extensively used to support surveillance and response. Tools for diagnosis, treatment and prevention need to be continually developed, laboratories for testing and field sites for their evaluation need to be upgraded and maintained on long-term basis. All this would require a very close interaction and bonding between the research community on one hand and the public health, agriculture and animal husbandry on the other. The importance of understanding the factors that increase contact between wild-life and humans in developing predictive approaches to disease emergence cannot be over emphasized. There is also a critical need for health monitoring and identification of new potentially zoonotic pathogens in wild life populations, as a forecast measure for emerging infectious diseases.

Research efforts should be supported that would guide public policy specially for rational use of drugs in humans, animals and agriculture. Likewise research on impact of environmental changes and climatic variability on the emergence of microbes which will inform policy discussions needs to be encouraged. All this cannot be achieved unless there is a national plan to strengthen health system and health research systems including human resource development. Adequate finances would need to be allocated to build and sustain appropriate infrastructure.

In October 2007, the Government of India has created a new Department of Health Research (DHR) within the Ministry of Health and Family Welfare Setting up of this new Department is a reflection of Government's intent of moving research to centre stage of health development. Amongst the allocation of business of this Department is to provide technical support for dealing with epidemics and investigation of outbreaks due to new and exotic agents and development of tools for prevention. This step is likely to give authority, direction, and boost to health research in this area. It is expected that DHR would play a conductor's role in orchestrating an effective health research response involving all players in emerging infectious diseases.

Should a Rapid Respond Fund to fight emerging infection be created it will go a long way in meeting the immediate financial requirements for travel, purchase of diagnostics, reagents, vaccines or equipments in emergencies. A chain of laboratories with appropriate biosafety would need to be set-up rapidly so that new and exotic agents can be handled confidently without posing threat to people and the environment.

The centres of excellence within various Ministries, Departments, Universities, research institutions in the country would need to be networked with strong linkages, based on mutual trust, confidence and respect. It would make more economic sense to share rather than duplicate cost intensive infrastructure. The way international scientific community came together at time of SARS, should be a lesson for Indian scientists for sharing experience, expertise and infrastructure for a common cause. Every time, we take two step towards successfully engaging an emerging infection, a new one erupts pushingus one step back in our efforts to combat emerging infections. Let's hope that new impetus to health research in India would help us take longer strides forward and shorter steps back.

HIV/AIDS; Growing concern

India is one of the largest and most populated countries in the world, with over one billion inhabitants. Of this number, it's estimated that around 2.4 million Indians are currently living with HIV. HIV emerged later in India than it did in many other countries. Infection rates soared throughout the 1990s, and today the epidemic affects all sectors of Indian society, not just the groups—such as sex workers and truck drivers—with which it was originally associated. In a country where poverty, illiteracy and poor health are rife, the spread of HIV presents a daunting challenge.

At the beginning of 1986, despite over 20,000 reported AIDS cases worldwide, India had no reported cases of HIV or AIDS. There was recognition, though, that this would not be the case for long, and concerns were raised about how India would cope once HIV and AIDS cases started to emerge. One report, published in a medical journal in January 1986, stated: "Unlike developed countries, India lacks the scientific laboratories, research facilities, equipment, and medical personnel to deal with an AIDS epidemic. In addition, factors such as cultural taboos against discussion of sexual practices, poor coordination between local health authorities and their communities, widespread poverty and malnutrition, and a lack of capacity to test and store blood would severely hinder the ability of the Government to control AIDS if the disease did become widespread."

Later in the year, India's first cases of HIV were diagnosed among sex workers in Chennai, Tamil Nadu. It was noted that contact with foreign visitors had played a role in initial infections among sex workers, and as HIV screening centres were set-up across the country there were calls for visitors to be screened for HIV. Gradually, these calls subsided as more attention was paid to ensuring that HIV screening was carried out in blood banks. In 1987 a National AIDS Control Programme was launched to co-ordinate national responses. Its activities covered surveillance, blood screening, and health education. By the end of 1987, out of 52,907 who had been tested, around 135 people were found to be HIV positive and 14 had AIDS. Most of these initial cases had occurred through heterosexual sex, but at the end of the 1980s a rapid spread of HIV was observed among injecting drug users in Manipur, Mizoram and Nagaland—three north-eastern states of India bordering Myanmar (Burma).

At the beginning of the 1990s, as infection rates continued to rise, responses were strengthened. In 1992 the government set-up NACO (the National AIDS Control Organisation), to oversee the formulation of policies, prevention work and control programmes relating to HIV and AIDS. In the same year, the government launched a Strategic Plan for HIV prevention. This plan established the administrative and technical basis for programme management and also set-up State AIDS bodies in 25 states and 7 union territories. It was able to make a number of important improvements in HIV prevention such as improving blood safety.

By this stage, cases of HIV infection had been reported in every state of the country. Throughout the 1990s, it was clear that although individual states and cities had separate epidemics, HIV had spread to the general population. Increasingly, cases of infection were observed among people that had previously been seen as 'low-risk', such as housewives and richer members of society. In 1998, one author wrote: "HIV infection is now common in India; exactly what the prevalence is, is not really known, but it can be stated without any fear of being wrong that infection is widespread... it is spreading rapidly into those segments that society in India does not recognize as being at risk. AIDS is coming out of the closet." In 1990 there had been tens of thousands of people living with HIV in India; by 2000 this had risen to millions.

In 2006 UNAIDS estimated that there were 5.6 million people living with HIV in India, which indicated that there were more people with HIV in India than in any other country in the world. However, NACO disputed this estimate, and claimed that the actual figure was lower. In 2007, following the first survey of HIV among the general population, UNAIDS and NACO agreed on a new estimate—between 2 million and 3.6 million people living with HIV. The figure was confirmed to be 2.4 million in 2008. This puts India behind South Africa and Nigeria in numbers living with HIV. In terms of AIDS cases, the most recent estimate comes from August 2006, at which stage the total number of AIDS cases reported to NACO was 124,995. Of this number, 29% were women, and 36% were under the age of 30. These figures are not accurate reflections of the actual situation though, as large numbers of AIDS cases go unreported.

Overall, around 0.3% of India's population is living with HIV. While this may seem a low rate, India's population is vast, so the actual number of people living with HIV is remarkably high. There are so many people living in India that a mere 0.1% increase in HIV prevalence would increase the estimated number of people living with HIV by over half a million. The national HIV prevalence rose dramatically in the early years of the epidemic, but a study released at the beginning of 2006 suggests that the HIV infection rate has recently fallen in southern India, the region that has been hit hardest by AIDS. In addition, NACO has released figures suggesting that the number of people living with HIV has declined. Researchers claim that this trend is the result of successful prevention campaigns, which have led to an increase in condom use.

The HIV/AIDS situation in different states

The vast size of India makes it difficult to examine the effects of HIV on the country as a whole. The majority of states within India have a higher population than most African countries, so a more detailed picture of the crisis can be gained by looking at each state individually.

Map of India showing the worst affected states

The HIV prevalence data for most states is established through testing pregnant women at antenatal clinics. While this means that the data are only directly relevant to sexually active women, they still provide a reasonable indication as to the overall HIV prevalence of each area. Data for six states are also available from a survey of the general population.

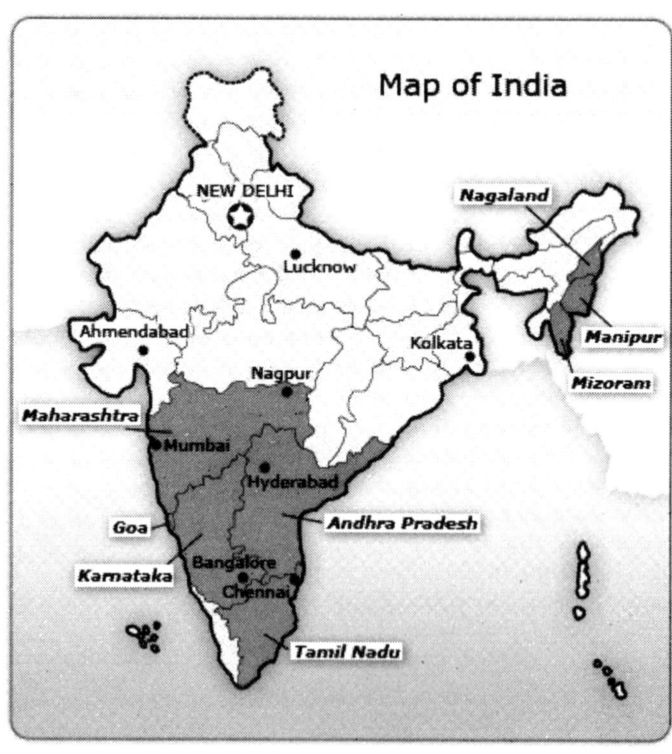

The following states have recorded the highest levels of HIV prevalence at antenatal and sexually transmitted disease (STD) clinics over recent years.

Andhra Pradesh

Andhra Pradesh in the southeast of the country has a total population of around 76 million, of whom 6 million live in or around the city of Hyderabad. The HIV prevalence at antenatal clinics was 1.26% in 2006—higher than in any other state—while the general population prevalence was 0.97% in 2005-06. The vast majority of infections in Andhra Pradesh are believed to result from sexual transmission. HIV prevalence at STD clinics was 24.4% in 2006.

Goa

Goa is a very small state in the southwest of India, and is best known as a tourist destination. Tourism is so prominent that the number of tourists almost equals the resident population, which is about 1.3 million. The HIV prevalence at antenatal clinics was found to be 0.50% in 2006. Prevalence at STD clinics was 8.6% in 2006, indicating that Goa has a serious epidemic of HIV among sexually active people.

Karnataka

Karnataka—a diverse state in the southwest of India—has a population of around 53 million. In Karnataka the average HIV prevalence at antenatal clinics has exceeded 1% in all recent years. Among the general population, 0.69% were found to be infected in 2005-06. Districts with the highest prevalence tend to be located in and around Bangalore in the southern part of the state, or in northern Karnataka's "devadasi belt." Devadasi women are a group of women who have historically been dedicated to the service of gods. These days, this has evolved into sanctioned prostitution, and as a result many women from this part of the country are supplied to the sex trade in big cities such as Mumbai. The average HIV prevalence among female sex workers in Karnataka was 8.64% in 2006, and 19.20% of men who have sex with men were found to be infected.

Maharashtra

Mumbai (Bombay) is the capital city of Maharashtra state and is the most populous city in India, with around 20 million inhabitants. Maharashtra is a very large state of three hundred thousand square kilometres, with a total population of around 97 million. The HIV prevalence at antenatal clinics in Maharashtra was 0.75% in 2006, and surveys of female sex workers have found around 20% to be infected. Similarly, high rates are found among injecting drug users and men who have sex with men. The 2005-06 survey found an infection rate of 0.62% in the general population of Maharashtra. This state is home to around one in five of all people living with HIV in India.

Tamil Nadu

When surveillance systems in the southern Indian state of Tamil Nadu, home to some 62 million people, showed that HIV infection rates among pregnant women were rising—tripling to 1.25% between 1995 and 1997—the State Government acted decisively. Funding for the Tamil Nadu State AIDS Control Society (TANSACS), which had been set-up in 1994, was significantly increased. Along with non-governmental organisations and other partners, TANSACS developed an active AIDS prevention campaign. This included hiring a leading international advertising agency to promote condom use for risky sex in a humorous way, without offending the many people who do not engage in risky behavior. The campaign also attacked the ignorance and stigma associated with HIV infection.

The HIV prevalence at antenatal clinics in Tamil Nadu was 0.25% in 2006, though several districts still have much higher rates. The general population survey of 2005-06 found a rate of 0.34% across the state. Prevalence among injecting drug users was 24.20% in 2006—the highest of all states and union territories.

Manipur

Manipur is a small state of some 2.2 million people in the northeast of India. The nearness of Manipur to Myanmar (Burma), and therefore to the Golden Triangle drug trail, has made it a major transit route for drug smuggling, with drugs easily available. HIV prevalence among injecting drug users is around 20%, and the virus is no longer confined to this group, but has spread further to the female sexual partners of drug users and their children. The HIV prevalence at antenatal clinics in Manipur has exceeded 1% in all recent years. The 2005-06 survey found that 1.13% of the general population was infected—the highest of all states surveyed.

Mizoram

The small northeastern state of Mizoram has fewer than a million inhabitants. In 1998, an HIV epidemic took off quickly among the state's male injecting drug users, with some drug clinics registering HIV rates of more than 70% among their patients. In recent years the average prevalence among this group has been much lower, at around 3-7%. HIV prevalence at antenatal clinics was 1% in 2006.

Nagaland

Nagaland is another small northeastern state, with a population of two million, where injecting drug use has again been the driving force behind the spread of HIV. In 2006, the HIV prevalence at antenatal clinics was 0.93%, and the rate among female sex workers was 16.40%.

Who is affected by HIV and AIDS in India?

People living with HIV in India come from incredibly diverse backgrounds, cultures and lifestyles. The vast majority of infections occur through heterosexual sex, and most of those who become infected would not fall into the category of 'high-risk groups'—although members of such groups, including sex workers, men who have sex with men, truck drivers and migrant workers, do face a proportionately higher risk of infection. See our page on affected groups in India for more information.

HIV prevention

Educating people about HIV/AIDS and how it can be prevented is complicated in India, as a number of major languages and hundreds of different dialects are spoken within its population. This means that, although some HIV/AIDS prevention and education can be done at the national level, many of the efforts are best carried out at the state and local level.

Each state has its own AIDS Prevention and Control Society, which carries out local initiatives with guidance from NACO. Under the second stage of the government's National AIDS Control Programme, which finished in March 2006, state AIDS control societies were granted funding for youth campaigns, blood safety checks, and HIV testing among other things. Various public platforms were used to raise awareness of the epidemic—concerts, radio dramas, a voluntary blood donation day and TV spots with a popular Indian film-star. Messages were also conveyed to young people through schools. Teachers and peer educators were trained to teach about the subject, and students were educated through active learning sessions, including debates and role-playing.

The next stage of the National AIDS Control Programme will see US$2.5 billion spent on fighting HIV and AIDS, most of which will be spent on prevention. Aside from the government, this money will come from non-governmental organisations, companies, and international agencies, such as the World Bank and the Bill and Melinda Gates Foundation.

The government has announced that this campaign will place a strong focus on condom promotion. It has already supported the installation of over 11,000 condom vending machines in colleges, road-side restaurants, stations, gas stations and hospitals, and plans to increase this number to 100,000 by the end of 2007. With support from the United States Agency for International Development (USAID), the government has also initiated a campaign called 'Condom Bindas Bol!', which involves advertising, public events and celebrity endorsements. It aims to break the taboo that currently surrounds condom use in India, and to persuade people that they should not be embarrassed to buy them. In one unique scheme, health activists in West Bengal are attempting to promote condom use through kite flying, which is popular before the state's biggest festival, Durga Puja: "The colorful kites carry the message that using a condom is a simple and instinctive act... they can fly high in the sky and land at distant places where we cannot reach."

This initiative is an example of how HIV prevention campaigns in India can be tailored to the situations of different states and areas. In doing so, they can make an important impact, particularly in rural areas where information is often lacking. Small-scale campaigns like this are often run or supported by non-governmental organisations, which play a vital role in preventing infections throughout India, particularly among high-risk groups. In some cases, members of these risk groups have formed their own organisations to respond to the epidemic. The government has however funded a small number of national campaigns to spread awareness about HIV/AIDS to complement the local level initiatives.

On World AIDS Day 2007 India flagged off its largest national campaign to date, in the form of a seven-coach train. The train, which will visit 23 states, stopping at over 180 stations, will offer education, counseling, an exhibition and symptomatic treatment.

Testing

The general consensus among those fighting AIDS worldwide is that HIV testing should be carried out voluntarily, with the consent of the individual concerned. This view has been supported by the Indian government and NACO, who have helped to establish of hundreds of voluntary counselling and testing (VCT) centres in India. By the end of 2005 there were 873 VCT centres in India, compared to just 62 in 1997. These centres tested 225,600 people for HIV during 2005.

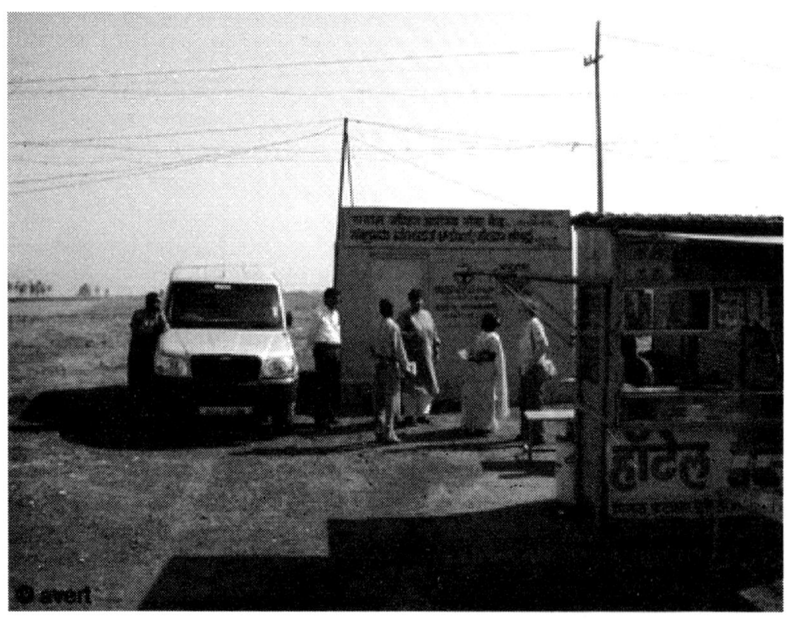

Health Clinic near Sangli, India, 2005

Although voluntary testing is officially supported in India, some states have tried to implement policies that would force people to be tested for HIV against their will. In Goa, the state government recently planned to make HIV tests compulsory before marriage, and in Punjab it has been proposed that all people wishing to obtain or retain a driver's license should be tested for HIV. Neither of these plans has come to pass, but they have concerned activists, who argue that HIV testing should never be imposed on people against their wishes.

Unfortunately, cases of people being tested without their consent or knowledge are common in Indian hospitals. In one 2002 study, it was suggested that over 95% of patients listed for surgical procedures are tested against their will, often resulting in their surgery being cancelled. Hospital staff and health professionals, much like the rest of the Indian population, are often unaware of the facts about HIV. This leads to unnecessary fears and, in some cases, causes them to stigmatise HIV positive people and discriminate against them, including testing them without consent.

Treatment for people living with HIV

HAART—a form of treatment involving antiretroviral drugs (ARVs), which significantly delays the progression from HIV to AIDS—has been available in richer countries since 1996. Unfortunately, as in many poorer countries, access to this treatment is severely limited in India, with only about 95,000 people (less than 15% of those in need) receiving ARVs in India by the end of 2006. Some people manage to access the drugs through private health facilities, which dominate India's healthcare sector, but the vast majority of people cannot afford to buy treatment privately. While the coverage of treatment remains unacceptably low, improvements are being made. The government has started to expand access to ARVs in a number of areas, and the national number of ARV centers increased from 25 to around 70 in 2005 alone.

In 2008, India's National Aids Control Organisation (NACO) began to roll out government funded second-line antiretroviral treatment. Second line ARV's are needed for people who's HIV has become resistant to the effects of their medication, necessitating a change in their antiretroviral regime.

NACO's initial one-year goal aims to provide second-line ART for the estimated 3,000 people in India who have become resistant to first-line drugs 47. Although welcome news, NGO and charity workers have voiced concern over that 3,000 people is a small target number, stating that this figure only represents a tiny percentage of those in need of the drugs. "Time is of the essence to save these lives, and NACO's announcement, although long-awaited, is short on urgency and on the scale required." Chinkhola Thangsing, M.D., Asia pacific Bureau Chief for the AIDS Healthcare Foundation, based in New Delhi. In 2009 select health centers across eight states rolled out second line treatment after the scheme was piloted in Chennai and Mumbai.

There are also plans to improve the provision of nevirapine to pregnant mothers with HIV, which can significantly reduce the risk that they will pass infection on to their child. It has been reported that, even where treatment to prevent mother-to-child-transmission is available, some women do not request it because of the stigma surrounding HIV.

The large scale of India's epidemic, the diversity of its spread, and the country's lack of finances and resources all present barriers to India's programme. Ironically, India is a major provider of cheap generic copies of ARVs to countries all over the world.

"It is a sad irony that India is one of the biggest producers of the drugs that have transformed the lives of people with AIDS in wealthy countries. But for millions of Indians, access to these medicines is a distant dream" Joanne Csete, Director of the HIV/AIDS programme at Human Rights Watch.

Stigma and discrimination in India

In India, as elsewhere, AIDS is often seen as "someone else's problem"—as something that affects people living on the margins of society, whose lifestyles are considered immoral. Even as it moves into the general population, the HIV epidemic is misunderstood and stigmatized among the Indian public. People living with HIV have faced violent attacks; been rejected by families, spouses and communities; been refused medical treatment; and even, in some reported cases, denied the last rites.

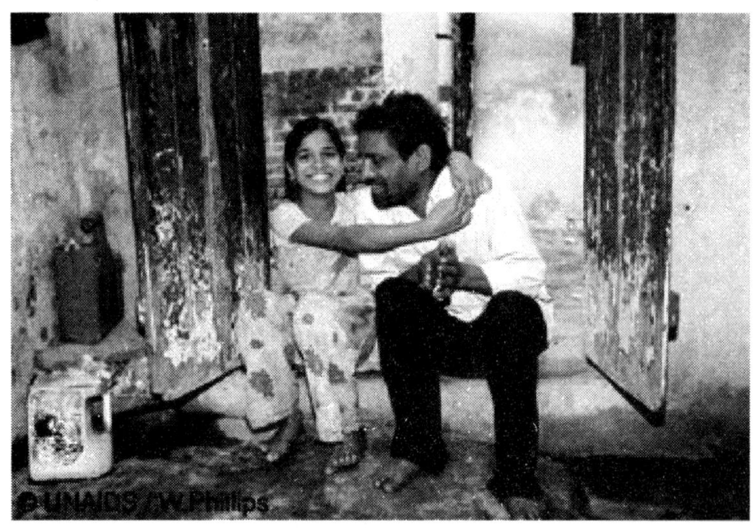

A schoolteacher fired after testing HIV-positive is embraced by daughter

As well as adding to the suffering of people living with HIV, this discrimination is hindering efforts to prevent new infections. While such strong reactions to HIV and AIDS exist, it is difficult to educate people about how they can avoid infection. AIDS outreach workers and peer-educators have reported harassment, and in schools, teachers sometimes face negative reactions from the parents of children that they teach about AIDS.

Discrimination is also alarmingly common in the health care sector. Negative attitudes from health care staff have generated anxiety and fear among many people living with HIV and AIDS. As a result, many keep their status secret. It is not surprising that among a majority of HIV positive people, AIDS-related fear and anxiety, and at times denial of their HIV status, can be traced to traumatic experiences in health care settings.

"There is an almost hysterical kind of fear . . . at all levels, starting from the humblest, the sweeper or the ward boy, up to the heads of departments, which make them pathologically scared of having to deal with an HIV positive patient. Wherever they have an HIV patient, the responses are shameful."

A 2006 study found that 25% of people living with HIV in India had been refused medical treatment on the basis of their HIV-positive status. It also found strong evidence of stigma in the workplace, with 74% of employees not disclosing their status to their employees for fear of discrimination. Of the 26% who did disclose their status, 10% reported having faced prejudice as a result. People in marginalized groups—female sex workers, hijras (transgender) and gay men—are often stigmatised not only because of their HIV status, but also because they belong to socially excluded groups.

The future of HIV and AIDS in India

Various groups have made predictions about the effect that AIDS will have on India and the rest of Asia in the future, and there has been a lot of dispute about the accuracy of these estimates. For instance, a 2002 report by the CIA's National Intelligence Council predicted 20 million to 25 million AIDS cases in India by 2010—more than any other country in the world. India's government responded by calling these figures "completely inaccurate", and accused those who cited them of "spreading panic." The government has also disputed predictions that India's epidemic is "on an African trajectory", although it claims to acknowledge the seriousness of the crisis. Indeed, recent surveys do suggest that national HIV prevalence has probably fallen slightly in recent years. This trend is mainly due to a drop in infections in southern states; in other areas there has been no significant decline. "In the north-east, the dual HIV epidemic driven by unsafe sex and injecting drug use is highly concerning. Moreover, there are many areas in the northern states where HIV is increasing, particularly among injecting drug users," said Sujatha Rao, Director General of NACO. Even if the country's epidemic does not match the severity of those in southern Africa, it is clear that HIV and AIDS will have a devastating effect on the lives of millions of Indians for many years to come. It is essential that effective action is taken to minimize this impact.

"The challenges India faces to overcome this epidemic are enormous. Yet India possesses in ample quantities all the resources needed to achieve universal access to HIV prevention and treatment... defeating AIDS will require a significant intensification of our efforts, in India, just as in the rest of the world" Peter Piot, Director of UNAIDS.

References

ActionAid (2003), 'The sound of silence: difficulties in communicating on HIV/AIDS in schools (experiences from India and Kenya)'.

Baria F. et al., India Today (15th March 1997), 'AIDS—striking home'.

Bhupesh M. (1992) 'India Disquiet About AIDS Control', the Lancet, Vol. 240, No. 8834/8835. NACO website, 'About NACO, National AIDS Control Programme Phase 1 (1992-1999)', accessed 4/7/06.

Bonilla-Chacin, Maria Eugenia and Jeffrey S. Hammer (1999), "Life and Death among the Poorest", World Bank Economist's Week.

Bureau of Hygiene and Tropical Diseases (1986) 'AIDS newsletter' Issue 1, January 30th.

Cassel C.K. ICD-9 code for palliative or terminal care. *N Engl J Med* 1996;335:1232-4.2.

Cassileth, Vickers, Magill. (2003). Music therapy for mood disturbance during hospitalization for autologous stem cell transplantation: a randomized controlled trial (abstract). PubMed, NCBI. Retrieved on March 7, 2006.

Census of India 2001: Provisional Population Totals.Registrar General and Census Commissioner, GOI.

Central Bureau of Health Intelligence.Directorate General of Health Services, Ministry of Health and Family Welfare. Health Information of India 2000-01.

Changing the Indian Health System—Draft Report, ICRIER, 2001

Chaudhury, Nazmul and Jeffrey S. Hammer (2005), "Another Paper on Poverty in India in the 1990's: Evidence from the National Family Health Surveys", World Bank, processed.

CLIP: Current Learning in Palliative Care. Online tutorials. Help the Hospices. Retrieved on March 7, 2006.

Committee on Emerging Microbial Threats to Health in 21st Century 2003 *Microbial threats to health in the United States: Emergence, defection and response* (eds.) M.S. Smolinski, M.A. Hamburg and J. Leaderberg (Washington DC: National Academy Press).

Das, Jishnu and Jeffrey S. Hammer (2005), "Which Doctor?: Combining Vignettes and Item Response Theory to Measure Doctor Quality", Journal of Development Economics, Vol. 78, pp. 348-383.

———(2007), "Money for Nothing: The Dire Straits of Indian Health Care", Journal of Development Economics, Vol. 83, No. 1, pp. 1-36.

Das, Jishnu, J. Hammer, S. Devarajan and L. Pritchett (2006), "Will a Wealthier **India** be a Healthier India?" presented at NBER/NCAER Conference on Growth in India, New Delhi.

———(2008), "Chronically Misinformed: Information, Income and Illness in Delhi."

David Alimi *et al.* (2003). Analgesic Effect of Auricular Acupuncture for Cancer Pain: A Randomized, Blinded, Controlled Trial. *Journal of Clinical Oncology*. Retrieved on March 7, 2006.

Deaton, Angus (2002), "Policy implications of the gradient of health and wealth", Health Affairs, March/April.

——— (2004), "Using food consumption to improve measures of wealth", World Bank

Deaton, Angus and Valerie Kozel (eds.), (2006), The Great Indian Poverty Debate, Macmillan India, New Delhi.

Disease Control Priorities Project, (2007) The World Bank, Washington, D.C.

Duggal, Ravi. Operationalizing Right to Healthcare in India. Right to Healthcare, Moving from Idea to Reality. CEHAT, Mumbai, 2003.

Earthtimes (2007) 'NACO Bows to Activists' Pressure on AIDS Treatment in India, Says AHF', 22 November.

Fauci A.S. 2001. Infectious diseases: consideration for 21st century; *Clin. Infec. Dis.* 32 675–685

Filmer, Deon and Lant Pritchett (2001), "Estimating Wealth Effects without Expenditure Data—or Tears: An application to enrollments in states of India", Demography.

Ganzini L., Goy E.R., Miller L.L., Harvath T.A., Jackson A., Delrot M.A. Nurses' experiences with hospice patients who refuse food and fluids to hasten death. *N Engl J Med* 2003;349:359-65.

Ghosh T.K. (1986), 'AIDS: a serious challenge to public health', *Journal of the Indian Medical Association,* January; 84(1):29-30

Grealish L., Lomasney A., Whiteman B. (2000). Foot massage. A nursing intervention to modify the distressing symptoms of pain and nausea inpatients hospitalized with cancer (abstract). PubMed, NCBI. Retrieved on March 07, 2006.

Gwatkin, Davidson, S. Rutstein, K. Johnson, R. Pande and A. Wagstaff, (2000) "Socio-economic differences in health, nutrition and population: 45 countries", World Bank.

Hammer, Jeffrey, Yamini Aiyar and Salimah Samji (2007), "Understanding Government Failure in Public Health Services", *Economic and Political Weekly,* October.

"HIV Sentinel Surveillance and HIV Estimation, 2006", *NACO,* 2007.

Human Rights News (2002) 'AIDS in India: Money won't solve crisis, Rising violence against AIDS-affected people', November 13.

Human Rights Watch (August 10th 2006), press release, 'AIDS Conference: Drive for HIV Testing Must Respect Rights, WHO, UNAIDS Policies Must Link Testing to Consent, Counseling and Treatment'.

InfoChange (August 2003) 'HIV/AIDS in Manipur: the need to focus women'.

Integration of behavioral and relaxation approaches into the treatment of chronic pain and insomnia. NIH Technology Assessment Panel on Integration of Behavioral and Relaxation Approaches into the Treatment of Chronic Pain and Insomnia. *The Journal of the American Medical Association* (archives), (1996). Retrieved on March 7, 2006.

International Institute for Population Sciences and ORC Macro. National Family Health Survey (NFHS-II) 1998-99. India.

International Institute for Population Sciences. Facility Survey, 1999.

International Institute for Population Sciences. RCH-RHS, India, 1998-99.

Jones K.E., Patel N., Levy M.A., Storeygard A., Balk D., Gittleman J.L. and Darzak P 2008 Global trends in emerging infectious diseases; *Nature (London)* 451 990–993.

Kaisernetwork.org, (September 5th 2004), Daily Report, 'India primarily to promote condom use in its HIV prevention programs, health minister says'. *The Hindu* (September 16th 2006), 'Shhhh not anymore!' Agence France Press (September 19th 2006), 'India takes condom campaign to the skies'.

Kakar D.N. and Kakar S.N. (2001), 'Combating AIDS in the 21st century Issues and Challenges', Sterling Publishers Private Limited, p. 31.

Kakar D.N. and Kakar S.N. (2001), 'Combating AIDS in the 21st century Issues and Challenges', Sterling Publishers Private Limited, p. 32.

Kiefer, Philip and Stuti Khemani, (2003) "Democracy, Public Expenditures and the Poor", World Bank Policy Research Working Paper Series No. 3164.

Kremer, Michael, Nazmul Chaudhury, Jeffrey S. Hammer, Karthik Muralidharan and F. Halsey Rogers (2006a), "Missing in Action: Teachers and Health Worker Absence in Developing Countries" Journal of Economic Perspectives, Vol. 20, No. 1.

Kremer, Michael, Nazmul Chaudhury, Jeffrey S. Hammer, Karthik Muralidharan and F. Halsey Rogers (2006b) "Is There a Doctor in the House?: Absenteeism among health workers in India", Harvard Conference on Health in India and China, New Delhi.

Kumar R., Jha P. *et al.* (2006), 'Trends in HIV-1 in young adults in south India from 2000 to 2004: a prevalence study', *The Lancet,* Vol. 367:1164-1172.

Lopez, Alan, and Christopher J.L. Murray (2007), Global Burden of Disease and RiskFactors, Oxford UP.

Mahal A. www.worldbank.org

Mahal, Ajay, *et al.*, (2002) "Who Benefits from Health Care Subsidies in India?", World Bank, Health, Population and Nutrition Working Paper Series.

Malavade J.A.B. *et al.* (2002) 'Ethical and legal issues in HIV/AIDS counseling and testing', Abstract ThPeE7902, the XIV International AIDS Conference.

Matching Services to needs. Copenhagen, WHO Regional Office for Europe, 2002 (document EUR/RC50/10).

Misra, Chatterjee, Rao. India Health Report.Oxford University Press, New Delhi.2003

Morbidity and Treatment of Ailments. NSS Fifty second round. Government of India, 1998.

NACO (2006), 'UNGASS India report: progress report on the declaration of commitment on HIV/AIDS'.

NACO (2007) 'Annual HIV Sentinel Surveillance Country Report 2006'.

NACO (April 2006), HIV/AIDS epidemiological Surveillance and Estimation report for the year 2005.

Nath L.M. (1998), 'The epidemic in India: an overview', in Godwin P. (Ed.), 'The looming epidemic', Mosaic books/New Delhi, p. 28. NACO, Annual Report 2002-2004.

National Coordination Committee for the Jana Swasthya Sabha. Health for All, NOW. 2004.

National Crime Records Bureau. Ministry of Home Affairs. Accidental Deaths and Suicides In India, 2000.

National Family Health Survey (Indian Institute of Population Studies) (1993, 1999) National Summary of Results, New Delhi and Bombay.

National Family Health Survey (NFHS-3) 2005-06, September 2007.

National Intelligence Council (2002) 'The Next wave of HIV/AIDS: Nigeria, Ethiopia, Russia, India and China', September, p. 3.

National Sample Survey Organisation. Department of Statistics. GOI. 42nd and 52nd Round.

Ottawa Charter for Health Promotion (http://www.who/int/hpr/NPH/docs/ottawa_charter_hp.pdf). Ottawa, WHO, 1986 (accessed 4 March 2004).

Pai M. *et al.* A high rate of Cesaerean sections in affluent section of Chennai, is it a cause for concern? *Nat Med J India,* 1999, 12:156-158.

Panda S. (2002), 'The HIV/AIDS epidemic in India: an overview', in Panda S., Chatterjee A. and Abdul-Quader A.S. (Eds.), 'The epidemic and the response in India', p. 20.

Peter Piot, speech at the launch of the 2005 AIDS Epidemic Update, New Delhi, 21st November 2005.

Phadke A. Drug Supply and Use. Towards a Rational Policy in India. Sage Publications New Delhi. Ministry of Chemicals and Fertilizers.

Planning Commission, Government of India (2004), Mid-term evaluation of the 10th plan, New Delhi.

Planning Commission, Government of India. Tenth Five Year Plan 2002-2007. Volume II.

Probe Qualitative Research Team (2002), Health Care Seeking Behavior in Andhra Pradesh, Bombay.

Quill T.E., Lo B., Brock D.W. Palliative options of last resort: a comparison of voluntarily stopping eating and drinking, terminal sedation, physician-assisted suicide, and voluntary active euthanasia. *JAMA* 1997;278:2099-104.

See Existential pain—an entity, a provocation, or a challenge? in *Journal of Pain Symptom and Management*, Volume 27, Issue 3, Pages 241-250 (March 2004).

Shariff Abusaleh. India Human Development Report.Oxford University Press, New Delhi.

Sivaram S. (2002) 'Integrating income generation and AIDS prevention efforts: lessons from working with devadasi women in rural Karnataka, India', Abstract MoOrF1048, The XIV International AIDS Conference. Tamil Nadu State AIDS Control Society, official website.

SRS Bulletin. Government of India, 1998.

Sullivan A.D., Hedberg K., Hopkins D. Legalized physician-assisted suicide in Oregon, 1998-2000. *N Engl J Med* 2001;344:605-7.

TB India 2003. RNTCP Stats Report. Central TB Division.DDHS GOI. Health Survey and Development Committee, GOI, 1946 (Bhore Report).

The Guardian (May 2006), 'Doubt over India's HIV claims' Sexually Transmitted Infections (2007) 'Interview with Peter Piot' Volume 83(6).

The International Society for Quality in Health Care. Alpha and accreditation (http:/ /www.isqua.org.au/isquaPages/Alpha.html). Victoria, Isqua, 2003 (accessed 4 March 2004).

The Times of India (2007) 'Red Ribbon Express to create AIDS awareness', 23 November.

The Times of India (2008) 'Fresh hope for HIV+: 2nd line treatment begins', January 24.

The Times of India (2009) 'Eight more states to offer second line treatment for HIV', January 5.

Time Asia (May 30th 2005), 'When silence kills', Perry A. Prasada Rao J.V.R *et al.* (2004), 'India's response to the AIDS epidemic', The Lancet, Vol. 364, No. 9442, October 9-15, 2004.

Time magazine (1986, 1st September), 'Public health: Nowhere to Run, Nowhere to Hide'. NACO (2006), 'UNGASS India report: progress report on the declaration of commitment on HIV/AIDS'.

UNAIDS (2000) 'Report on the global HIV/AIDS epidemic 2000'. July, p. 13.

UNAIDS (2001) 'India: HIV and AIDS-related discrimination, stigmatization and denial'.

UNAIDS (2007), '2.5 million people in India living with HIV, according to new estimates', press release.

UNAIDS (2008), Report of the global AIDS epidemic.

UNAIDS (2008), Report of the global AIDS epidemic. *NACO* (April 2006), HIV/AIDS epidemiological Surveillance and Estimation report for the year 2005.

UNAIDS (2008), Report of the global AIDS epidemic. *NACO* (August 2006), Monthly updates on AIDS.

UNAIDS (2008), Report of the global AIDS epidemic. The Lancet (2003) 'Spreading the word about HIV/AIDS in India', Vol.361, May 3.

UNDP (2006), The Socio Economic Impact of HIV and AIDS in India.

UNICEF (28th June 2005), press release, 'Reducing Mother-to-Child Transmission of HIV/AIDS in India'.

Vienna Recommendations for Health Promoting Hospitals (http:/Iwww.euro.who.int/ document/IHB/hphviennarecom.pdf) (accessed 4 March 2004).

Walker, Walker *et al.* (1999). Psychological, clinical and pathological effects of relaxation training and guided imagery during primary chemotherapy (abstract).. PubMed, National Center for Biotechnology Information (NCBI). Retrieved on March 7, 2006.

Walsh D., Gombeski W., Goldstein P., Hayes D., Armour M. (1994). "Managing a palliative oncology program: the role of a business plan." *J Pain Symptom Manage* 9(2): 109. PMID 7517428.

WHO (17th April 2007), 'Towards Universal Access: Scaling up priority HIV/AIDS interventions in the health sector'.

WHO Regional Office for Europe. Health Promoting Hospital, (http://www.euro.who.int/healthpromohosp). Copenhagen, WHO Regional Office for Europe, 2002 (accessed 4 March 2004).

WHO South-East Asia Regional Office 2005 *Combating emerging* ***infectious diseases*** (SEA-CD-139) Woolhouse M.E. and Gowtage-Sequeria Sonya 2005 Host range and emerging and Re-emerging Pathogens; *Emerg. Infect. Dis.* 11, 1842–1847 *e*Publication: 15 October 2008.

WHO Standards Working Group. Development of standards for disease prevention and health promotion. WHO, Meeting on standards for disease prevention and health promotion, Bratislava, 14 May 2002.

World Bank (1995), India: Policy and Financing Strategies for Strengthening Primary Health Care Services, Report No. 13042-IN.

World Bank (1998), Reducing Poverty in India: Options for More Effective Public Services, Washington.

World Bank (2003), World Development Report 2004: Making Services Work for PoorPeople, Oxford University Press.

World Bank 'South Asia Region (SAR)- India' Regional Updates. *NACO* website, 'Information, Education, Communication and Social Mobilization', accessed 4/7/06.

World Health Organisation. The World Health Report, 2003.

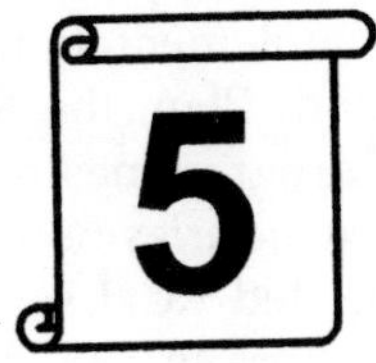

Reproductive and Child Health Programme

I. GENESIS

The Universal Immunisation Programme (UIP), aimed at reduction in mortality and morbidity among infants and younger children due to Vaccine Preventable Diseases, was started in 1985-86. The Oral Dehydration Therapy (ORT) was also started in view of the fact that diarrhea was a leading cause of deaths among children. Various other programmes under Maternal and Child Health (MCH) were also implemented during the Seventh Plan. The objectives of all these programmes were convergent and aimed at improving the health of the mothers and young children and to provide them facilities for prevention and treatment of major disease conditions. While these programmes did have a beneficial impact, the separate identity for each programme was causing problems in its effective management and this was also reducing somewhat the outcomes. Therefore, in the Eighth Plan, these programmes were integrated under Child Survival and Safe Motherhood (CSSM) Programme which was implemented from 1992-93.[1]

The process of integration of related programmes initiated with the implementation of the CSSM Programme was taken step further in 1994, when the International Conference on Population and Development in Cairo recommended that the participant countries should implement unified programmes for Reproductive and Child Health (RCH). The RCH approach has been defined as "People have the ability to reproduce and regulate their fertility, women are able to go through pregnancy and child birth safely, the outcome of pregnancies is successful in terms of maternal and infant survival and well-being and couples are able to have sexual relations free of fear of pregnancy and of contacting diseases." This concept is in keeping with the evolution of an integrated approach to the programmes aimed at improving the health status of young women and children, which has been going on in the country. It is obviously sensible that the integrated RCH Programme would help in reducing the cost of inputs to some extent because overlapping of expenditure would no longer be necessary and integrated implementation would optimise outcomes at the field level. During the Ninth Plan, the RCH Programme, accordingly, has integrated all the related programmes of the Eighth Plan. The concept of RCH is to provide to the beneficiaries need-based, client-centred, demand driven, high quality and integrated RCH services. The RCH Programme is a composite programme incorporating the inputs of the Government of India as well as funding support from external donor agencies including the World Bank and the European Commission.[2]

The RCH programme incorporates the components covered under the Child Survival and Safe Motherhood Programme and includes two additional components, one relating to sexually transmitted diseases (STD) and the other relating to reproductive tract infection (RTI). The main highlights of the RCH Programme are:

(i) The Programme integrates all interventions of fertility regulation, maternal and child health with reproductive health of both men and women.

(ii) The services to be provided will be client-centred, demand-driven, high quality and based on the needs of the community arrived at, through decentralised participatory planning and a target free approach.

(iii) The programme envisages upgradation of the level of facilities for providing various interventions and quality of care. The First Referral Units (FRUs) being set-up at sub-district level will provide comprehensive emergency obstetric and new born care. PHCs will be substantially upgraded.

(iv) The Programme will improve access of the community to various services which are commonly required. It is proposed to provide facilities for MTP at the PHCs, counseling and IUD insertion at SCs in a phased manner.

(v) The Programme aims at improving the outreach of services, particularly for the vulnerable groups of population who have till now substantially been let out of the planning process:

- Special programmes will be taken up for urban slums, tribal population and adolescents.
- Non-Governmental Organisations will be involved in a much larger way to improve out-reach and make it people's programme.
- Skills of practitioners of ISM will be upgraded by training and research and development in ISM will be supported to improve the range of the RCH services.

- Panchayati Raj system will have a greater role in planning, implementation and assessment of client satisfaction.

Ninth Five Year Plan has mentioned the following features of RCH Programme:

- Effective maternal and child health care,
- Increased access to contraceptive care,
- Safe management of unwanted preganancies,
- Nutritional services to vulnerable groups,
- Prevention and treatment of RTI/STD,
- Reproductive health services for adolescents,
- Prevention and treatment of gynecological problems, and
- Screening and treatment of cancers, especially that of uterine cervix and breast.

For over 30 years Family Welfare Programme was known for its rigid, target-based approach in contraceptives. The performance was measured by the reported numbers of the four contraceptive methods-Sterilisation, Intrauterine device, Oral pills. and Condoms. This was widely criticised for being a coercive approach.

The 1994 Cairo International Conference on Population and Development (ICPD) formulated a growing International consensus that improving reproductive health and family planning is essential to human welfare and development.

A growing body of evidence and the Cairo consensus suggest "Numerical method specific contraceptive target and monetary incentives" for providers to be replaced by a broader system of "programme performance goals" and measures focused on a range of reproductive health services.

We can say in brief that Reproductive and Child Health Services is equivalent to:

- Family Planning, to focus on fertility regulation,
- Child Survival and Safe Motherhood Programme,
- Treatment of Reproductive Tract Infections and Sexually Transmitted Infections and prevention of AIDS through—
  1. Client-Oriented/Mother-Friendly/user-specific, family welfare Services, and
  2. High quality services.

The specific programmes under Reproductive and Child Health Services are:

1. Prevention and management of unwanted pregnancies,
2. Maternal care:

   (a) Ante-natal services,
   (b) Natal services,
   (c) Post-natal services,
3. Child Survival, and.
4. Treatment of Reproductive Tract Infections (RTI) and Sexually Transmitted Infections (STI)

The following definition of reproductive health, approved in April 1994, by the WHO Global Policy Council, provides the basis for action in this field.[3]

"Reproductive health implies that people are able to have a responsible, satisfying and safe sex life and that they have the capability to reproduce and the freedom to decide if, when and how often to do so. Implicit in this last condition are the right of men and women to be informed of and to have access to safe, effective, affordable and acceptable methods of fertility regulation of their choice, and the right of access to appropriate health care services that will enable women to go safely through pregnancy and childbirth and provide couples with the best chance of having a healthy infant."[4]

Reproductive health must address, as its basic elements, sexual behaviour, family planning, maternal care and safe motherhood, abortion, reproductive tract infections (including sexually transmitted diseases and HIV/AIDS, and certain reproductive tract malignancies such as cervical cancer.

II. THE PACKAGE OF REPRODUCTIVE AND CHILD HEALTH SERVICES

The different services provided under RCH programme are:

1. For the Mothers

- TT Immunization
- Prevention and treatment of anaemia
- Ante-natal care and early-identification of maternal complications
- Deliveries by trained personnel
- Promotion of institutional deliveries
- Management of Obstetric emergencies
- Birth spacing

2. For the Children

- Essential newborn care
- Exclusive breast feeding and weaning
- Immunization

- Appropriate management of diarrhea
- Appropriate management of ARI
- Vitamin A prophylaxis
- Treatment of Anaemia

3. For Eligible Couples

- Prevention of pregnancy
- Safe abortion

4. RTI/STD

- Prevention and treatment of reproductive tract and sexually transmitted diseases.

Principles and Approach

The guiding principles and approach of reproductive health care are to a great extent different than those of the existing dominant approach of MCH and FP programme.[5] A glimpse of the shift in approach and principle can be studied from the Table 5.1.

The guiding principles of reproductive health care are those of human rights, ethics, equity, quality of care, universal access, participation, partnership, integration, optimal use of resources and sustainability. Partnerships and sharing of responsibilities between government, governmental organisations and the private sector are important in stimulating new ideas and approaches and ensuring service coverage and quality of care. These principles are the same as the principles of primary health care.

We must keep in mind that reproductive health is a crucial part of general health and is central to human development. It affects everybody; it involves intimate and highly valued aspects of life. Not only is it a reflection of health in infancy, childhood and adolescence, it also sets the stage for health beyond the reproductive years, for both men and women, and has effects from one generation to another. Reproductive health includes sexual health care, for maintaining and enhancing the functions of the reproductive system, and the prevention and management of RTls, HIV/AIDS and infertility. Reproductive health care is an integral part of primary health care. The guiding principles and the approaches of reproductive health care are similar to the delivery of primary health care. These are:

- education concerning prevailing health problems and the methods of preventing and controlling them;
- promotion of food supply and proper nutrition;
- an adequate supply of safe water and basic sanitation;
- maternal and child health care, including family planning;

- immunisation against the major infectious diseases;
- appropriate treatment of common diseases and injuries; and
- provision of essential drugs.

TABLE 5.1

Principles and Approach of Existing MCH/FP Programme and of RHC Programme

Existing MCH/FP Programmes	*Reproductive Health Programmes*
Targets population is primarily women	Target population is both women and men.
Vertical programmes	Integrated and inter-sectoral programmes
Top-down planning and implementation	Bottom-up planning responding to local reproductive health needs within socio-cultural and economic milieu and decentralized implementation
Focus on individual cases	Public Health approach with family and community focus
Pregnancy—based approach	Life cycle approach
Medical approach: health needs identified by providers; reliance on medical solutions	Communty-based approach: respect women's knowledge and definition of their health needs; reliance on holistic solutions that take into account the social, biological and psychological factors determining health.
Provider centred: prescribe fertility control methods	Client centred: provide information and enable women to choose the methods they wish to adopt.
Method specific information provided	Apart from information on all methods of fertility regulation, provide knowledge on sexuality and reproduction.
Emphasis on achieving output targets	Emphasis on coverage and quality of services
Services provided in a clinical atmosphere	Provide services in a humane and caring setting
Vague general health rights	Respect specific reproductive health rights

Source: WHO: SEARO, Essential Reproductive Health Care, New Delhi, p. 5.

Advantages of the Scheme

RCH can avoid the problems prevalent in earlier family planning programme and can improve the coverage and quality of services provided the RCH programme is implemented as scheduled.

1. Target-free Approach can make the Programme Flexible

The achievements of family planning programme were judged simply on the completion of targets fixed from above. It was found that the top down approach is not realistic and based on field situations. Thus, the users preference is not reflected in the targets. A major feature of the target-free approach in its emphasis on the promotion of modem spacing methods. The approach intends also to achieve a greater participation of males in the family welfare programme. Moreover, in the absence of method-specific targets, the grass root level workers including the ANM and the Multipurpose Health Workers (both male and female) are expected to work closely with the community and arrive at an estimate of the various family welfare activities required in the area/population covered by them. The male health workers, in particular, are made responsible for motivation for vasectomy and condoms. These activities are expected to result in an improvement in the knowledge of modern temporary methods as well as male methods of contraception; and an improvement in the proportion of spacing as well as male methods in the contraceptive method-mix.[6]

2. Target-free Approach can make the Reporting Honest and Reliable

Field Staff used to do false reporting in order to prove the progress to avoid disciplinary action. This approach has made the reporting realistic and thus can help in effective policy-making and planning.

Earlier, we had malpractices of performing sterilisation/vasectomy upon ineligible persons. All such cases and practices would be avoided.

3. New Programme can Ensure Forward and Backward Linkages

The RCH programme can promote linkages to make it effective towards positive health. Since it is not merely a family planning programme, it is a total package covering the total health of women and children, a very positive view.

4. Over-head Cost can be Reduced

Costs incurred in managing programes in an integrated way can reduce a lot of cost as overhead cost can be reduced.

5. Effective Maternal and Child Health

At the village level, the Auxiliary Nurse Midwife is responsible for rendering maternal and child health services alongwith family welfare services. She is supposed to register pregnant women and assess their health throughout pregnancy, by at least three visits. Regular height and weight checkup, blood pressure test, urine test as well as providing tetanus toxoid injections and iron and folic acid tablets constitute important aspects of any antenatal checkup. Another responsibility of the ANM is to refer pregnant women who have symptoms of abnormal pregnancy or labour, or who have gynecological problems that are beyond her level of competence, to the Primary Health Centre.

At the instance of the Ministry of Health and Family Welfare, Government of India, New Delhi and as a part of monitoring and evaluation of the performance of the family welfare programme under the new target-free approach, the Population Research Centre, J.S.S. Institute of Economic Research, Dharwad, undertook a rapid survey in the rural areas of Belgaum District, Karnataka state during the last two weeks of December 1997 and first two weeks of January 1998. Using a simple and short questionnaire, the survey interviewed a total of 1,000 currently married women age 15-44, from 50 villages, at the rate of 20 women per village. Apart from several background characteristics of women, the survey collected information on utilization of ante-natal care, place of delivery, and assistance during delivery, child immunizations, knowledge and practice of family planning, visits by the ANM and services received from her; health problems of the women including side-effects of family planning methods, and respondents ratings on various aspects of quality of care provided by the nearest PHC, sub-centre or the ANM.

(a) While the provision of tetanus toxoid injections and iron/folic tablets is better, other components of antenatal care such as monitoring the weight and blood pressure, and urine tests were not carried out for the majority of women during their pregnancy by multi-member females.
(b) Overall, 51 per cent of the deliveries which occurred during the five years preceding the survey took place at home, 30 per cent in private hospitals or nursing homes, and little less than one-fifth in government health facilities. Of the births that took place at home, the majority (62 per cent) were attended by untrained persons including relatives, friends and neighbours.
(c) Little less than one-quarter of women in the rural areas of Belgaum District have an unmet need for family planning, that is, they are not using contraception even though they do not want any more children or want to wait at least two years before having their next child. The unmet need for spacing (11 per cent) is almost the same as that for limiting births (12 per cent). If all the women with an unmet need were to use family planning, the contraceptive prevalence rate would increase from 62 per cent to 85 per cent.
(d) Among the three registers (Eligible Couple register, ANC register, and immunization register) examined, the EC register was found to be relatively more complete and accurate than the other two registers.

In another study, a rapid research survey was conducted in rural areas of Dharwad District in Karnataka during February-April, 1997 to check the coverage, quality of services and client satisfaction under the new strategy of 'target-free' approach. The analysis of service statistics for the district showed that removal of targets appears to have made no significant impact on the total number of annual acceptors. However, it had a favourable impact on method mix as sterilizations have come down slightly while acceptors of IUD and Pill have gone up from that of the previous year.

The unmet need for contraception was estimated to be 10 per cent, 6 per cent for limiting and 4 per cent for spacing.

It was found that immunization levels are yet to become universal. About 70 per cent of pregnant women had two doses of Tetanus toxoid vaccination and only half of the children were fully immunized.

Measurement of weight and blood pressure, as well as urine tests mwere reported rarely. Only 40 per cent of deliveries were attended by trained persons. On record maintenance, it was observed that EC register was better maintained than ANC and immunization registers. Some of the important policy recommendations emerging from the study are:

1. Improve ANM services, especially make them visit women with unmet need for contraception, and past acceptors of sterilization.
2. As a large number of sterilization acceptors complain about method side effects, a special health campaign for sterilized men and women should be launched by multipurpose workers female. In order to safeguard future levels of acceptance, past acceptors should be made to feel that they are looked after well by programme functionaries.
3. It should be ensured that sub-centres have adequate supply of drugs, and attempts should be made to reduce waiting time and provide free services at primary health centres. The guilty should be punished.
4. A television set could be placed in PHC waiting room and also a VCP to disseminate information and messages on health and family welfare and facilities in sub-centres.
5. Concerted attempts should be made to raise immunization levels by workers as they appear to have reached a point of stagnation before acquiring universality.[7]

Let us mention the role of Apex institution-National Institute of Health and Family Welfare in Promoting RCH activities.

National Institute of Health and Family Welfare (Role in RCH)

History and Need

The National Institute of Health and Family Welfare came into being with effect from 9 March, 1977, by the amalgamation of the erstwhile institutes, namely, the National Institute of Family Planning and the National Institute of Health Administration and Education. It has been established as an autonomous body (registered under the Societies Registration Act, 1860) and its object is to act as an apex technical institute for promoting the Health and Family Welfare Planning Programme in the country through education, training, services, research and evaluation. The overall objective of the Institute has been to playa leading role in orienting training and research in health administration and education to the newer concepts of administration and education and thereby strengthen and accelerate India's health and family welfare programmes.

Organisation

The Institute is governed by a General Executive Council with the Union Minister for Health and Family Welfare as the President! Chairman. The day-to-day activities are administered by the Director. The Institute is supported in its activities by International Agencies such as WHO/SEARO and UNICEF. Closer contacts and collaboration exist between the Institute and numerous other organisations in the country. The finances for the functioning of the Institute are provided by the Government of India through grants-in-aid.

Structure

As health administration is based on the concept of 'multi-disciplinary' approach, the Institute has departments embracing various disciplines. These are the departments of Public Health Administration, Hospital Administration, Family Welfare, Maternal and Child Health Programme Planning, Evaluation, Social Sciences, Epidemiology, Health Education, Public Administration, Biostatistics, Education and Training, Field Training, Public Health Nursing and Field Services. A field practice area in the Rohtak District of Haryana State exists for experimentation and field training exercises of the participants of the institute. Research in the field of Health Administration is reckoned to be a key factor for the development of the activities of the Institute and is therefore, an integral part of the functioning of all departments of the Institute. The new Institute has been renamed as the National Institute of Health and Family Welfare.

Activities

The main activities of the Institute are:

(a) Education and Training
(b) Research
(c) Evaluation of Health Programmes
(d) Consultation Services
(e) Clearing House Functions
(f) Publications and Documents.

Objectives in the Context of RCH

(i) To organise, co-ordinate and monitor training in the country.

(ii) To upgrade the competence of family welfare personnel and managers to provide technically sound client centred and gender sensitive RCH services.

(iii) To create mass awareness of RCH and population stabilization issues by holding orientation training programmes.

(iv) To involve other government departments in promotion of RCH programme by team training for convergence of services.

SPECIFIC OBJECTIVES

(a) To co-ordinate: (i) training financed by the Family Welfare Department in RCH management, clinical and interpesonal counselling skills and communications (IEC), and (ii) awareness generation and community mobilization (including convergence of related programmes such as ICDS) as requested by MOHFW.

(b) To co-ordinate the development and or adaptation, as necessary, of model training curricula, facilitators, guides, and prototype manuals/materials, and provide such materials to collaborating centres and training centres for local adaptation and use.

(c) To assist MOHFW in the development of clinical management protocols for safe motherhood, fertility regulation methods, reproductive tract infections and sexually transmitted diseases and child survival as specified in the essential package of RCH services and ensure that such protocols are integrated into training.

(d) To assist MOHFW and national procurement support agency for appointment of suitable collaborating institutions from Government, NGO and private/corporate sector in accordance with World Bank Guidelines and to organise training of trainers of these institutions.

(e) To review the work of the collaborative institutions annually and to assist the MOHFW in determining suitability of the institution to continue as a collaborating institution.

(f) To assist states, districts through collaborating institutions, in formulation of integrated training plans at State and District-levels so as to: (i) avoid unnecessary duplication; (ii) ensure there are no critical gaps in the training plans; and (iii) coordinate scheduling of training with other programme inputs such as equipment, civil works, IEC and NGO activities.

(g) To assist States in the establishment of system of proficiency certificate award to trainees and monitor and report on state specific achievements on the project performance.

The RCH Programme should take care of the following factors before formulation, implemation and evaluation strategy:

(a) according to the topography of the District,
(b) according to the priority needs of the people,
(c) linked properly with the objectives and goals of District planning,
(d) fitted into the overall economic and social development of the country,
(e) properly linked with projects in the allied area, and
(f) able to achieve useful and permanent results.

Let us now analyse the factors which impede the effective functioning of RCH programme. It is based on author's study in Punjab and Kamataka. We have also given suggestions to improve RCH programme.

Let us mention the schedule of operation of RCH programme in Punjab and Karnataka (See Tables 5.2 and 5.3). We may also mention the facilities required in A, Band C categories of Districts. The project has not so far been implemented fully. However, we discuss our observations and findings on the basis of the experiments done so far.

TABLE 5.2

Punjab-Year-wise Category of Districts

Category	*Year-I*	*Year-II*	*Year-III*
A			
B	Hoshiarpur	Jalandhar	Faridkot
	Patiala	Ludhiana	Rupnagar
	Moga	Kapurthala	Bathinda
		Gurdaspur	Muktsar
		Amritsar	Nawanshahr
		Sangrur	
C	Firozepur	Mansa	
	Fatehgarh Sahib		

Though it is desirable that the entire package of services indicated above is made available to all those who need it, it will not be possible to immediately implement such a comprehensive package on a nation-wide basis. Hence, it is envisaged that improvement in quality and coverage of services over and above the existing level will be attempted in all states in an incremental manner so that maternal and child health indices improve.

After consultation with experts, a package of essential reproductive

TABLE 5.3

Karnataka-Year-wise Category of District

Category	*Year-I*	*Year-II*	*Year-III*
A	Dakshin Kannada	Kodagu (Coorg)	
	Mandya		
B	Uttar Kannada	Hassan	Shimoga
	Chikmaglur	Bangalore (R)	Chitradurga
	Dharwad	Tumkur	
		Mysore	
		Belgaum	
C	Bijapur	Bellary	
	Bidar	Raichur	
	Gulbarga		
	Bangalore		

health services for nation-wide implementation at various levels of health care has been identified. Essential components recommended for nation-wide implementation include:

- Prevention and management of unwanted pregnancy.
- Services to promote safe motherhood.
- Services to promote child survival.
- Prevention and treatment of RTI/STD.

Most of the services are already included in the Family Welfare Programme. However, there are wide variations in the quality and coverage of services not only between various states, but also between various districts in the same state. The focus is therefore on the improvement in the quality and coverage of the services. A project preparation workshop held in Sept. 1995 discussed the issues and problems in implementation of essential RCH package and recommended the reproductive and child health services, that should be made available at community, sub-centre, PHC and FRU/District Hospital.

Implementation schedule of Punjab and Karnataka is given in above Tables.

The Ministry of Health and Family Welfare has got the research conducted on the impact of RCH programme in these districts. Analysis of the reports indicates that:

(a) Infrastructure facilities are non-existent.
(b) Personnel responsible for RCH lack motivation.
(c) Lack of effective supervision.
(d) Slackness in work.

(e) Non-availability of funds.
(f) Lack of team work.
(g) Not following the work as scheduled.

The study on RCH conducted in some districts in Punjab State revealed that there has not been much impact of the new RCH programme. The personnel responsible lack motivation and interest. Because of financial crisis, normal functioning of the health department is at a standstill. Besides, there is no supervision, resulting into absentism and irregularity. Let us mention various factors responsible for this state of affairs and also desired remedial action:

1. Lack of Adequate Facilities in the Institutions Responsible far the Provision of RCH Services

After the project is formulated, the project manager must ensure the availability of necessary inputs. It has been generally observed that the projects are delayed because of the absence of timely availability of all the inputs simultaneously. In one of the projects, the health personnel had no work to do because of the non- availability of vaccine. Obtaining resources is a process that takes place periodically throughout the life of the project. It was revealed that failure to obtain resources simultaneously in time is the most common cause of delay in implementation. The project manager must begin the process of procuring resources immediately after the formulation stage. Sometimes, the process may be started quite early if the resources are scarce and not easily available. The absence of one resource would inflate the cost of the project as the other resources would remain idle. The project manager must take the following steps:

(a) Working with the relative administrative units in preparing a time-table of administrative steps to be taken to obtain the planned resources.
(b) Monitoring this time-table to ensure that the administrative steps are being completed in time.
(c) Taking corrective action as and when necessary.

In spite of all these precautions, there is a possibility of not getting the resources in time. What can be done under such critical situation? Most of the experts indicated that the whole project staff remains idle for months together. This is very serious in big projects. It is suggested that project officers may be delegated powers to purchase the inputs locally or employ persons, if not available from the agency as planned. This would ensure that the project is on schedule.

2. Lack of Clarity among the Persons Responsible for Implementation of RCH Programme

There is a dichotomy between the personnel responsible for the formulation and the personnel responsible for the implementation of the RCH project. The latter are not clear about the implications of the project. Because of lack of identity, they develop low morale resulting into poor management. It was mentioned by a number of persons working on these projects that, "they are thrown into the fields to operate the RCH project without proper briefing about the project and its rationale in the total system. Besides, the supervisors, at the head-quarters, never guide them about their role in the projects."

3. Poor linkages Among the Allied Projects

In a particular geographical or functional area, a number of projects are being implemented to improve the standard of living of the people. Most of the projects are complementary and supplementary. Because of the poor coordination among the various departments at the state level, the projects are implemented in the area without developing linkages with each other. For example, a project for the agriculture development to grow more food can be beautifully linked with the health projects on nutrition. Population control has many dimensions and needs the co-operation of many agencies. Thus, there is a need of area planning and developing an integrated area approach, where different projects may develop linkages to have optimum benefit.

4. Absence of the Full Involvement of the Beneficiaries in the Formulation and Implementation of Projects

The success or failure of the RCH project ultimately depends upon the acceptance of these projects by the people. If the people are not taken into confidence during the formulation and implementation of RCH projects, these would be less successful. People's participation would provide extra nuclear energy to the success of the RCH projects. Most of the beneficiaries contacted by the writer were of the view that they are not treated as equal partners in the process of formulation and implementation of projects. The failure of the scheme is because of the absence of identity of the people with the programmes. It is essential for the experts to motivate and encourage the people to participate in the formulation and implementation of projects. Although people's participation in affairs governing !heir lives dates back to the beginning of human society, the concept has taken a new dimension as societies have grown in size and complexity. This is partly because the management has become more and more a specialized enterprise, an area for technocrats and trained general administrators and political leaders. Although they officially advocate and preach people's involvement, in practice, they bring them into picture only after the major decisions have been made. Hence, they often leave the ordinary citizens to follow their pre-determined paths. Peter Drucker agrees with this contention when he says that "the overwhelming majority of these people have little or no opportunity to influence policy,, and their perspectives on the situation are systematically ignored by almost all theorists. For them the problem of development is one of the everyday life."

5. Local Communities are Treated as Passive Participants in Improvement and Bettering of their Lives

Most of the project personnel working in the villages return to the cities after their duty hours. The villagers cannot make their views known to them in cities. The result is lack of communication between them. When the project fails, it is intentionally ascribed to the obstinacy, fatalism, illiteracy or apparent irrationality of the poor people. The potential for community involvement has been seriously underestimated. We must encourage people's participation through all methods to promote development.

6. Absence of Satisfactory Monitoring System to Measure the Regulated Performance during Implementation

Project control is the managerial function that helps the managers to keep the project functioning as scheduled. It is possible only if the realistic advance targets of output are fixed before implementation. This is not being done as is evident from the perusal of the most of the projects studied. Monitoring, if properly designed, can help the managers in keeping the process of implementation as scheduled. The project performance is compared at different intervals of time with the control indicators. Whenever deviations are located, causes of deviations are examined, solutions are found to correct the deviations. The following are the general causes of deviation:

(1) "Excessive optimism on the part of the project planners, resulting in unrealistic estimates with respect to:
   - the time, funds, manpower or other resources required to do an activity, and
   - the possibility of achieving the expected results.

(2) Unfrozen resistance from or changes in the environment of the project (natural disaster, political changes, etc.).

(3) Decisions at higher, managerial levels to change the planned resources inputs of the project (change of a staff member).

(4) Inefficient administrative procedures.

If there is any unavoidable deviation beyond the control of the project authorities, we can think of alternative proposals immediately without wasting the future resources. If such timely action is taken, the developing countries can be sure of the success of the projects. More safe design of the control system would require specifying who reports what to whom and when.

7. Unscientific Manpower Planning and Insufficient Utilisation of Project Personnel

The success of the project depends upon the quality and quantity of personnel associated with it. It was observed that in many projects, the projects personnel have their utilisation time as low as 20 per cent. This is highly serious as the resources are being consumed by the establishment rather than invested in the RCH programme. Because of the absence of manpower planning, personnel of the project utilize very little time. People in the area remarked about the workers appointed to motivate people to adopt family planning norm: "They are not available at all. They rarely devote any time for this work. They remain away from their work." It is essential to see through proper manpower planning that only needed persons are appointed and they are utilised to increase the over-all productivity, efficiency and effectiveness. The projects should be so administered as to lead to over-all improvement in its performance.

8. Lack of Clarification of Authority, Responsibility and Relationships

In the developing world, the persons responsible for implementation of the project do not work as a team, as there is no clarification of authority, responsibility and relationships amongst them, i.e. the roles of the various participants are not often mutually understood. This results in friction among these persons. Most of the time of these persons is spent in solving their mutual disputes. It becomes very difficult for them to devote their whole hearted attention to the project.

9. Private Sector Engaged only in Curative Services

Ninth Plan suggested the Private Sector participation in RCH. It is estimated that the private sector accounts for more than three quarters of all health care expenditure in India. Private sector provides MCH and family planning services also, but to a lesser extent. It is increasingly recognised that the private sector represents an untapped potential for increasing the coverage and improving the quality of reproductive and child health services in the country. The challenge is to find ways and means to optimally utilise their potential. The major limitations in the private sector include the following:

(a) the focus so far has been mainly on curative services;
(b) the quality of services is often variable; and
(c) as the users have to pay for the services, the poorer sections of population cannot afford these services.

Some of the initiatives could be through collaboration between public and private sector in providing health care to the poorer segments of population, who cannot afford to pay for health services. While organising the involvement of private medical practitioners in RCH care, it is essential to provide orientation training to all and ensure utilisation of their services in a cost-effective and sustainable manner.

Private/voluntary organisations providing health care to women are relatively small in number but they could play an effective role in the delivery of reproductive and child health care services at affordable cost, especially in certain specific locations such as urban slums. We need to give the private sector and voluntary organisations appropriate incentives to broaden the range of activities and improve the quality of reproductive and child health-related services they offer. Continued collaboration, training and technical assistance by governmental agencies to private medical practitioners and private/voluntary organisations may help in strengthening reproductive and child health services in remote or underserved areas.

10. Previous Implementation Experience of the Completed Projects not Referred to

It was a great surprise to learn that there are no records of past experiences in implementation of earlier projects. One can always learn from the mistakes of others. Some of the project personnel remarked that "they do not know anything about the difficulties encountered by the project personnel and the causes of the failure of the project undertaken earlier." It is beneficial to examine how major projects have been managed in the past. It would also be better to identify those approaches which have been most successful. \ye can keep a record of good and bad points of the past project and this cumulative experience may be passed on to the present project managers. In this way, many of the difficulties likely to be encountered would vanish.

Frank A. Wilsoh in his article, "Planning for Project Management" in the *Journal of Administration Overseas* (July 1979) has rightly mentioned that, "Disappointing and inefficient project performance is a fact of life. .Ex-post evaluation of existing projects can be the means by which we can systematically seek to analyse the potential for improving project management. Evaluation Studies give the opportunity for developing a greater understanding of the way projects are managed and implemented."

11. Faulty and Cumbersome Administrative Procedures

Whenever a project is formulated, we do not pay much attention to the problems of communication, co-ordination, headquarters field relationship, supervision, etc. The purpose of these procedures is to help in the smooth functioning of the project. Without proper procedures, most of the project personnel remain engrossed in preparing unnecessary reports. These procedures should be clarified in the initial stages of project management, so that no confusion arises later on. If there are already set procedures in a particular organisation, these may be adopted, otherwise new procedures should be outlined and made known to the project personnel. It must be clear that administrative procedures are an aid to help the efficient functioning of the project. The meticulous applications of these procedures may result into red-tap ism and inefficiency.

The Five Year Plan (1978-83) has also indicated the technical, administrative and managerial problems which affect project efficiency. These are mentioned below:

(a) Inadequate investigation and data collection as a result of which the project appraisal, even when it is sought to be done in a systematic way, has to be carried out on the basis of wholly inadequate information, thus leading to wrong investment decisions.

(b) Inadequate detailed planning of projects in terms of their time schedule, input resource requirements and skills needed for project implementation.

(c) Lack of delegation of authority to subordinate organisation levels.

(d) Delays in issuing sanction, approvals, fund authorisations and releases.

(e) Organisational weaknesses in planning and implementation at various levels.

(f) Lack of specific assignment of responsibility and accountability for results.

(g) Problems of industrial relations and inadequate motivation of personnel, lack of proper career planning and incentives and commitment to results.

(h) Inadequate share of representation of the weaker sections in elected bodies in the village, district and block levels and agencies.

We can improve the management. of projects, if we keep these difficulties or problems or obstacles in mind and try to reduce these to negligible proportions. Besides, there is a need of training project personnel in the art of project management.

Empowerment of women is one of the most important key factors for the welfare and development of any society. Of late, the government has also subscribed to the idea that without empowering women, the development of society is not possible in the right direction and at a desired pace. So, the government has started many Women Empowerment Programmes (WEPs) at national as well at state level.

Empowerment of women is a slow but continuous process. Women must come up to play their role in planning, decision-making and implementation. The scenario has been changing slowly in cities but the same has not been happening in rural areas and urban slums. For making WEP's successful at gross root level, in rural areas and urban flums, where it is required the most, the most important factor is that the PHYSICAL HEALTH as well as MENTAL HEALTH of the Women. In this chapter, we shall discuss about Women's Health and Development followed by Reproductive and Child Health.

One more very important fact, requiring the attention of NGOs and other implementing agencies for WEPs, is that there are two big segments amongst the women. One segment is that women. One segment is that which is aware of its rights but closes its eyes towards its duties. And another bigger segment of women is that which knows its duties without asking for its rights and thus suffering silently. This gap has to be bridged. Unless and until a balance between rights and duties is struck, WEPs cannot be successful. (In chapter 5-Reproductive and Child Health)

Approach during the tenth plan

During the Tenth Plan, the paradigm shift, which began in the Ninth Plan, will be fully operationalised. The shift was from:

- demographic targets to focussing on enabling couples to achieve their reproductive goals;
- Methods specific contraceptive targets to meeting all the unmet needs for contraception to reduce unwanted pregnancies;
- Numerous vertical programmes for family planning and maternal and child health to integrated health care for women and children;
- centrally defined targets to *community need assessment and decentralised area specific microplanning* and implementation of program for health care for women and children, to reduce infant mortality and reduce high desired fertility;
- quantitative coverage to *emphasis on quality and content of care;*
- predominantly women centred programmes to *meeting the health care needs of the family with emphasis on involvement of men in planned parenthood;*
- supply driven service delivery to *need and demand driven service; improved logistics for ensuring adequate and timely supplies to meet the needs;*
- service provision based on providers' perception to *addressing choices and conveniences of the couples;*
- The population growth rate continues to be high due to the large size of the population in the reproductive age-group (accounting for an estimated 60 per cent of the total population growth);
- higher fertility due to the unmet need for contraception (contributing to around 20 per cent of population growth); and
- high wanted fertility due to the prevailing high Infant Mortality Rate (IMR) and other socio-economic reasons (estimated contribution of about 20 per cent to population growth).

The Tenth Plan will fully operaanalise efforts to:

- assess and meet the unmet needs for contraception;
- achieve reduction in the high desired level of fertility through programmes for reduction in IMR and maternal mortality ratio (MMR); and
- enable families to achieve their reproductive goals.

If the reproductive goals of families are fully met the country will be able to achieve the National Population Policy goal of replacement level of fertility by 2010. The medium and long-term goals will be to continue this process to accelerate the pace of demographic transition and achieve population stabilisation by 2045. Early population stabilisation will enable the country to achieve its developmental goal of improving the economic status and quality of life of the citizens.

Reductions in fertility, mortality and population growth rate will be major objectives during the Tenth Plan. Three of the 11 monitorable targets for the Tenth Plan and beyond are:

- reduction in IMR to 45 per 1,000 live births by 2007 and 28 per 1,000 live births by 2012;
- reduction in maternal mortality ratio to 2 per 1,000 live births by 2007 and 1 per 1,000 live births by 2012; and
- reduction in decadal growth rate of the population between 2001-2011 to 16.2.

CONCLUSION

The new RCH programme needs to be designed scientifically, keeping in view the minor details meticulously. The programme is certainly better than the earlier Family Planning and maternal and child health programmes aimed at specific activity.

However, with the overall policy made by the Ministry of Health and Family Welfare, each district should design its own programme keeping in view the needs, resources, topography, quality of the people, facilities and infrastructure available as well as plan strategy of implementation and evaluation to inject flexibility, as situations differ from district to district.

Radhakrishna Rao in his Article, "Towards controlling the Numbers" in *The Daily Tribune* (31st January, 2000) rightly suggests that a target free approach has now become a part of the population control drive. To what extent this approach will contribute to the success of population control, no one is sure as yet. Sociologists, however, are clear in their perception that when literacy, health, hygiene and economic improvements get high priority, family planning stands a better chance of success.

The document prepared for the International Conference on Population and Development has recognised in its programme of action that "the main message for improving individual well-being comprises two elements: to provide contraceptive methods within the broader reproductive health services and to advance women's equal participation in education, health and economic opportunities."

Notes and References

1. Annual Report, Ministry of Health and Family Welfare, 1998-99, pp. 7-9.

2. State Family Welfare Bureau, DH and FWS, Reproductive and Child Health, Bangalore, July, 1988, p. 1.
3. WHO, May-June, 1994, p. 30.
4. State Family Welfare Bureau, Bangalore, *op. cit.*, pp. 19-20.
5. WHO, SEARO: Managing Essential Reproductive Health Care, New Delhi, p. 5.
6. B.M. Ramesh, S.B. Ganiger and D.G. Satihal "Family Welfare Programme under Target Free Approach: A Rapid Survey in Belgaum District, Karnataka, 1998, Population Research Centre, J.S.S. Institute of Economic Research, Dharwad.
7. P.N. Mari Bhat, Target Free Approach to Family Planning Programme: A Rapid Survey in Dharwad District in Karnataka, 1997, Population Research Centre, J.S.S. Institute of Economic Research, Dharwad, pp. i-iii.

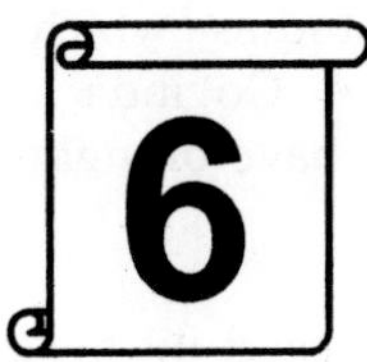

Information, Education and Communication (IEC)

The creation of awareness is integral to the process of social development. The possibility for the power of communication to liberate the minds and potential of people to critical awareness is real in every field linked to human development, and the generation of public will hinges on effective communication of information and ideas that relate to people's needs, aspirations and capacities for progress in thought and action. In this sense, getting the development process started is largely the task of information, education and communication.

The communication aspect of a national family planning programme is generally termed as IEC-Information, Education and Communication. The Year Book (1986-87) of Family Welfare Programme in India has rightly mentioned that the success of the Family Welfare Programme depends primarily upon the voluntary and widespread acceptance of the concept of small family and delayed marriages and well spaced and properly linked births are an effective way of achieving this objective. Mass education and Media activities, accordingly, were given multi-dimensional and integrated thrust through Information-Education-Communication activities in the form of a comprehensive package of social transformation to bring behavioural and attitudinal changes in the people so as to enable them to adopt family planning as a way of life. In brief, we can simplify it, and can call it simply as communication function. Sometimes, the activities under IEC are also referred to as "Mass Communication", "Mass Education", "Mass Education and Media."

Donald J. Bogue[1] has rightly said that IEC is a term widely used to identify the activities of family planning programme to inform. the public and stimulate them to adopt contraception. In every technical component of the Family Planning Programme provided by family planning workers, there exists a corresponding educational aspect, which has to be imparted more or less simultaneously, so as to enhance the continuing usefulness of the services provided at the time of need. This would have permanent value.

An added importance of communication in family planning resulted from the experience and studies which indicated that pure clinical approach did not bear fruit. A. Govindachari has mentioned some of the findings of the studies, which have brought to notice the limited impact of clinical approach. These are:

(i) The population reached by the clinics was very limited;
(ii) Education on family planning in the clinics was mostly through individual contacts. There was no organized community education;
(iii) The educational efforts were mostly directed towards women, since the clinics normally have female social workers. Husbands, who are important from the point of view of making in family planning, especially in an Indian cultural context, were not given due attention;
(iv) Couples felt shy to visit clinics for fear of identification by their friends and neighbours;
(v) The working hours of the clinics were found to be inconvenient, especially for the low income groups;
(vi) There was a lack of social support for the programme due to inadequate involvement of the community;
(vii) People generally prefer to obtain contraceptives in an informal way which does not involve formal recording procedures and publicity. This was not possible in a clinic situation; and
(viii) There was very little involvement of other supporting staff, like. the village level workers, extension officers, etc. in the family planning programme.[2]

Today, Family planning programmes around the world are applying a broad range of service delivery and communication strategies. To make family planning services and supplies more accessible, conventional clinic-based programmes have been supplemented by innovative approaches to services delivery. These include community-based outreach, social marketing through commercial outlets at subsidized prices, and employment-based programmes organized or supported by employees or Unions. Extensive communication campaigns, combining a variety of modem and traditional mass-media are spreading family planning awareness and encouraging more people to seek out family planning services.[3]

Nature

The Information, Education, Communication (IEC) component of

National Family Welfare programme is mainly to create an effective communication strategy, to inform the masses about the means and measures of Family Welfare Programme, educate them about the perils of over-population and motivate and persuade them to adopt small family norm, 'using all possible channels of media.[4]

In a Family Planning organisation, external communication is very important in the implementation of its programme, as information about the utility and means· of planned parenthood through appropriate choice and correct use of contraceptives by the eligible married couples is important. Moreover, communication being two-way process brings to the attention of the management the needs, reactions and complaints of the people concerned for necessary initiative or remedial actions. The external communication process needs to be guided by considerations of relevance of information, the choice of communication channels and the existing understanding capacity (education, etc.) of the people concerned outside the organisation. Moreover, it should not by any means be only one sided, i.e. from the organisation to the people. The reverse flow of information from the people to the organisation would make the latter to judge the impact of the programme as well as provide the basis for any changes in the strategies of the Programme. Here again, barriers and disruptions in the two-way communication process have to be dealt with appropriately.

Broadly speaking, communication is the means by which intentions of the programme are classified to ensure fruitful results. It may even be looked upon as the means by which special information inputs are fed into social systems. It is the means by which behaviour of the personnel engaged in the programme is modified; change is effected, information is made productive and goals are achieved.[5] Barnard has aptly viewed it as the means by which people can be linked together in an organisation to achieve the objectives of the programmes.[6] Communication is a universal phenomenon among living beings. Newman and Summer have viewed communication as an exchange of facts, ideas, opinion, or emotions by two or more persons?

Family Planning Communication implies a number of actions starting with identifying the audience, assessing needs and channels for response identifying specific messages especially in areas of resistance to change in attitude and behaviour, selecting complementary media for optimal combination, producing communication materials and refining message and techniques after pre-testing, revision and re-testing, dissemination of communication, continuous support through stages of programmes implementation mainly to ensure community involvement and participatory monitoring and evaluation. Since, Family Planning is a challenging and arduous task, communication technology must be well planned. A successful communication effort blends the use of traditional communication media with the modem, brings together the channels of government communication with those of the community and of voluntary organisations and a variety of other groups. Family Planning ideology can be registered in the minds of the people not simply by providing the information on Family Planning, but because people can told that they exist, shown that they work and encouraged (and empowered) to try them and make them work for themselves. This is the nature of the support which communication lends to a family planning programme.[7]

ESSENTIALS AND ASPECTS OF MASS MOTIVATION CAMPAIGN

Essentials

Dr. John Hubley quoted by Gloria Gorden in his Article, "Let's Communicate" in *World Health,* January-Feb. 1989) has rightly described the essentials of Communication.

Promote actions which are realistic and feasible within the constraints faced by the community. Build on ideas, concepts and practices that people already have. Repeat and reinforce information overtime, using different methods. Use existing channels of Communication such as songs, drama and story-telling, and be adaptable.

Entertain and attract the attention of the Community. Use clear, simple language with local expressions and emphasize short-term benefits of action.

Provide opportunities for dialogue and discussion to allow learner participation and feedback on understanding and implementation.[8]

Use demonstrations to show the benefits of adopting practices. E.M. Rogers mentions the following essentials:

(i) Family Planning Communication campaigns should be preceded by extensive planning of the strategies to be followed.
(ii) A Consumer Orientation in family planning communication activities will be more effective in achieving the objectives of the National Family Planning Programme.
(iii) A new family planning communication approach should be launched on a small scale pilot project basis.
(iv) Social research can perform an important function in more effective family planning .communication, (a) by providing feedback for the design of communication messages through pre-testing; and (b) by yielding evaluative data about the efforts of communication activities.[9]

Channels of Communication

(a) Radio

Radio has been in use since long. It has been effective as a means of communication. Since the start of the programme on a regular basis, May 1967, on All-India Radio, there have been many challenges as it was a new and sensitive issue. All types of methods have been tried on Radio and even today the importance of Radio as a means of popularising F.P

Programme is enormous. To quote G.K. Mathur, "It is through this common sense and realistic approach that All-India Radio is trying to create a massive awareness base which may serve as a take-off platform for ever widening acceptance of actual family planning methods. In all our programmes we have stressed that the family planning campaign is a people's programme, for the total well-being of the family. It is from this angle that a distinction has been made between the programmes directed directed scarcely populated areas, like hill areas, desert areas, of shore islands, etc., and programmes meant for over-crowded cities and densely populated areas. In order to avoid any possible resistance to the broadcast of family planning programmes on a fixed-time basis, they introduced the family planning themes in between various programmes, thus taking the listener unawares."

All India Radio produces and broadcasts in different formats such as group discussions, interviews, spot recordings, features plays, etc. in different languages and areas. The Commercial Broadcasting Services (CBS) have been broadcasting the programme 'Haseen Lambe' regularly, as well as one minute spots over various channels in Hindi and regional languages.

(b) Television

Television has become very popular. In fact, the potential impact of television, as a means of informing the people, is greater than that of any other means of mass communication. With television, as with the motion picture film, we can hear what is to be done, can see it done and can see the results. Unlike the motion picture, television conveys the feeling of immediacy. In this sense, it combines radio's intimate quality with the motion pictures' ability to magnify the smallest detail which all can see.

(c) Films

Government of India, Publicity Division has been making documentary and other films on various themes of F.P. activities. Parmod Pati has mentioned that, "The Films Division has produced so far a number of films on subjects relating to family planning. A good number of films are now under production. A large number of news-reels have already exhibited slogans relating to family planning. Only a few of these are purely informational, for they are factual and principally of interest value without any attempt in conveying a specific educational message. They focus attention on food problem or housing *vis-a-vis* the rise in population. They talk of education facilities or employment and rise in population. But most of the remaining films are designed primarily to motivate, to encourage and inspire the audience to particular action in accepting new ideas and changing attitudes in accepting the norm of a small family or a means to space children or even to accept methods to completely limit further procreation. Some of the films help to put information about a particular means of contraception in the right perspective while the others keep on emphasising the massage "if you have two that would do." Not all these films {:an be claimed to be outstanding. While an occasional film is made with a festival jury in mind, most of these films meet the needs of the communicator fully so far as family planning education is concerned.

An integrated IEC strategy, mixing inter-personal communication with multi-media contents was developed. Activities were given multi-dimensional and integrated thrust to increase the outreach and impact of Reproductive and Child Health and Family Welfare messages with the objective of bridging the gap between awareness and acceptance.

As part of the new strategy to utilise the services of eminent film makers, the Ministry has assigned eminent directors, Shri Arnol Palekar and Shyam Benegal's two feature films, i.e. 'Kairee' and 'Teri Godi Hari Bhari Rabe' respectively.

(d) Advertising and Visual Publicity

The Directorate of Advertising and Visual Publicity (DA VP) releases press advertisement and arranges exhibitions at various centres throughout the country. Special attention is given to the places of intensive multi-media campaigns.

(e) Song and Drama Division

To educate the masses about family welfare issues, Song and Drama Division organises live entertainment programmes like puppet shows, dance, dramas, folk recitals, mythological recitals, traditional plays, magic shows, etc. Special Programmes to sensitise people regarding the Pulse Polio Immunisation programmes are also being organised by the field units, so that greater number of people can bring their children up to the age of 5 years for the extra doses of Polio drops. More than 15,000 variety shows are organised every year.

(f) Press Information

PIB conducts field visits of journalists for the coverage of family welfare activities. It organises special briefing and seminars for journalists. A Scheme to sensitizes 'Opinion Leaders' by holding one day session on various aspects of family welfare issues, was instituted in 1993-94. Under this scheme, 10421 opinion leaders of various categories including members of Zilla Panchayats, Panchs, private practitioners, teachers, etc. are exposed to family welfare issues. Now, it is proposed to be implemented through State Regional Health and Family Welfare Training Centres.

(g) Personal Communication

Changes in knowledge, attitudes, behaviour, habits and customs can be brought about by personal as well as impersonal methods of FP education. These methods have certain advantages and disadvantages. While personal methods involve face-to-face interaction the impersonal methods do not require such a close personal contact. Personal methods are indeed more convincing and generally more successful. However, the success of personal methods greatly depends on the establishment of a good rapport between the FP educator and his recipients. The impersonal methods are relatively simpler and even less time-consuming. The radio, the newspapers, the posters, and the pamphlets, etc., can all play an important role in imparting FP education .. Experience with personal and impersonal methods of FP education have revealed that if both the methods are used simultaneously one can obtain better results than simply using one or the other method. The most important aspect in the adoption of the programme is the use of inter-personal relationships.

Mr. Manu N. Kulkarni has rightly said that the information transfer among the poor household takes place through indirect mechanisms like gossip among men in tea and bidi shops and gossip sessions of the women when they gather around a village well, pond, bathing ghats and temples. The health matters affecting poor women like pregnancy, maternity, child spacing, family planning, etc. are not talked out openly. When Public Health advertisement makes such information 'open', a sense of shyness and distrust is shown by these poor women and the "closeness" of information is lost. Unfortunately, this does not work when it comes information sharing on private health. Private health is not like DDT spraying for malaria eradication. The chances of Private health information sharing are better when it is shared through informal gossip sessions, inter-personal communication, folk media or street theatre. Commercial advertisements cannot penetrate the antenna of the poor and the deprived."[10]

Thus, we see that communication, i.e. dissemination of information is only one important element in FP education. The adoption or acceptance may not take place simply by communicating FP information. A study conducted by United States Public Health Services has revealed that "Unfortunately knowledge alone does not motivate a person to act in accordance with it. He may well know the correct answers to questions without really believing and accepting such information as the basis for his own action."

Dr. Gisela Gastrin, a Finnish physician mentions in his article, "How Education Helps"? "People can be motivated to adjust their outlook towards health and disease, but before this can happen their negative attitudes have to be countered with factual information .... Education needs to be a part of a comprehensive programme in which responsibilities involving the health authorities and others are clearly delineated and resource allocated."[11]

It was mentioned by Dr. E. Berthat in his article, "A New Role for Teachers" that besides information and motivation, action is indispensable. He said that "Information and motivation are not enough; it remains for governments to ensure that a good health infrastructure is available to all the people. Health education has to convince the men and women wo are responsible for taking decisions that health is a basic raw material for their country's eventual social and economic development."[12]

A Family Planning educator as a persuasive communicator can make the best possible use of the personal methods of FP education. But he has to see that the messages which he is delivering get mentally registered with his recipients. Actually, he can present his message and then wait until he gets the requisite response from his recipients. D.F. Skinner has distinguished between two types of approaches to the learning situation, as 'operant behaviour' and 'respondent behaviour'. The two situation, as also been described as involving instrumental learning and conditional learning. In 'instrumental learning situation', which involves 'operant behaviour', the FP educator will present his message and then wait for the receiver to make a correct response. When the receiver makes this response the FP educator will attempt to fix the response by the appropriate award or reinforcement. On the other hand, in 'conditioned learning situation', which involves 'respondent behaviour', the FP education presents his message in such a way that he elicits the response that he wants from his recipients and thus the stimulus that originally served to elicit the response becomes the reinforcing or rewarding element in conditioning. Undoubtedly, conditioning is much more efficient than instrumental learning. It is, however, necessary for the FP educator to be aware of both kinds of situations since the condition for using 'respondent behaviour' may not be present in the persuasive situation. The FP educator has to be aware that the recipients of his messages differ in the ways in which they learn a given response. They may give different responses essentially in the same situation because of certain specific reasons.

Educational methods to promote family planning currently used by Health and Family Planning workers are often dialectic in character, prescribing "do's" and "don'ts" and are not a convenient medium for structured learning. Doubts have been raised about their effectiveness. They do not provide a learning environment within which people can examine whether the recommended procedures fit into their culture, are feasible in terms of cost and of lifestyles, and are not socially and psychologically counter-productive. In addition, family planning workers often use in appropriate and unrelated visual aids, which have been prepared without keeping in mind the local perceptual patterns of population groups or with insufficient regard to the relevance of these materials to the objectives they are intended to serve.

Everett M. Rogers has maintained that most family programmes have taken too narrow a view of communication in the past. They define the province of family planning communication in terms: (1) of only mass-media 'channels, and (2) of only the communication skills of producing family planning messages. Both functions, of course, are indeed the responsibility of the communication specialist. But, he should do much more, by engaging in activities that include: (1) inter-personnels, channels; and (2) the formation of communication strategies based upon social scientific understanding of behavioural change.

We know that the goals of family planning programmes cannot be reached by using mass-media channels alone. The audiences for such channels are too limited, the attention-getting powers are inadequate, and the motivating and persuading abilities of the mass media are severely restricted. Research investigations consistently indicate that interpersonal channels are necessary to convince most individuals to adopt family planning methods. So, the province of family planning communication whould include word-of-mouth interaction from peers who have previously adopted. By family planning communication, we do not just mean mass-medial channels, they are often mediated and interpreted by opinion leaders to be a large audience of receivers. So, mass media and interpersonal channels are impossible to separate in their functions and effects, even if we tried to do so.

(h) Local Community Groups

In this strategy, the doubts and misgivings hampering the promotion of family welfare measures are dispelled and popular support for the programme enlisted. Andreas Fuglessang, while admitting the role of information in motivating group action, has warned the need of guarding against Pseudo information. To quote him:

> "If genuine change is desired it will occur only through the social mechanisms for change which the community has established and to which it is accustomed. People are eager to change behaviour if they perceive the change as beneficial. . . . It is the fallacy of modernity that we believe, we communicate through bonds of mutual confidence. It is the prime task of the health communicator to facilitate a state of communal trust and also avoid Pseudo information."[13]

Mothers' Clubs in Korean villages play an important role: (1) in facilitating family planning communication, (2) in the general community development of these villages, and (3) in contributing toward women equality. Local community groups could be important in reaching national family planning goals in other nations.

Mother's clubs for family planning communication are also being tried out on a pilot project basis in the Philippines and in Bangladesh, and are widely used in Colombia. Other types of local community groups can also be used for family planning communications, such as agricultural cooperatives, local units of political parties, farmers' associations, etc. Or, as in the "Extra Drive" approach used since 1971 in the province of East Java in Indonesia, strong local leadership in the village is used as a motivational force; here a local group with regular meetings is not used, but a temporarory, once-only meeting of all target couples performs a similar function. The "group planning of births" in the People's Republic of China also depends for its success on encouraging the adoption of family planning methods and lowering fertility, on a once-a-year public meeting followed by continuous peer pressure to encourage parental implementation of the group birth plan.

All these examples illustrate a general proposition: that local community groups can be an essential tool in family planning communication by providing motivation for the adoption of family planning methods and for their continued use to reduce fertility. In most Asian nations, there is presently no government development apparatus that reaches to the local level of social organisation in village. Local groups provide a mean for government to deliver services to the mass population and to change strongly-held beliefs and behaviour.

We must popularise such clubs in India and make trade unions, Mahila Mandals, Youth Organisations and students' associations active in this direction, as has been the experience, in many other countries.

Donald J. Bogue rightly says that taking all factors into account, the group meeting in which some entertainment such as a film or film strip is shown, followed by group discussions, or comment by local leaders, combines many desirable features and is probably one of the best ways (if not the best) to bring information in family planning to a village or neighbourhood.

(i) Mahila Swasthya Sangh

Greater emphasis is being laid on inter-personal communication to encourage community participation, particularly for the womenfolk through Mahila Swasthya Sangh (MSS) in villages with a population of over 1000 or 200 households in plain areas and for population of 500 or more in hilly terrain, including the North Eastern States. The Auxiliary Nurse Midwife (ANM) is the member Secretary of MSS. The MSS comprise five grass-root level functionaries and 10 prominent women from the village community. The field level functionaries of education are also the members of MSS. MSS are being constituted since 1990-91 at village level. A nominal amount of Rs. 1,200 per year is allocated for arranging its monthly meetings.

We can, thus safely say that in order to ensure the success of family planning programmes, the IEC activities must make use of all the communication skills and technology. P.T. Piotrow has rightly said that to enable couples to make informed choices, information about family planning methods must come through many media, leading ultimately to person to person contacts between clients and providers.[14]

(j) Media Advocacy Through NGOs

Indian Association of Parliamentarians on Population and Development (IAPPD) Education

The project Involvement of Elected Representatives for Advocacy on Population, Reproductive Health, HIV/AIDS, Reproductive Rights and women empowerment being implemented by Indian Association of Parliamentarians on Population and Development was launched in

November 1999. The project was to cover Madhya Pradesh and Rajasthan initially for a period of two years. The goal of the project is to sensitize/ mobilize and to involve elected representatives towards effective population stabilization approach, reproductive health programme including awareness of HIV/AIDS, etc. at district level. Twenty-four such sensitization workshops of elected representatives have been held. Renewal of this project, extended is under consideration in the next country programme of UNEPA.

(k) National Population Education Programme

Since its launch in 1980, the National Population Education Programme has been working to attain the institutionalization of Population Education in the education system of the country. In pursuance of this strategy, four projects of Population Education with UNFPA assistance, three through the Department of Education, M/o HRD and one through DGET, M/o Labour, are under operation. All the four population Education Projects are under consideration on a limited scale in the next country programme of UNFPA (2003-07).

(i) Population Education in the School Sector (NCERT)

The Population Education Programme in School Stream project has been implemented as "Population and Development Education in School." The overriding objective of the project has been the institutionalization of re-conceptualized population education, the content and process of school education. The project has been implemented by NCERT at the national level and SCERTs/State Institute of Education at the State/UTs Levels.

(ii) Population Education in the Higher Education System (UGC)

Seventeen Population Education Resources Centres (PERCs) covering 186 universities and 1400 colleges, in over 32 States and UTs are functioning, with emphasis on national capacity building, adolescence education and improved management system.

(iii) Adult Literacy Programme (DAE)

Phase III of the project on Adult Literacy, in operation since 1987,has been implemented now by the Diet of Adult Education at the national, level and State Resource Centres (SRCs), Regional Resource Centers (PRCs) in States. The project has covered around 450 Total Literacy Campaign (TLC) districts spread over 28 states and seven UTs. The number of participants covered in these districts was 140 million in the 9-35 years age group, of whom around 60% were women.[15]

(l) Training of IEC Personnel

The IEC Division organized a series of capacity building programme for IEC personnel at Central, States and district level. The IEC officers working at Centre/States attended a two-week capacity building communicator workshop in November 2002, which was organized by Administrative Staff College of India, Hyderabad in collaboration with Johns Hopkins University, at their campus on behalf of the Department. The awareness generation training coordinated by the National Institute of Health and Family Welfare for health functionaries of the State and district level included a module on interpersonal communication.

Ninetieth Report of Department-related Parliamentary-standing committee on Ministry of Health and Family Welfare observes that:

To quote 101 reports;

The committee has been given to understand that during the year 2001-02, IEC activities, based on the communication strategy, especially in demographically weak districts, will be intensified. Greater emphasis would be laid on a more judicious media-mix based on local specific media forms and need-based inter-personal communication schemes. More stress would be given at grass root level and the segments not reached by conventional mass media channels for effectively transmitting population-related values and messages. Remote areas would be covered by adopting multi-media strategy. Greater emphasis is to be given to training and strengthening of Mahila Swasthya Sanghs and other grass-root level functionaries. The Department has also informed that as part of the new lEe strategy in tune with the Reproductive and Child Health Programme, it has been decided to utilize private professional agencies for creating audio-visual and visual software and designing advertising campaigns for the Mass Media. The Committee appreciates that the Department has decided to intensify its activities in demographically weak districts. However, the Committee feels that unless local administration is involved and representatives of local people associate themselves with the family welfare programmes, the benefits of these programmes cannot be fully realized. The Committee recommends that the Department should take necessary measures in this regard.

CONCLUSIONS AND RECOMMENDATIONS

Without evaluating the impact of FP education programmes on the bulk of the people, one cannot possible identify positive as well as negative aspects of the programme. An objective evaluation of the FP education programme alone can help one improve guidelines for future action. Cost-benefit analysis should be an integral part of this evaluation, so that one may assess how available resources have been utilized. Through objective evaluation, one may also be able to curtail mass production of ritualistic' FP education material as produced by various FP education bureaus. The amount thus saved can be effectively utilized for a more purposeful and meaningful health education programme.

FP education is the most difficult task as habits, usages and customs are deeply entrenched. But, FP educator would fail in its purpose, if it could not produce social change, as it is easier to destroy our villages than to change our customs. Professional training helps the FP experts to deal with the health changes effectively. Their pharamcopoeia in both fields must be strong in order to translate the findings of biological investigations to social application. So over and above each technical act, there is a corresponding education function which doubles the value of the act, increases its efficiency and endows it with real human and social value.[16]

We now give some concrete suggestions, which can enable effective communication and information:

1. Strengthen Media to Cover Populous Areas through Audience Segmentation

A recent study conducted by Monis Raza has indicated that the couple protection rate varies from 62 to 68 in different areas. Therefore, there is a need to segment the population areas so that more attention can be paid to low acceptability areas. To quote E.M. Rogers, "We conclude that audience segmentation strategies, which delineate sub-categories of the total audience and aim special messages at them, offer important potential for family planning communication effectiveness."

Joung Whang rightly stresses that sound communication strategies at the grass-roots level require segmentation of individual clients of the community into specific categories, according to geographical and social accessibility, kind of media available to identified clients, particular language and symbols familiar to them, level of understanding, motivation already attained, level of aspiration, etc. There is a need Audience research to get feedback, ready reference and analysis for programme planners on various aspects pertaining to audience composition, its habits, tastes, preference, exposure, extent of coverage, impact of the programme.

2. Adequate and Reliable Information based on Research in Bio-medical Aspects of Family Planning

The National Perspective Plan For Women (1988-2000 AD) has rightly stressed the need to educate and inform the people about Family Planning on the basis of genuine research and findings so that they can choose right methods. To quote the Perspective Plan:

> "It is unfortunate that the family planning policy is oriented towards fertility concerned with providing a means for women and men to have control on their own bodies. . . . Research studies have shed light on the fact that the knowledge regarding Family Planning/ Methods is low despite the huge amounts of money spent on propaganda. The only method known to all is sterilization. The high of abortion show the desire and need of the women for family planning and the failure of the family planning information and services to reach them in time. Laproscopic operations are being performed in several family planning camps without proper care and

follow-up. Consequent problems tend to create apprehension among people. More intensive propagation of spacing methods together with innovative strategies for delivery of supplies has to be taken up and spread of information about temporary methods should *be accorded* high priority."

B.L. Raina has rightly mentioned that it is essential: (a) to understand human reproductive processes, (b) to find out means for modification adaptation and control of these processes; (c) to know the complexity of human behaviours and its consequences; and (d) to mobilize our knowledge so gained for achievement of our social aims. The knowledge on reproductive processes is still limited. Species differences make problem the more difficult.

3. Research to make Mass Communication More Effective

There is a need of continuous research in the areas of FP Programme Communication activities. Reliance on mass media can reach only to those few who constitute the elite group. If the family planning programme was based only on elite participation, the public relations tools could have some utility because the rest of the population did not matter. But when the success of F.P. Programme is based on total participation, the public relations tools have got to be redevised. There has been no organized attempt to find out new tools and techniques of Public Relations based on a scientific study of the nature of the Public to be reached. The problem calls for intensive research programme to delineate channels of communication for reaching the public. To quote Dinesh Chandra Dubey and Kamla Gopal Rao, "With no pretence of giving a comprehensive review of needed research in mass communication for popularizing family planning, the foregoing review only seeks to highlight some of the important areas of research. While most of research findings in mass communication have been extracted from studies in highly urbanized, modem, western cultures, the authors feel strongly that the insights derived from these studies need to be tested out for their validity in the transitional societies and in developing societies."

4. Impart Training Programmes for Family Planning Education

Bharara has nicely said that 'The population programme essentially has multi-disciplinary and multi-dimensional characteristics. These disciplines fall within four categories, viz., (i) demography and statistics, (ii) biomedicine, (iii) social and behavioural sciences, and (iv) administration and programme planning. Accordingly, the personnel engaged in the family welfare programme are drawn from these disciplines and are demographers, statisticians, doctors, nurses and other paramedical workers; social scientists, social workers and extension educators; arid planners, administrators, supervisors, evaluators, etc. Each discipline represented must be integrated into the whole of the programme in the most effective and efficient manner. Personnel from these disciplines have to be available in adequate number at the front line of action, as well as at other levels of administration, supervision and planning. It necessarily implies that the roles and responsibilities of these personnel will vary according to the level at which they function, even though the ultimate goal remains very much the same. All the personnel, therefore, become co-ordinated parts of a machinery, working as a team, in co-operation with each other, by fully synchronizing their activities. This is what a training programme has to cater to, and produce personnel who will be able to function accordingly.

The roles for each group of functionaries at different levels being so varied, training programmes have to develop correct role perceptions among the workers and, accordingly correct role!expectations among their supervisors and those higher up in the echelons of administration. The higher the degree of role consensus, the lesser the chances of role conflicts, job dissatisfaction and frustrations.

5. Develop Effective Public Relations

One of the important functions of family welfare administrators is the development of cordial, equitable and harmonious relationships with the beneficiaries to ensure their welfare and participation. The public relations is the establishment of a climate of understanding. The purpose of public relations is not only to supply information, but also to encourage an understanding and co-operation between the social scientists, soda workers and beneficiaries.

The management of any public agency should not only employ competent media specialists—those who handle press contacts, prepare news releases, write radio scripts, and carryon other information activities—but it should also create a favourable image of help both! and outside the agency.[17] The family welfare programmes have not desired publicity through the publicity media. Our inquiries have shown that the poor coverage was not due to apathy of the press or other of publicity but due to lack of communication and inadequate release of information on the subject. Publicity is very useful or even essential not only to highlight the programmes and achievements of the organisation but to enlist the cooperation of a large number of employees and the goodwill of public, in the implementation of family welfare programme. Many well intentioned and technically sound family welfare programmes, aimed at solving family welfare problems, have been frustrated by lack of popular acceptance and community participation. To quote a WHO Report, "It has been observed that such programmes are either not actively associated or passively ignored because they do not belong to the population they are designed to help; they are rather seen by the population as imposed external programme that belong to the government and consequently deserves and require little, if any, of the population's attention, action, or other response."[18]

Some of the measures which are suggested for improvement of, relations are:

- A publicity sub-committee may be constituted at all levels. This committee may look after the publicity programmes of the family welfare organisations;
- Personal contacts should' be maintained with the local press, specially by arranging meetings and press conferences from time to time;
- The help of local office of the press information bureau may be utilize to release photo-features from time to time; Local stations of All-India Radio be persuaded to include talks and discussions of family planning work specialists in the field of family welfare. Sometimes, discussions have much better effect than straight talks;
- It is desirable to celebrate "Family Welfare Day" in the country every year during which, on a selected theme, publicity can be given through all available media of publicity. "Family Welfare Day" should be observed by all agencies in the field of family planning work from the village to union level on committed basis; and
- It may be worthwhile introducing printed "news letter" by every State, which can be sent to all State Boards, the Central Board and voluntary organisations concerned, highlighting the major events or developments in the field within their states during the month.

Another dimension of Public Relations in the area of Family Welfare is counselling the people and also those implementing Family Welfare Programmes. Primary Objective of all family welfare services is to ensure that every individual becomes a well adjusted and productive member of a society. Effective delivery of these services depends, not merely on the material resources or well conceived programmes, but also on the quality of the personnel implementing them. So, there is a need of developing good rapport with the personnel responsible for implementation through counselling. "Counselling" is defined in the "Encylopaedia of Social Work of India" as a professional activity associated with the process of helping individual or groups with their various problems and extending to developmental ends.

Successful Field Counselling depends on the following factors:

The counsellor should be a mature person, with broad outlook; wide interest and sensitiveness to the behavioural pattern and needs of the persons he/she deals with. These qualities are essential for development of a positive relationship, which is an indispensable tool, in addition to knowledge and counselling skill. A field counsellor should have faith in voluntary and State action and their capacity to effectively render family welfare services.

A field counsellor is a dynamic and constructive leader with keen sensitivity to the community needs, feelings and attitudes and the capacity to stimulate the agency and the community to work towards goals, established through mutual and continued interaction between the two. He should be a catalytic agent of planned change, rather than a victim of the system.

Effective field counselling requires that the counsellor has knowledge of relevant family planning welfare activities of minimum standards for their family of other social services of National, State and Local levels and of Field Counselling Technique.[19]

Thus, public relations including counselling can help in promoting Family Welfare activities. Due care should be taken that the public relations should not degenerate into a propaganda machinery. "Public relations activities must be honest, truthful, open, authoritative and responsible, they must be fair and realistic; and they must be conducted in the public Interest." Due safeguards are therefore necessary to make public relations effective for two-ways and authentic communication nerves of family welfare agencies. This traffic can be best organised by professional public relations men, but at the lowest levels of administration, the administrative personnel must do their own public relations. According to E.C. Gera, "It is not enough for mass media to be blaring forth statement in Governments policies and programmes. There must be deliberate and organised attempts also to assess the needs of people to listen to their grievances and to redress them. And the people, particularly the uneducated people must be treated' with courtesy instead of being shouted at and compelled to shell out bribes."[20] All this requires dedicated, scientific and well-conceived public relations work.

6. Understand the Area of Operation

Before launching any F.P. programme, the family planning personnel must assess the local problems and must possess the knowledge about the beliefs, conceptions and misconceptions which the people have formed about family planning activities. It needs to be stressed that the cusltural context of F.P. education programme is of the greatest importance in the Indian situation. The social scientists can help the family planning workers through their studies and research.

7. Effective Administrative Machinery to Impart Family Planning

There is a lot of wastage and corruption in the conduct of mass Education in F.P. Programme. Some activities like Drama, Folk Songs, Puppet shows remain only on the paper and thus the huge amount meant for the purpose is either wasted or embezzled. Vehicles supplied for this purpose are wrongly used. After independence, the family welfare administrative machinery of India advanced considerably both in magnitude and direction. Administrative efficiency is the most urgent demand of the day. Most of the grievances of the citizens are because of the apathy of the administration and lack of dynamic administration. An international group of public administration experts has also stressed upon this, "Dysfunctional and inapplicable administrative structures, systems, and practices must be replaced. Nothing less than dynamic organisations, resourceful management and streamlined administrative processes will suffice . . . the tortrous the consuming routines, special privileges, corruption, indolence and insolence often encumbering any governmental bureaucracies and civil services have no place in development administration. This calls for continuous action to foster honesty and integrity and to weed out corruption as well as to develop p measure."[21]

8. Develop Attractive Mass-Media Material

No doubt, a vast majority of our people is still unable to read and write. But, literacy is definitely spreading. More importantly, the printed word influences the literate opinion leader in the village like the teacher, panchayat chief, etc. who will be amongst the first to adopt family planning and who will be able to influence his untutored brethren.

9. Motivate Extension Personnel

The quality of the F.P. operations run by Government would be dependent to a great extent upon the quality of extension workers engaged in their operation. Personnel move the administrative machinery. To quote Mrs. Indira Gandhi: "If Government has to do more for the people, its employees must play a more dynamic and more creative role, as the instrument for implementing government policies and programmes."[22]

An extension group cannot work with their heart init unless they are adequately motivated with reasonable remuneration and prospects of advancement. The emoluments paid to F.P. personnel have been less than those paid to professionals in comparable pursuits, while the task of successful extension is one of the most difficult. If the Extension workers are motivated, this would generate loyalty, co-operation and team work, essential for the achievement of the goals of P.P. Programmes.

Whenever there is a failure of the family planning programme, we generally attribute it to the illiteracy, ignorance and irrational attitudes of the people. On the other hand, we should make a fresh assessment of what the obstacles to family planning success actually are. In order to tackle these problems, IEC can help a great deal in promoting positive attitudes. The obstacles should not be considered as insurmountable barriers. Within each State and Union Territory, there is a need to set-up communication research project to provide information needed to replan the IEC activities to tide over the difficulties. Lyle Saunders has suggested the following change in IEC activities in future.[23]

(i) Family Planning communicators in the future are likely to be more focused on communities as audiences are more concerned with trying to change collective beliefs and values than with informing individuals;

(ii) They may find it necessary to spend more time providing information demanded by more strongly committed political leaders, justifying and defending the spread of sterilization and abortion and developing public support for ideas· and activities that may be initially unpopular;

(iii) They will be concerned with explaining new kinds of contraceptives and a variety of incentive and disincentive measures;

(iv) They will find themselves working more closely with other special interest communicators in efforts to integrate development programmes and trying to maximize the accuracy and reliance of family planning information provided by communicators with other major interests;

(v) They will have a role to play in changing the image of family planning as a health matter and may both contribute to and learn from the promotional activities of those on the commercial sector who are distributing contraceptives;

(vi) They will be helping to formulate and implement new communication strategies; and

(vii) They may have some new interesting tools to work with its current trends on communication technology.

10. Multi-disciplinary Integrated Approach to Promote Communication

12th joint conference of central council of health and family planning suggested that the revised strategy predicates on multi-disciplinary integrated approach. Addressing the areas beyond family welfare and mobilizing all development agencies and sectors of society directly interfacing with the people to join in the task of family welfare promotion is a *sine-quo-non* for its success. The communication support for this work will now accordingly have to be through a multi-dimensional integrated thrust.

This requires a far broader vision for family welfare than has prevailed so far. On the one hand, family welfare communication, will need to be embedded in primary health care messages and on the other, form an organic part of a core package of social development issues; particularly those relating to female, literacy, employment status, age of marriage and child survival:

(i) Therefore, it is necessary that the State Family Planning organisations and State Education Health Bureau make more coordinated use of manpower and material to put out programmes and messages of health and family wefare in an integrated fashion, integration where possible and in any case functional co-ordination of these two units must be done immediately. Along side efforts must be initiated to ensure that health and family welfare IEC efforts link up and co-ordinate with the media efforts for women and child development, adult and non-formal education and youth activities. The budget for Health and Family Welfare IEC must be substantially enhanced.

(ii) The gap between widespread awareness and limited practice of family welfare also calls for different communication approaches which concentrate on effecting behavioural changes more rapidly. Therefore, at the present stage of the programme, greater use must be made of all inter-personnel channels and appropriate training and orientation of all developmental workers to bring about their involvement with family planning. Equally, the reorientation of Health and Family Welfare workers to enable an internalization of the broader perspective is important.

(iii) With the country presently going through a communication revolution, all media channels must be fully utilized to create an enabling ethos for the programme and as a means to vault the barriers of illiteracy and ignorance. Greater family welfare acceptance is noted where there is greater exposure to media. Towards this end, the Council recommends urgent steps to be taken to ensure greater access to television and radio for the most critical target groups, who presently form the media-deprived class. This is to be done through promotion of group listening and community viewing situations. A pooling of resources for all departments to create such an access must be considered. The greater use of television, film, radio and traditional media must be encouraged to create a synergy between mass media and inter-personal channels. In the case of television, which is a government medium, maximum support must be ensured to health and family welfare issues by earmarking minimum time for programmes on health and family welfare; weaving of appropriate messages in the regular serials and other sponsored propagation of public service messages on health and family welfare at prime time.

(iv) Altogether, information must move to another plane from general to the specific, giving the how and why on what is required to be done so as to empower people to act on their own behalf. The spirit of family planning communication has to communicate information, not publicity and propaganda. The States may, therefore, like to ensure that the budget for media work are more effectively utilized on developing information, education and communication materials.

(v) As a part of the effort to bring about total mobilization of society and wider involvement of everyone in the programme, strenuous efforts must now be made to secure free publicity and promotion of the family planning programme and its objectives through every possible source. Free display at sports stadiums, bus panels and other commercial channels should be actively solicited and engineered.

(vi) All communication materials and messages must be protested before application in the field. The pretesting should be done through quick and ready methods so that material can be corrected at appropriate stage.

(vii) Some immediate administrative measures are necessary to revitalize the IEC programme. There are large number of vacancies in the State media set-ups, particularly at the field level. These must be filled in the shortest possible time. The media staff working in the States should be utilized for intensifying IEC programmes, instead of deputing them for routine clerical jobs.

An efficient extension F.P. service, capable of winning people's confidence as their friend, philosopher and guide, takes decades to build up. Careful selection and training, morale-building, service conditions, rational organisation-these are the bricks and mortars of the extension officers. Close co-ordination with research, input supply, marketing and guidance, and employment of an effective combination of communication techniques are prerequisites for the successful functioning of the F.P. service. Various management tasks involved in building up such extension service need strengthening.

Notes and References

1. Donald J. Bogue, "A five year Information-Education Communication Perspective to meet the Population, Health, Food Crises, 1975-1980", in *Family Planning Resumed*, p. 117, Vol. I, 1977, No. 1.
2. A. Govindachari, 'The Role of Extension Education in Family Planning', in *Aspects of Population Policy in India*, New Delhi, 1969, pp. 124-25.
3. Population Reports, Series Number 35, November 1987, p. 2.
4. Annual Report of the Ministry of the Health and Family Welfare, 1998-99, p. 73.
5. H. Koontz and E. O'Donnell, "Principles of Management: An Analysis of Managerial Functions", London: McGraw Hill, Kogakusha Ltd., 1972, pp. 53840.
6. Chester, I. Barnard, "The Functions of the Executive", Cambridge; Harward University Press, 1968, pp: 226-27.
7. W.H. Newman and C.E. Summer, "The Process of Management Concepts Behaviour and Practice", Englewood, Cliffs, N.J., Prentice Hall, 1961, p. 59.
8. *World Health*, Jan.-Feb. 1989.
9. E.M. Rogers in Joung Whang, ed., pp. 130-31.
10. *The Economic Times*, March 9, 1989.
11. WHO, *World Health*, Nov. 1975, p. 14.
12. *Ibid*., May, 1979, p. 25.
13. Andreas Fuglesang, "Fold Wisdom and Pseudo Information", in *World Health*, Jan.-Feb. 1989, pp. 6-7.
14. E.M. Rogers, Management of Family Planning IEC Activities, in Joung Whang, (ed.), pp. 116-17.

15. Population Reports, Series L Number 35, Nov. 1987, p. 16.
16. WHO Technical Report Series, 1954, No. 89, p. 4.
17. Felix, Nigro A., Modem Public Administration, *op. cit.*, p. 205.
18. *WHO Chronicle*, 30 (1976), pp. 177-78.
19. Central Social Welfare Board, Field Counselling Service, A Pilot Project, 1974, New Delhi, p. 13.
20. F.C. Gera, "Need for Public Relations in Administration" in *IJPA Journal*, Vol.. XXI, July-Sept. 1975, pp. 545-56.
21. United Nations Public Administration in the Second United Nation Development Decade, *Ibid.*
22. Presidential Address by Mrs. Indira Gandhi delivered on October 22, 1971, at the Annual Meeting of *IJPA*, New Delhi.
23. Lyle Salmders, Family Planning Resource, Vol. 1, No. 1, pp. 30-31.

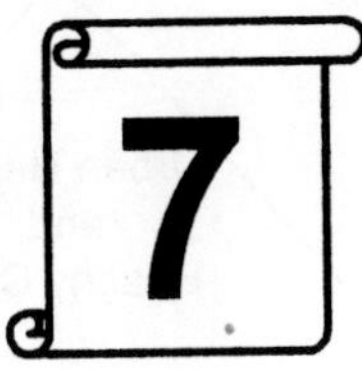

Urban Health: Healthy Cities

> Cities are the locus of productive economic activities and hope for the future, yet they face growing environmental problems and increasing poverty. . . 'It is clear that, in the short-term, the bright lights of the city have dimmed and are, for many urban households, extinguished.'
>
> —*(World Bank, 1991)*

In the beginning of 20th century, there was only 10 percent of the population in the world living in urban areas, which increased to 80 percent, the population increased to about 50 percent. This largest movement of human beings from rural to urban area in the known history of human kind, has indeed necessitated a relook into our settlement development perspectives. Today, we have 21 mega cities with more than 10 million inhabitants in each of them. Seventeen among these are in the developing countries. The process of urbanization appears to be irreversible at least in the near future.

V. Suresh, and P. Jayapal in their article, "Towards an Inclusive City in the New Millennium" in *Shelter* rightly says:

> "Today's city presents a scenario of paradoxes. On the one hand, the city exhibits considerable potential with economic vibrancy and on the other; it presents a scenario of declining opportunities for the teaming millions. Whereas this centre of prosperity is resulting in the improvement of quality of life of large number of population, it is also turning into an agglomeration of poverty, with even more population living in conditions which are unacceptable, while the city has created peaks of affluence, it has also created depths of poverty and despair. And, even while it acts as the centre of cultural synthesis, it also presents a scenario of 'hollow of conscience' with crimes against women and children rising to unbelievable heights. The

CHART 7.1

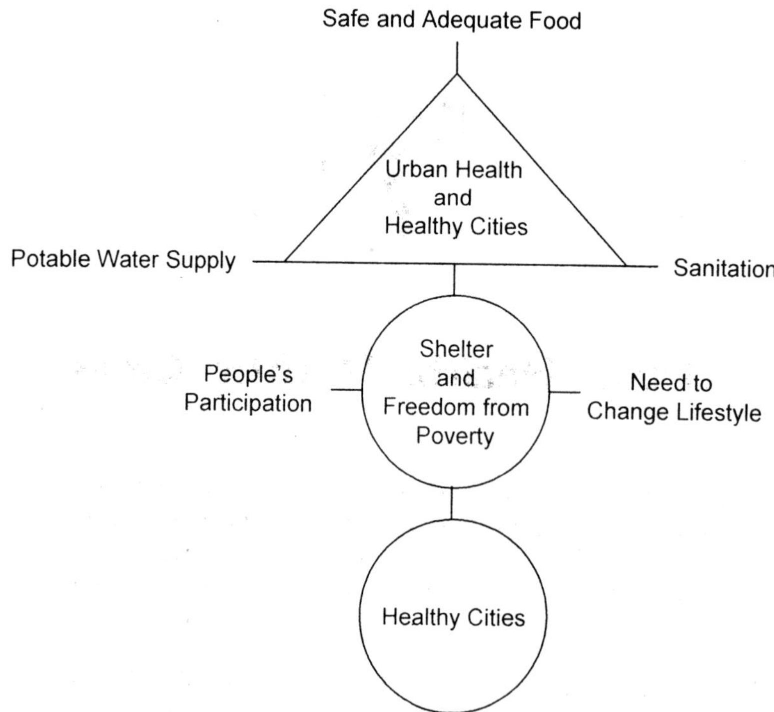

increasing difference in the levels of income and quality of life of the people as reflected in the economic marginality, has resulted in the discernible demarcation of the 'have's and haven'ts' in terms of spatial, economic, cultural components in the city fabric."[1]

Surveys have revealed that there were 27 women in the urban areas, among one lakh, who are suffering from breast cancer while in rural areas the number is as low as eight. that Draft Status Paper—1995 of Government of Punjab, has observed that[2] Urbanization has been considered as an index of development but in case of developing countries like India, urbanization is not the outcome of merely the growth potential generated by urban settlements. It has been largely due to people work relationship in rural areas, in which land is the essential medium and which is right now so critically balanced that even small addition to population is pushing people out of agriculture to non-agricultural occupations. Thus, by and large, in India urbanization is emerging as merely a process of transfer of rural poverty to urban environment, which only results in concentration of misery. This has resulted in the malfunctioning of most of the urban settlements leading to emergence of number of imbalances and problems. Thus, most of these settlements suffer from improper and haphazard development, absence of basic infrastructures and services, uncontrolled and unchecked growth of slums, lack of housing, high degree of visual and environmental degradation and uncontrolled traffic. The cumulative effect of these factors is the degradation of quality of life in urban settlements and huge amount of subsidies required to keep them going. These facts are more evident in case of larger cities especially metros and super-metros.[2]

Urban areas in the past have not received much attention in terms of their planning, development and management despite the fact that cities and economic development are inextricably linked. Because of high productivity of urban areas, economic development activities get located in cities. Accordingly it is desirable that human settlements are provided with necessary planning and development inputs so that their orderly growth and development in ensured. This would also be necessary for ensuring efficient functioning of human settlements for improving their productivity and for providing desirable quality of life to its residents in order to cater to their both economic and physical and metaphysical needs. The urban development strategy for any state thus assumes importance for not only its economic emancipation but also its physical well-being. All these factors and circumstances affect the health of the people.

Ninth Five Year plan has analyzed the urban health situation. To quote the plan:[3]

> "Nearly 30% of India's population lives in urban areas. Urban migration over the last decade has resulted in rapid growth of people living in urban slums. The massive inflow of the population has also resulted in the deterioration of living conditions in the cities. From the data it would appear that the urban population has better health facilities and health indices than the rural population. However, in many towns and cities the health status of urban slum-dwellers is worse than that of the rural population. The urban health facilities provide health care, especially tertiary care to both the urban and rural population. The available urban health care infrastructure is insufficient to meet the health care needs of the growing urban population."

Realizing this the municipalities, State Governments and the Central Government have tried to provide funds for building up urban health care. Unlike the rural health services, there have not been any well-planned and organized efforts to provide primary, secondary and tertiary care services in geographically delineated areas in urban health care. As a result, there is either non-availability or substantial under over-crowding at secondary and tertiary care centers.

Slums Urban development. is accompanied Krishna Gowada and others have rightly observed that the growth and problems of slums are a consequence of city development.[4]

The growth of slums in any city is considered as a sign of environmental degradation. Yet the slums keep on proliferating as a result of the pressure of population growth and housing shortage. Slums give rise to problems relating to health, sanitation, land use and even crime. It has been observed that the intermediary zone has the largest number of slums compared to the city centre and the periphery in Bangalore. Slums are identified in some parts of the central area. Presence of slums in the central area in Cotton pet and Kalsipalyam areas has resulted in unwholesome and improper utilization of valuable land and has added chaos to the already congested areas of the city. The slums with their associated problems like insanitary conditions; social pathology, juvenile delinquency, etc. have become a nuisance to the smooth functioning of commercial activities. Besides these, there are a number of clusters of residential areas, which may also be grouped under slums on account of overgrowing, dilapidation, lack of ventilation and which are thus detrimental to health and safety of the residents. Through the Slum Board, community toilets have been provided, but the people use them very badly. Access to toilets and availability of adequate water are the major problems. These areas have been using streets and conservancies as latrines, wastes are let out into open drains and stinking cesspools are created resulting in health hazards.

John Ashton in his Article, "Healthy Cities" defines the concept of Healthy Cities.[5] to quote:

> "Defining the healthy city is not an easy task. Certainly a healthy city is more than one, which simply has good health services. The idea implies that the city, as a place, which allows scope for human possibility and experience, has a crucial role to play in determining the health of those living in it. Yet each city own personality."

A healthy city has been defined as one, which is continually expanding and creating opportunities for people to live life to the full and to support each other. Central to such a definition is the social implication that, in a healthy city, there is some kind of common field of play and the broadly speaking the citizens are striving towards the same goal. Yet conflict and its creative resolution are also part of a healthy city.

At its most fundamental a city is unhealthy if it cannot provide its citizens with these basic resources for health:

- Safe and adequate food,
- A safe water supply,
- Sanitation,
- Shelter, and
- Freedom from poverty.

However, it is clear that these alone are insufficient, and that a range of environmental prerequisites (economic, physical, social and cultural) are part of what most people expect for themselves and their families if they are to enjoy full health in the city.

It has seven main elements:[6]

1. The establishment of an inter-pectoral committee for the city, which brings together the key decision-makers from the different agencies and bureaucracies to take a strategic view of health in the city.
2. A parallel technical group to carry out a community diagnosis, which is wide-ranging and has a particular focus on inequalities in health within the city.
3. The creation of a great debate within the city about the nature of current health problems—what can and needs to be done about them.
4. The formulation of city plans for health, which are action-based and inter-sectoral in nature.
5. The development of models of good practice representing the different entry-point priorities of the different cities. These may range from major environmental action to support for better individual lifestyles or the formation of self-help groups, and will illustrate the principles of health promotion, particularly public participation.
6. Monitoring and research into the effectiveness of models of good practice on health in cities; this will involve higher educational institutions in meaningful collaboration with their host communities.
7. Mutual support, cultural exchange, collaboration and learning between cities.

Urban health studies and projects have been done by multilateral and bilateral agencies, World Bank, WHO, UNICEF, USAID, etc. have been providing great assistance to developing world to improve urban health. At present in India, World Bank is assisting 6 states of Indian Union to improve secondary health care in urban areas with a total assistance of about 3000 crores. In cities, the health system is totally disorganized as it encompasses primary, secondary and tertiary care as well as assistance by Government, Private, and Voluntary institutions. We find too many doctors, too many medicine shops and still people suffering from poor health. There is no co-ordination resulting in duplication, overlapping and wastage of resources. What can be done to make cities healthy? What can be done to keep cities clean? How can we provide good health care? How can we interlink health with other urban development services? Let us now discuss the facts and suggestions to improve health care system, which can provide decent health services to all the people. (Refer Chart 7.2)

I. Need of Change of Lifestyles

People in urban areas lead sedatic life, which is compounded by the habits of gambling, drinking, smoking and prostitution, etc. All these add

CHART 7.2

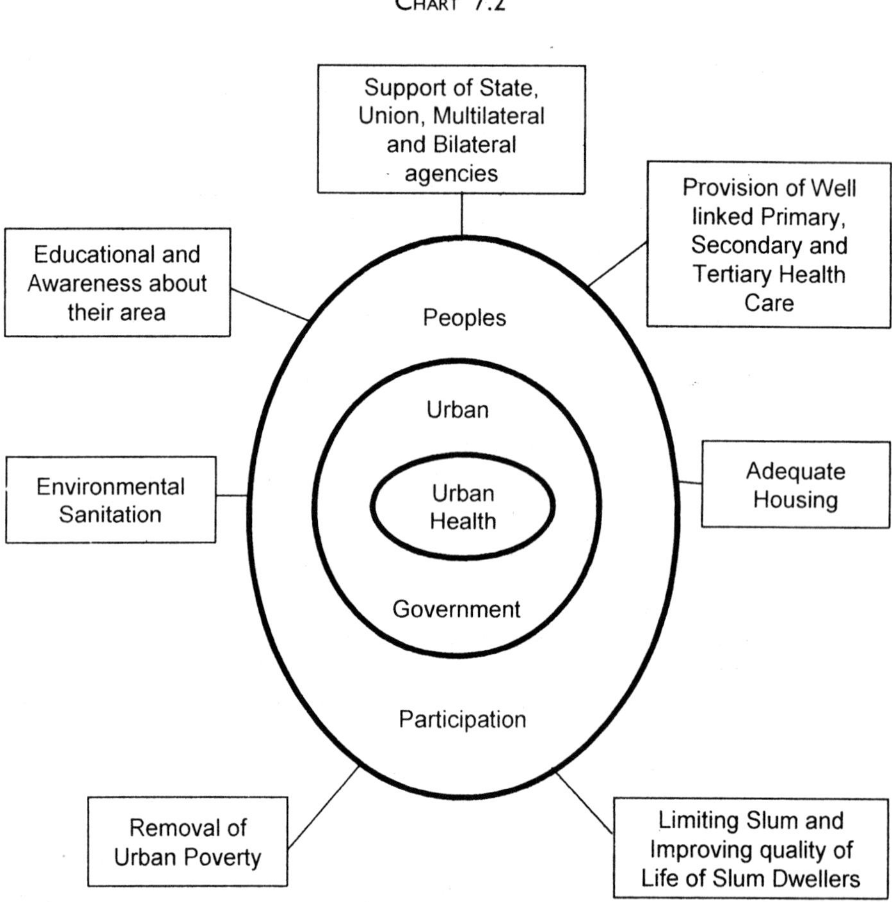

to poor health. Since availability of transport has become easy, they easily fall prey to coronary diseases, diabetes, hypertension, etc.

Rene Dcekstra[7] has rightly said that the rapid social changes in many parts of the world especially taking the form of over-urbanization, have brought about important changes in values, family structure and community experience, which in turn interfere with some of the important psycho-social and health needs of human beings. The shrinking of the extended family and the disintegration of communities have resulted in less effective social support networks and less likelihood of giving or receiving emotional support; in less responsibility for local affairs; in fewer opportunities for cooperative small group interaction and action; and in fewer activities in general that stimulate a sense of personal involvement, belonging, comradeship and responsibility. Gripped by a sense of isolation or alienation, young people particularly, in their search for group membership and values worth identifying with, that is, in quest of a sense of belonging and responsibility, simply cannot satisfy those needs in healthy ways. They become all the more subject health risk behaviours like addiction, or to manipulation or abuse by political and criminal organisations. Besides, there is a need to change to Active lifestyle by urban-dwellers to keep metabolism active.

2. Need of Improving Environmental Sanitation and Avoid Environmental Pollution

Urban life is progressively deterioration on account of unplanned industrialization, uncontrolled migration of population, lack of management of trade waste and human waste. Existing conditions in cities/towns are marked by congestion, overcrowding, lack of adequate drainage and poor arrangements for solid waste disposal. Various types of industries have come up in close proximity of the urban areas and within residential localities. This has resulted in discharge of obnoxious wastewater on to the fields, dumping of solid industrial waste nearby and emission of poisonous fumes and smoke in the atmosphere. Housing stock, which is a dominant element of physical environment, is of very poor quality.[8]

At present, there is no sanitation worth the name for 52 per cent of the urban population. The sewerage system covers only 35 per cent of the population of Class IV cities and 75 per cent of the population of Class I cities. About 34 percent of urban population does not have any arrangement even for drainage of rainwater around its habitats. 60 per cent of the municipal bodies in India collect less than 40 per cent of the urban waste, which is allowed to decompose and putrefy on the roadside and around houses and factories. Quite a substantial portion of it goes into the drains, choking them and creating slush and stink all around, besides providing breeding ground for pests, files and mosquitoes and cockroaches.

Urban settlements also suffer from inadequate piped water supply and underground sewerage facilities. No sewage treatment plant has been installed in most of the towns with the result that sullage is disposed of onto land or into nullahs causing land, air pollution and under ground water pollution. Storm water drainage has hardly been provided in any town. Stagnation of water along the roads and within the residential areas result in breeding of mosquitoes/files causing nuisance and health problems. Refuse is indiscriminately thrown into lanes and backyards while squatters defecate in the open causing serious health hazards. Traffic congestion is a common problem in all-urban settlements. Due to vehicular emissions the air is also polluted. Noise pollution is constantly increasing due to heavy traffic. Recreational facilities such as parks and playgrounds are least provided in urban areas. Government is fully aware of the environmental problems and is keen to provide for good health and well-being of the citizens but action is lacking.

Health problems of big towns and cities are closely related to environmental conditions, due to overcrowding, inadequate and poor housing, lack of adequate safe drinking water supply, lack of drainage, non-collection of waste, water, and its improper disposal, untreated discharge of industrial waste discharge of smoke and toxic gases into atmosphere, etc. lead to pollution of air, water and land in urban towns and cities to a degree much greater than in rural areas. The environmental degradation leads to high prevalence of both communicable and non-communicable diseases in an urban society (Rao and Chakraborty, 1976).

In addition to above problems, the ever-increasing trends of urbanization are mounting tremendous pressures on civic amenities and on health and other services. The unprecedented growth in urban population has also been witnessed by most of the urban areas, which resulted in deterioration in the standard and quality of public life. In almost every urban center, irrespective of its size and class, the availability of core civic services have been found to be scarce (NIUA, 1989).

To achieve the objective of Environmentally Sustainable Development of urban centers, it is suggested that:[9]

(i) Efforts would be made to minimize migration from rural to urban areas by creating appropriate level of infrastructure and opportunities for gainful employment in rural settlements. This would mean planned development of rural areas and promoting cottage and other industries, which are agro-based.

(ii) In order to achieve maximum growth of small and medium towns and to induce desired level of population therein, it is proposed to distribute socio-economic activities in small and medium towns. More investment would be made in these towns for creating more economic opportunities for gainful employment in such centers.

(iii) It is proposed to prescribe a certain minimum limit of area to be earmarked as green cover in each human settlement. Concept of city forests would be given a fair trial for ensuring appropriate level of environment.

(iv) All community open spaces would be planned, developed and managed in close cooperation with the people so as to ensure its optimum utilization with minimum of investment.

(v) Ribbon development along important highways and roads would be checked in order to ensure free flow of men and material.

(vi) Planning of human settlement would be done in such a manner that it minimizes the travel needs of the people living therein. Plans would encourage and give precedence to pedestrian movement, cyclists, two-wheelers and motorcars in that order of preference. Minimizing travel and use of vehicle would lead to creation of human settlements, which are highly energy efficient and would have minimum pollution due to reduced use of petrol driven vehicles.

(vii) Informal sector would be considered an essential part of human settlements because of its considerable contribution to city economy and capacity to provide gainful employment to its work force. Thus, informal sector would be properly planned and its requirements duly catered for in the planning and developmental process.

(viii) Burning of agro-waste as an industrial fuel would be banned, so as to minimize pollution. Appropriate mechanism and safeguards would be provided to check this growing menace.

(ix) Planning of trees on large scale along with roads, within the open spaces provided in the urban area and around the human settlements would be undertaken to help in preserving proper environment in urban areas. People would be educated and encouraged to plant more trees in the available open spaces.

(x) Segregation of inter and intra-city traffic would be done on priority and all through traffic would be discouraged to enter urban areas. This would considerably reduce the environmental pollution and improve equality of life along the major roads.

(xi) Historical monuments and heritage buildings and areas would be properly planned, conserved and preserved by making them an integral part of city developmental process.

(xii) Tree preservation order would be made applicable in all urban areas so as to stop illegal hopping, lopping, chopping and topping of trees. All existing trees would be declared as protected trees and would not be removed without prior permission.

(xiii) Visual pollution in urban areas would be checked by using the mechanism of advertisement control.

(xiv) All future industries to be set-up in urban areas would be closely scrutinized so far as their environmental hazards are concerned and only non-polluting or industries having sufficient environmental safeguards would be permitted urban areas.

(xv) In order to preserve the environment in residential areas all industrial areas would be sealed from residential areas by providing a green belt having trees, which would minimize pollution.

(xvi) It would be made mandatory for all industrial units to use a part of their plot area for planting trees.

(xvii) Environmental Impact Assessment in case of certain categories of large industries would be carried out more scientifically.

(xviii) State would discourage the setting up of highly polluting, hazardous, chemical and other units so as to minimize adverse impact on urban environment. Eco-friendly units would be given priority and would be permitted to be set-up as part and parcel of urban settlements.

(xix) All environment-related laws would be made more simple and effective and would be strictly enforced for minimizing pollution in the State.

(xx) In order to make all urban areas environmentally sustainable, cities and towns would be planned on the basis of their holding capacity in terms of population, economic activity, etc. Growth of over-sized and metrocities would be discouraged. Emphasis would be laid on the growth and development of small and medium towns.

3. Health Promotion in Urban Areas: Need of Improving Health Services in Urban Areas especially in Slums and Deprived Sections of the Urban Areas

At present, there are health facilities, which are not functioning well. We find long lines and rush but no facilities. That is why, private doctors are fleeing the people.

During the Ninth Plan period, efforts will be directed to evolve a well-structured organisation of urban primary health care to remedy the existing situation. A health care delivery system aimed at providing basic health and family welfare services to the population within 1-3 kms. of their dwelling will be made available by establishing Urban Health and Family Welfare Centres manned by medical and para-medical persons.

These centres will have:[10]

1. adequate out-patent facility;
2. inpatient facility (at least 10 beds of which four will be for maternity care and the remaining beds will be for medical, surgical and paediatric care);
3. supportive services including laboratory and radiology facilities and pharmacy; and
4. provision for referral/transport of patients.

The essential services, to be provided, will include:

1. medical and surgical services including eye and ENT care;
2. obstetric care and new-born care and child health;
3. counselling for reproductive health and contraception;
4. dental services;
5. emergency and trauma care; and
6. prevention and control of communicable and non-communicable diseases.

For effective integration of health-related services the urban health centers will coordinate with other assigned social sector activities of Nagarpalikas especially for provision of safe drinking water and sanitation.

An overview of all the facilities available in a defined geographical area will be undertaken and appropriate linkages between primary, secondary and tertiary care centres in the area will be established so that provision of basic minimum health services and optimal utilization of the available health care facilities for referral services will be ensured. Earmarked funds under BMS and a ACA for BMS will be effectively utilized to fill the critical gaps in health manpower and infrastructure in urban areas also so that the performance of both health and family welfare programmes improve.

4. Removal of Urban Poverty

Urban poverty is the root cause of all problems including health. A.K. Neog in his Article, "Urban Poverty" mentions:

> "Urban poverty is more visible in the slum and depressed areas where public utilities like health and sanitation services, water supply, etc. are utterly inadequate. So on the health front also an urban poor faces hazards, which affect his efficiency. In a caste-ridden, status conscious society, an urban poor is likely to face more sociological and psychological problems than a rural poor."[11]

Urban poverty is not always a by-product of rural poverty. Those urban-dwellers who fail to cope with the struggle for development may also fall into poverty trap. In the areas where urbanization is more due to administrative expansion (as in North-East India) than industrialization, many households, which cannot win the race for development may have to pin join those below the poverty line. Displacement, land alienation, etc. aggravate the situation. Hence, the urbanization process itself may generate poverty. Thus, urban poverty can be distinct from rural poverty and presents itself as a subject of investigation and study.

Ministry of Urban Affairs and Urban Development, GOI, New Delhi, in its Annual Report, 1998-99, mentions the efforts of Government of India to alleviate urban poverty.

In a decision of far reaching consequences, the Union Cabinet on 5th August 1997 approved the Swarna Jayanti Shahari Rozgar Yojana (SJSRY). The SJSRY has been launched as replacement for Nehru Rozgar Yojana (NRY). Urban Basic Services for the Poor (UBSP), and Prime Minister's Integrated Urban Poverty Eradication Programme (PMIUPEP) on 1.12.97. The SJSRY seeks to provide gainful employment to the urban unemployed or underemployed poor through encouraging the setting up to self-employment ventures and provision of wage employment.

The Swarna Jayanti Shahari Rozgar Yojana is funded on a 75: 25 basis between the Centre and States.

The Scheme consists of two special schemes, namely:

(a) The Urban Self Employment Programme (USEP); and
(b) The Urban Wage Employment Programme (UWEP).

Salient Features

The Swarna Jayanti Shahari Rozgar Yojana rests on foundation of community empowerment. This programme relies on establishing and promoting community organisations and structures to provide supporting and facilitating mechanism for local development. Towards this end community organisations like Neighbourhood Groups (NGs), Neighbourhood Committees (NCs), and Community Development Societies (CDSs) are set-up in the target areas based on the UBSP pattern. The CDSs is the focal point for purposes of identification of beneficiaries, preparation of application, monitoring or recovery, and generally providing whatever other support is necessary to the programme. The CDSs is to identify viable projects suitable for the particular area.

The CDSs, being a federation of different community-based organisations, shall be the nodal agency for this programme. It is expected that they will lay emphasis on providing the entire gamut of social sector inputs to their areas including, but not limited to, health, welfare, education, etc. through establishing, convergence between schemes being implemented by different line departments within their jurisdiction.

5. Need of Multilateral and Bilateral Assistance to Improve Urban High

Since the resources and expertise in the developing world is limited, therefore, there is a need of support from multilateral and bilateral agencies. Forty-fourth World Health Assembly in its resolution 27 identified six imperatives for improvement of health.

The resolution specifically requested WHO to:

- Strengthen its information base for the benefit of Member States and its own work in relation to the human and environmental aspects of urban development;
- Strengthen its technical cooperation with countries in order to increase awareness of the needs of the urban poor, develop national skills to meet these needs and support the extension of city networks worldwide; and
- Promote regional networks and inter-disciplinary panels of experts and community leaders, to advise on health aspects of urban development.

In encouraging participants to take a positive view and to identify opportunities for making a contribution to improving urban conditions and health, the Chairman of the Technical Discussions of the 44th World Health Assembly identified six personal imperatives:

1. To decentralize and put the emphasis for action at the municipal level.
2. To mobilize everyone who can help in city networks.
3. To invest in safe drinking water and waste disposal.

4. To help the poor to enhance their incomes and improve their housing.
5. To provide families with a range of sustainable health services in or near their homes with an emphasis on family planning as the centre piece.
6. To ask the poor to identify their own needs and priorities and expect surprises.

6. Need of a Well-defined Slum Policy

J.S. Saksena and P.N. Govindarajuler in their Article, "Health Care For Urban Slums with special reference to Bangalore City" have rightly sensed the problem. To quote them:

> "Slum-dwellers have the worst of both the worlds—urban and rural. On one side they suffer from economic hardships, lack of education and absence of health infrastructure like the rural population. On the other hand, they also suffer the ill-effects of over-crowding, pollution and rootlessness characteristic of large metropolitan cities."

They further add:

> "Most comforts and conveniences of the cities are sustained by the work done by slum-dwellers. As such, the affluent and the privileged have the moral responsibility to try to mitigate and alleviate their suffering. Rural population may be ignorant of the "goodies" they are missing, but a slum-dweller is painfully aware of the privations suffered by hum due to his constantly rubbing shoulders with urban affluence and conspicuous consumption with resultant frustration and resentment."

It is reported that the Union Urban Development Ministry is finalizing a draft National Slum Policy to deal with one of the most serious socio-economic problems threatening urban life in India in the form of an enormous growth of slums. Once believed to be an inevitable side effect of industrialization and the consequent migration of labour from rural areas, proliferation of slums has other causes too in India. They have grown within and on the peripheries of many towns and all the metropolitan cities, including the country's Capital.

The national policy is expected to provide a new approach to an old problem evolved in the recognition of the fact that slum-residents are a major and important contributor to city resources and form an indispensable sector, providing various kinds of skilled and unskilled services to enrich city life and facilitate its functions. A draft piece of legislation is also under preparation.[12]

To improve the quality of life of these residents, slum policy should contain clauses to enhance educational, health and moral standards. This requires coordination among ministries/department concerned.

Urban Development Strategy for Punjab suggests the following to minimize slum growth:

(i) Re-launching of the Integrated Urban Poverty Alleviation Scheme (IUPAS), which would include restructured existing urban poverty alleviation programmes providing for a package to urban poor.

(ii) Allocation and creation of a fund with annual contribution, for income generating activities and provision of infrastructure for urban poor.

(iii) Establishment of Urban Poverty Alleviation Fund in every municipality since slum-related issue are included in the Twelfth Schedule of 74th Constitutional Amendment Act, 1992.

(iv) Urban shelter-related programmes would be community-based so as to involve the users in the programme.

(v) Close monitoring of all the programmes by State-level agencies so as to ensure effective implementation.

(vi) Involvement of private sector and NGOs in the programme.

(vii) Keeping close watch on the growth and development of slums and to evolve appropriate strategies to minimize them.

(viii) To undertake shelter up-gradation programmes for slums on priority basis and to link it with the issue of gainful employment.

7. Need of Mass Education and Awareness

Education seems to be an important factor in achieving better health status as also for better utilization of health facilities. Particularly, as the weaker sections treat their children as an asset for earning more, they it seems, instigate their children to become school dropouts. Hence, in order to make them understand importance of education, adult literacy programme should be rigorously implemented. In these programmes, health education should be given due place to make them understand basic issues in health. More voluntary efforts are called for in this venture.[13]

8. Need of Linking Health with Other Sectors of Development

It is being realized widely now that the isolating therapeutic approach to civic health, hitherto in vogue, generally overlooks many critical variables determining the health of the communities and its members. The isolating approach, therefore, needs to be substituted by a broader, synchronized approach. For this, the linkages of health sector with other aspects like housing, education, income, environment, etc. are not only to be realized but also to be taken in account while ensuring an all round development. In the planning of municipal programmes, health sector should get a higher priority and larger outlay particularly to meet the requirements of the dovetailed plans.[14]

9. Need of Participation of People in Local Self-Government

Participation is essential to lubricate potential energy of the people into kinetic energy. Urban areas need the co-operation of the people to keep the city clean and healthy. K.S. Nesamani has beautifully explained the need of participation in urban development. To quote him:[15]

Participatory development is not an attempt to replace the top-down development approach with slum-dwellers/low income participation. Rather, it should stress the need for the government participation in terms of national-level economic planning and coordination of development planning and the demerits of widening disparities and worsening poverty inherent in slum-dwellers. Participatory development attempts to introduce a bottom-up style of development in order to remedy the government approach's shortcomings, . specifically by focusing on qualitative improvements in slum-dwellers' participation.

Participation of slum-dwellers can reduce the cost of the social programme which government often invests. It will give an idea to the government with a great deal of information on the social and economic needs of the population. It will help the government to identify the potential leader who can assist in the development process or at least disseminate information on government goals.

10. Need of Providing Adequate Housing with All Amenities is sine-qua-non for Good Health

The situation of Housing is very serious as one in five families live in slums. Even those who are living in urban areas are without good facilities; half of the urban population is without sanitation facilities. The Government is making efforts but without positive results.

The National Plan of Action, prepared by the Government of India for the Habitat Conference defined adequate shelter, in the Indian context as the one "which would include adequate living space with provision for incremental development and proper access to physical and social infrastructure and services including energy, fuel, potable water, waste disposal and sanitation services, and education, health and recreational facilities. It must have adequate privacy and security, as also lighting and ventilation. The location of the shelter must be suitable with reference turk place, markets, communication services, and social and cultural amenities. . . The endeavour of the government and the people of India would be to maintain the cost of such adequate shelter at an affordable level. . . The critical task is to ensure that access to adequate and affordable shelter is available to all, including people living in poverty, the vulnerable and the disadvantaged, either through the market or through well targeted and transparent subsides." (pp. 99-100, India Country Report).

There is a need to take rational decisions to ensure what is contemplated. Worlds written or spoken are of no use unless put to action.

11. Need of Efficient and Dynamic Local Administration

People both elected and permanent must conduct their business in a manner, which can help the urban areas to enjoy quality of life.

In the words of Jean Paul Jardel:[16]

> Action at the local level is also to be encouraged to the full. The Healthy Cities project is one example of the efforts being made to convince countries to put health firmly on the political agenda of communities and local governments. Once again, it's a matter of "thinking globally and acting locally." Local action is by far the most effective approach, all the more so if it takes place within a national, regional and even a worldwide framework.

The interdependence of human beings with their physical, social and economic environment must now more than ever be taken into account in health-related activities. Local power to act must therefore be reinforced, and local authorities must be convinced of the important role of health in development efforts. Furthermore, all sectors that have an influence on health must be integrated into a collaborative team. The planning and carrying out of strategies must be flexible, to take into account the wide diversity of towns, countries and situations. Enlightened leadership is called for, to encourage the participation of everyone. And, finally, it must never be forgotten that Health for All is a common, shared objective, which alone can allow us to hope for eventual justice and equity in ensuring the fundamental right of every human being: the right to health.

CONCLUSION

We may conclude in the words of Shri Jagmohan, "A World Bank Study has revealed that the polluted air in the Indian cities is causing premature death of about 40,000 persons every year. The extent of water pollution can be gauged from the state of our rivers which, for most part of the years, are hardly distinguishable from vast urban gutters. Noise is another factor that lowers the quality of life in our cities. According to the survey conducted by the National Physical Laboratory, Delhi, Mumbai and Calcutta are the noisiest cities in the world.[17]

Clearly, it is the march of unhealthy new realities has to be halted and these realities have to be replaced by another set of new realities—positive, productive and elevating, there has to be fundamental transformation of the institutional framework of urban India as well as that of the framework of the Indian mind and soul.

Notes and References

1. V. Suresh and P. Jayapal, Towards an inclusive city in the New Millennium, in *Shelter*, Vol. 2, Nos. 3 and 4, July-Oct. 1999, p. 9.

2. Government of Punjab, Department of Housing and Urban Development, Urban Development Strategy for Punjab, Draft Status Paper, 1995, pp. 5-6.
3. Government of India, Planning Commission, Ninth Five Year Plan, 1997-2002, New Delhi, p. 149.
4. Krishna Gowda, M.V. Sridhara, P. Raj Mamatha, "Planning for the 21st Century: A Case Study of Bangalore, *Shelter*, Vol. 3, No. 1, HUDCO Publication, pp. 7-8, January 2000.
5. John Asthon, Healthy Cities, in *World Health*, June 1988, pp. 9-10.
6. *Ibid.*, p. 11.
7. Rene Diekotra, City Lifestyles, in *World Health*, June 1988, p. 19.
8. Quoted in Shreekant V. Khandewala, Health Administration and the Weaker Sections in an Indian Metropolies, New Delhi, Devika, 1996, p. 4.
9. Urban Development Strategy for Punjab, *op. cit.*, pp. 37-38.
10. Ninth Five-Year Plan, *op. cit.*, pp. 149-50.
11. A.K. Neog, Urban Poverty in Urbanization and Development in North-East India, Ed. (J.B. Ganguly), New Delhi, Deep and Deep, 1995, p. 70.
12. S. Saraswati, "Towards National Slum Policy" in *The Daily Tribune*, February 1, 2000.
13. Khandewala, *op. cit.*, p. 203.
14. *Ibid.*, p. 209.
15. K.S. Nesamani, Participation of Slum-dwellers in Urban Governance, in *Shelter*, A HUDCO Publication, New Delhi, Vol. 3, No. 1 (Challenges for the New Millennium).
16. Jean Paul Jardel, Health in the City, *World Health*, March-April 1991, p. 3.
17. *The Sunday Tribune*, Specturm, June 11, 2000.

Urban Slums: Living Disasters

The recent report of Census of India reveals that urbanization has increased to 31.13% between 1991 and 2001 as compared to 16% in 1951 and 26% in 1991. It is expected to touch the mark of more than 40% in 2021. Thirty-five cities in the country have crossed a population of over one million. Greater Mumbai with a population of 163.38 lacs, Kolkata with a population of 132.16 lacs and Delhi with 127.91 lacs, occupy first three positions respectively in 2001. The Punjab, which is known for its villages, has 33.95% of its population living in urban areas as compared to the national average of 31.13%. Let us take the example of Punjab. The urban population in the State is distributed over 157 towns out of which 14 towns have more than one lac population in 2001 as compared to 10 in 1991. The increase in urban population has created a large number of problems for the Local Self-Government, which is already under great stress and strain. The problems faced by the urban local self-government do not merely limit themselves to traditional functions of providing basic services e.g., potable water supply, sewerage, waste disposal, etc. but extend to new and emerging problems of lawlessness, prostitution, rape, distress, thefts, crimes especially against women, unemployment, shelter, etc. Thus, administration of cities has become complex; hence require the co-operation of all including adequate finance and especially the people's participation and involvement.

Provisional data relating to slums in the 2001 Census throw some interesting light on the slum population. Nearly 28 million persons lived in the slums in 1981, accounting for 17.5 per cent of the urban population. The estimates for 1991 were 45.7 million slum-dwellers accounting for 21.5 per cent of population. According to the 2001 Census, there are 40.6 million persons living in slums in 607 towns/cities, and they account for 22.8 per cent of the population of these cities. However, the latest Census data also reflect the problems inherent in not having an accepted definition of slums and absence of proper listing of slum settlements in the urban offices concerned with slum improvement and civic amenities. The practice of notifying slums under relevant laws is not being followed, especially where the land involved belongs to Government or any of its agencies. As a result of these lacunae, these data are not definitive because towns with less than 50,000 population, and slum clusters, which are not formally or informally recognized if the population was less than 300 are these excluded.

Former Hon'ble Minister for Urban Development, GOI, Jagmohan, had rightly spelled out the existing and emerging problems of Local-Self Government as follows: ('City Lights', *Hindustan Times,* December 14, 2000). "Invariably, cultural and civilization contours get imprinted on the faces of cities. The city has many facets. As an economic entity, it is a set of business and industry; as a social organisation, it is a creator of community and collective action; as a political unit, it is a centre of power and government; and as a cultural force, it is a repository of old traditions, a fountain head of new ideas, an instrument of intellectual advancement, and a moulder of attitudes and thoughts. It is a spiritual workshop of the nation, a most imposing creation of its social, economic and cultural aspirations."

Urban policies, poverty, pollution, productivity, planning and pattern, and shortages (both physical and financial) are the crucial issues around which the machinery of urban governance in India revolves. The formidable nature of these issues has thrown this machinery in deep crisis. But this crisis is not merely of governance. It extends to the governed as well. It is a crisis of character, commitment, conscience, the creative and constructive sense of the community as a whole. This crisis has been with us for quite some time. But, of late, the degree of this crisis has undergone such a change that it has virtually become a new kind of crisis. This crisis is daily weakening the structure of urban governance in India is heading to the disaster that lies ahead.

Already, in every aspect of city life-density of population, availability of land, housing, slums and squatter settlements, municipal services, open spaces, and the scale and character of migration, employment, traffic and transport, energy, communication, crime, health and environment, civic set-up and finance—the prevailing conditions present a grim picture.

Take for example, the arena of municipal services and urban infrastructure. At present, there is no sanitation worth the name for 52% of the urban population. The sewerage system covers only 35% of the population of Class IV cities and 75% of the population of Class I cities.

About 34% of urban population does not have any arrangement even for drainage of rainwater around its habitats. 60% of the municipal bodies in India collect less than 40% of the solid waste generated daily. At least 28% of the urban waste is allowed to decompose and purify on the roadside and around residential areas and factories. On an average, the slum and squatter population is increasing at more than double the general growth rate of population of the cities. At present, at least 35% of the population of our cities is living in slum settlements. Both economy and technology are changing fast.

Their fallout, as well as let loose by globalization, cannot be fully anticipated and accounted for. But one thing, i.e. of fundamental importance is that the fate and future of our cities depend on the creativity and ingenuity, the vision and the will we bring to the task and the civilization and cultural underpinnings we would provide to it.

In addition the slum and squatters population is increasing at a fast rate causing a number of problems for Local-Self Government. The estimate of Census of 2001 is that about 35% of the city population lives in slums. The quality of life of the people in the city is poor. Krishan Gowda, M.V. Sridhar and Ms. Mamatha P. Raj, in their article, "Planning for the 21st Century: A Case Study of Bangalore", in *Shelter*, January 2000, draws our attention to the city of 21st century. To quote them: "We need to rethink or re-envision of city of the 21st century, i.e. one which is socially just, ecologically sustainable, politically participatory, economically viable and really capable of adaptation of future needs."

Inevitably this results in the uncontrolled physical expansion of the cities. City growth has leapt far ahead of city planning and management, to the point where development of structures and activities in the city life is simply haphazard. In the older "core areas" of city slums and in the relatively new built-up areas, the scene is one of overcrowding, lack of access roads, scarcity of drinking-water, ramshackle buildings, uncollected garbage, lack of sewers, inadequate air-space, and a housing environment littered with human faces. All of these are conducive to the spread of tuberculosis, pneumonia, influenza, threadworm, cholera, dysentery and other diarrhoeal diseases. Just as intensive planning activities prevent diseases and promote health, so the lack of planning, or its inadequacy, breeds diseases and contributes significantly to a high rate of mortality, especially among children.[1]

Slums are cancerous for urban life and no effort should be spared to eradicate them. No doubt, they are manifestation of socio-economic conditions prevailing in the country, but if no heed is paid to contain them, urban life will become not only miserable but also unbearable. A serious policy of urban development, based on sound principles of town planning and efficient administration, committed to the service of the humanity with vast financial resources and authority can only successfully combat the problems of slums.[2]

Slums are a bye-product of urbanization and industrialization. Slum-dwellers are the real architect of urban facilities but their own life is endangered with poor facilities made available to them. Because of the laxity on the part of the municipal government, these slums sprang up and later on become difficult to control.

GENESIS OF SLUMS AND MAGNITUDE OF THE PROBLEM

"Slum" is defined as that area where the buildings are in any respect unfit for human habitation; or by reason of dilapidation, overcrowding, faulty arrangement of buildings, streets, lack of ventilation, light or sanitation facilities or combination of these factors, are detrimental to safety, health or morals (Slums Improvement and Clearance Act, 1956). Approximately, 68.8% of the country's slums population is concentrated in the 300 Class I cities and less than 1/3rd of this population resides in the remaining 3300 urban centers.[3]

Slums are not fit for settlement and are a danger both for residents and the urban population living nearby. Roosevelt has rightly said that poverty anywhere is a danger to prosperity. Sh. Aditya Prakash, retired Principal of the College of Architecture, Chandigarh, has termed the growth of slums in the City Beautiful of Chandigarh, as a "planning failure." He says: "The slums should not have been allowed to sprout in the first place. The need of the hour is to solve poverty and shelter problems and it can be done through proper planning."

Evolution of Slums

Urbanization has been considered as an index of development but in case of developing countries like India, urbanization is not the outcome of merely the growth potential generated by urban settlements. It has been largely due to people work relationship in rural areas, in which land is the essential medium and which is right now so critically balanced that even small addition to population is pushing people out of agriculture to non-agricultural occupations. Thus, by and large, in India urbanization is emerging as merely a process of transfer of rural poverty to urban environment, which only results in concentration of misery. This has resulted in the malfunctioning of most of the urban settlements leading to emergence of number of imbalances and problems. Thus, most of these settlements suffer from improper and haphazard development, absence of basic infrastructure and services, uncontrolled and unchecked growth of slums, lack of housing, high degree of visual and environmental degradation and uncontrolled traffic. The cumulative effect of these factors is the degradation of quality of life in urban settlements and huge amount of subsidies is required to maintain them. These facts are more evident in case of larger cities especially metros and super metros.

Problems of Urban Areas Especially Human Settlements

Urban areas have not received much attention in terms of the planning, development and management despite the fact that cities and economic development are inextricably linked. Because of high productivity of urban areas, economic development activities get located in cities. Accordingly, it is desirable that human settlements are provided with necessary planning and development inputs so that the orderly growth and development is ensured. This would also be necessary for ensuring efficient functioning of human settlements for improving their productivity and for providing desirable quality of life to its residents in order to cater to their both economic and physical and metaphysical needs. The urban development strategy for any state thus assumes importance of not only its economic emancipation but also its physical well-being.

Concept of Slums[4]

The concept of slums and its definition vary from country to country depending upon the socio-economic conditions of each society. Irrespective of location, whether in the core of the city, in the form of old dilapidated structures or in the outskirts, in the form of squatting. Slums have often been characterized—

(a) Physically, an area of the city with inadequate housing, deficient facilities, overcrowding and congestion.
(b) Socially, slum is a way of life, a special character which has its own set of norms and values reflected in poor sanitation, health values, health practices, deviant behaviour and social isolation.
(c) Legally speaking, section 3 of the Slum Areas (Improvement and Clearance) Act, 1956 defines slums as areas where buildings:
  (i) are in any respect unfit for human habitation; and
  (ii) are by reason of dilapidation, over-crowding, faulty arrangements of streets, lack of ventilation, light or sanitation facilities or any combination of these factors which are detrimental to safety, health and morals..

The slum areas are declared by a notification in the official gazette, which require:

(a) repair,
(b) stability,
(c) natural light and air,
(d) system of dump,
(e) water supply,
(f) drainage and sanitary conveniences, and
(g) facilities for storage, preparation of cooking of food and disposal of waste water, the buildings deemed to be unfit if it is so ineffective in one or more of the said matter and not found reasonably suitable for occupation in that condition.

Slums a Great Danger to the Population

Jai Saksena and P.N. Govindarajuler in their article, "Health Care For Urban Slums with special reference to Bangalore City" have rightly sensed the problem. To quote them: "Slum-dwellers have the worst of both the worlds—urban and rural. On one side they suffer from economic hardships, lack of education and absence of health infrastructure like the rural population. On the other hand, they also suffer the ill-effects of over-crowding, pollution and rootlessness characteristic of large metropolitan cities."

They further add that "Most comforts and conveniences of the cities are sustained by the work done by slum-dwellers. As such, the affluent and the privileged have the moral responsibility to try to mitigate and alleviate their suffering. Rural population may be ignorant of the "goodies" they are missing, but a slum-dweller is painfully aware of the privations suffered by him due to his constantly rubbing shoulders with urban affluence and conspicuous consumption with resultant resentment."[5]

Growth of Slums

While demographic data on slum populations and on civic amenities to slum-dwellers from the Census are still awaited, there appears to be no change in the basic level or improvement in the features of slum settlements despite several decades of programmes for the environmental improvement and upgradation of slums. There is cause to wonder whether 'Cities without Slums' is a slogan about an objective, which, however desirable, is believed to be unreachable, or whether it is a serious planning and urban development concern. Certainly the degree of effort to upgrade slums to a more habitable level does not indicate a serious effort in this direction.[6]

Slums by and large are the creation of urbanization process, which necessitates the transfer of rural poverty to urban environment. Lack of resources with the local level agencies results in non-provision of basic services and accordingly large number of slums grow in cities. Percentage of population of slums increases in direct proportion to the population and size of the city of which they form part. Larger cities have more proportion of population in slums. World Development Report of 1994 prepared by the World Bank says that growth of slums in India is primarily due to inadequate infrastructures. It further says that though proportion of population living below the poverty line has shown a decline, number of people living in slums have, however, increased. Thus, growth of slums cannot be visualized as the product of poverty alone; infact number of other factors are responsible for the growth of slums. Government of India has launched a new scheme to prevent the growth of slums in urban areas. New Scheme provides alternative sites to existing slum-dwellers/EWS Families living in cities with population ranging between 5 to 20 lacs. House sites are allotted on a graded scale of 35 sq. mts., for cities in population range between 5-10 lac, 30 sq. mts. for population ranges between 15-20 lacs. However, scheme does not provide for slums in cities-dwellers belonging to EWS category with special emphasis on people below poverty line. These schemes are operational in few selected towns.

Growths of slums have become faster over the years and this problem has spread over all the settlements. Major problem in solving shelter-related issues of EWS or shelterless is the availability of land. It is proposed to create a Land Bank for the poor in all the urban areas, which would be funded by various financial institutions like HUDCO and other State level agencies. Further addition would be made to the Land Bank through the mechanism of earmarking 5% of total land developed under any scheme for EWS housing, which would be transferred to the Land Bank. Private colonizers would also contribute to the Land Bank. Similarly, all Town Development Schemes would earmark 5% of area for EWS housing. Thus, a large land pool would be created, which can be used for providing shelter to EWS.

The number and population of slums are always on the increase. Even many areas, in urban towns, have become so congested and short of basic services, that we can also call them slums. Life in these areas is miserable. If one has to visit old areas of Delhi, Ludhiana, Patiala, Calcutta, Bombay, for that matter, one finds that these are nothing but slums.

Life of People in Slums (See Chart 8.1)

A Survey on the health status of adolescent girls in Patiala, carried out by a team of expert lady doctors, has revealed that 92.5 per cent of girls in urban slums are anemic while the percentage of such girls in urban areas is 88.6 and 86% in rural areas. It was further found that 38.7 percent girls in urban slums were severely anemic.

Not only mental disorders but problems relating to physical abuse (15.2%), domestic violence (30.2%) and sexual abuse (10.2%) were seen in urban slums indicating poverty, illiteracy and low status of women in this category.[7] It is paradoxical situation that on the one hand they provide all services to urban population, on the other, they cannot meet their needs.

CHART 8.1

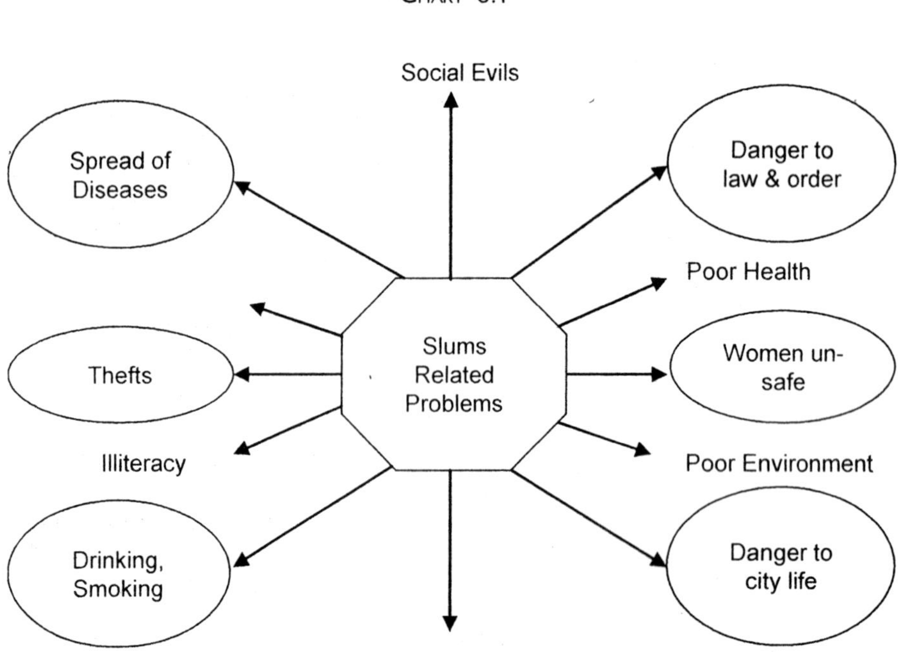

Over a period of time, slum-dwellers are beginning to see themselves as citizens contributing to the economy and, therefore, deserving their own place in the sun. It is the slum and pavement dweller, who provides the vast network of services that the middle and upper classes enjoy at cheap rates. These services include the entire food supply network (vegetables, milk, eggs, butter, bread, meat, poultry as well as restaurant services), clothing, laundry, vending and sales, transport, conservancy, communication, construction and domestic services for homes, offices. The slum-dwellers, if united, have the power to bring to a halt the entire urban system, so powerful is their role in urban economy.[8]

Most of the slum-dwellers are immigrants of villages or towns and then migrate to slums or another form of low-income urban housing. They move to the place after the migrant has established himself in the city with a job, a network of friends and some sort of understanding of the political and bureaucratic structure of the municipality. However, this pattern of movement from rural to slum is a very common one. Some move permanently. This usually happens when a migrant already has a well establishment network of relatives and friends living there. Some of migrants come not only from rural areas but also from other urban centres of the country. Others never settle permanently in the city but stay only long enough to take advantage of the economic opportunities available there before returning to their place of origin.[9]

Within the existing broad loose definition, following housing areas can be categorized as "Slum":

- (i) Inner city blighted areas;
- (ii) Squatter settlements on both private and public land;
- (iii) Illegal land sub-divisions (unauthorized colonies);
- (iv) Urban villages;
- (v) Resettlement colonies (like those in Delhi); and
- (vi) A squatter settlement improved under the environmental improvement scheme.[10]

Towards a National Slum Policy

The Draft National Slum Policy drawn up by the Department of Urban Employment Poverty Alleviation in the Ministry of Urban Development in April 1999, had been widely debated and many comments received. It needs to be finalized. A National Policy on slums is of great significance given the degree of wrong perception regarding the nature and extent of the slum problem. Such a policy can help bring an attitudinal change among the authorities and the people at large, including the urban poor and the slum-dwellers, regarding measures to improve their quality of life and make our cities free from the worst features of slums. Slums are generally treated as the inevitable outcome of continuing migration of unskilled labour, but, in fact, most slum-dwellers are permanent residents of the city. In many instances, families in slums span several generations.

The main objectives of a slum policy would be:

- To create awareness of the underlying principles that guide the process of slum development and improvement and the options that are available for bringing about the integration of these settlements and the communities residing there with the urban area as a whole.
- To strengthen the legal and policy framework to facilitate the process of slum development and improvement on a sustainable basis; to ensure that the slum population are provided civic services, amenities, and economic opportunities to enable them to rise above the degrading conditions in which they live.
- To arrive at a policy of affirming the legal and tenurial rights of the slum-dwellers.
- To establish a framework for involving all stakeholders in the efficient and smooth implementation of policy objectives.

Some Case Studies in Slums

In Ludhiana, a woman named Geeta about 20 years has four children. She got married at the age of 14. Her husband, a Rickshaw puller earns merely Rs. 30 per day, i.e. 600 per month, which he spends in drinking, smoking and gambling. Geeta works as maid in some houses leaving her children back, earning about 1500 per month. She has one room jhuggi with no privacy. Children are being neglected. She feels exhausted and tired of life.

In Jalandhar, a woman named Sarita about 23 years age old having three children was abandoned by her husband, as he got illicit relations with her sister who was living with them. She works as a rag picker hardly making both ends meet. She feels to commit suicide but because of children she is pulling her life.

In another case in Patiala, a woman about 25, with pale face and a mother of four children was suffering from HIV positive. Her husband alongwith his friends used to drink at night and all of them used to exploit her sexually. Her life has become miserable. She feels suffocated and cannot look after the children.

In another case in Ropar a man aged 50 has been living for the last 20 years with 3 children and his wife in small 2 rooms. Some persons in the area forced him to sell her daughters aged 13 and 15 to some persons aged 45 and 47. He resisted but could not do anything. He complained to the Police but no case was registered. He is feeling guilty and disheartened.

A Case Study of Chandigarh City Beautiful

Let us now mention about the growth of slums in the newly planned city beautiful, i.e. Chandigarh.

The city was planned on modern lines, has also been engulfed by slums, causing misery to the slum-dwellers as well as neighbouring population. Slums or so-called *bastis* are increasing at a fast rate. These *bastis* have become a danger to the inhabitants as well as to the residents of the city. Personal observations reveal the disgusting, pathetic and painful sights. Human beings are living like animals and these *bastis* are potential source of epidemics, malaria and other communicable diseases. Those responsible for creating these slums should be severely punished. If this is the state of affairs of a modern city, then what would be the condition of slums in Delhi, Bombay, Calcutta, Hyderabad and so on.

A survey was conducted by the Center for Indian Development Studies, for Municipal Corporation, Chandigarh, for the implementation of the Swaran Jayanti Shahari Rozgar Yojna (SJSRY) in the city, in 37 colonies of Chandigarh, of which 23 fall in the category of rehabilitated and 14 unauthorized ones on the government land, reveals that shortage of water, slushy conditions, lack of sanitation and drainage system, especially in unauthorized colonies, are the major problems ailing them.

We must take bold steps to save the city by providing alternate sites to the existing *bastis* and ban the creation of future slums.

An observation and case studies into the lives of people inhabiting slum areas reveal a pathetic scene, where it is difficult to watch horrible problems of people. These problems relate to the following areas:

1. Poverty.
2. Social evils like drinking, smoking, gambling, prostitution, etc.
3. Poor Health—Women mostly anemic, Children under developed, frequent pregnancies, poor health services.
4. Illiteracy—lack of education facilities, mostly illiterate.
5. Exploitation of women—Very low status of women, marriage mostly at the ages of 13-14-15, number of children high ranging from 3-5, works both for domestic services as well as maids to earn some money.
6. Poor housing causing tensions, lack of privacy, lack of safety of young girls, etc.
7. Lack of sanitation—Causing diseases and poor life.
8. Lack of potable water—They even do not get good waster to drink causing many water borne diseases.
9. Poor Environment—The all around environment has been poor causing many health problems.

We have seen that people in urban areas living in slums or slums like places are faced with a large number of problems concerning their life. How to overcome them? How to provide good life to them? What should be done to provide them basic facilities needed for human beings? What has been the role of Government, NGOs and other agencies in providing them good life? The answer to these questions is simple, i.e. People living in these areas need to come together, to locate problems, find solutions and put them into action with the support of municipal bodies. This is known as urban participatory development. It is based on the premises that people both men and women and especially women, have the potentiality to solve their problems.

There is a continuous tug-of-war between city level authorities and the slum-dwellers and the battle line is continuously redrawn in the form of regularization of unauthorized colonies. This causes considerable stress on the city administration including law and order problems leading to considerable costs and inconvenience to the city population as a whole. In many cases, such unauthorized colonies are demolished or upgraded incurring huge costs. The city authorities undertake a sort of fire-fighting salvage operation from time to time incurring large expenditure. This cost is estimated to be many times more than the cost involved in habitating them by proper planning by reserving pre-planned land for this group of population. Past experience indicates that no amount of legal and regulatory mechanisms could stop movement of people in search of economic upliftment. What, therefore, is there to be done? More specifically, what our local governments do? Never in the history have there been such large urban agglomerations. Future emphasis must be on working out ways and means for interdependence between national and local units and between local governments with one another. It is realized that the solutions to slum-dwellers' problems can be found together with them.[11]

It is worthwhile to examine how our governments, specifically the urban local governments are dealing with this situation after five decades. The growth of slum population in these growing cities is so prolific that, our local governments have lost control of the deteriorating urban decay. In other words, the government organisations have generally found themselves largely ineffective to forge authentic partnership with the urban slum people in solving habitat-related issues.[12]

Role of Government in Improving Slums

Various Central Government Schemes—National Slum Development Programme (NSDP), Swarna Jayanti Shahri Rozgar Yojana (SJSRY), VAMBAY, Night Shelters, Two Million Housing Scheme, Accelerated Urban Water Supply Programme (AUWSP), Low-Cost Sanitation—provide for a wide range of services to the urban poor including slum-dwellers. They include identification of the urban poor, formation of community groups, involvement of non-government organisations (NGOs), self-help/thrift and credit activities, training for livelihood, credit and subsidy for economic activities, housing and sanitation, environmental improvement, community assets, wage employment, convergence of services, etc. What is needed is to ensure that the task of meeting the needs of the slum-dwellers is better organized and effectively administered, and duly monitored at both State and Central levels. There are also many instances of successful implementation of urban poverty alleviation/slum upgrading and services programmes in the Indian situation.

Guidelines for Special Central Assistance to States for Slum Improvement

The Government of India has introduced Special Central Assistance to States for upgradation of urban slums with the following elements:

- The scheme should be applicable to all the States and Union Territories having urban population.
- Funds are allocated to States on the basis of Urban slum population.

Components

- Physical amenities (water supply, storm water drains, street lights, etc.)
- Community Infrastructure centres for pre-school education, non-formal education, primary health care center, etc.
- Social Amenities like Pre-school education, non-formal education, adult education, maternity, child health, etc.
- Convergence between schemes being implemented by different line departments.
- Shelter upgradation or construction of new houses (including EWS) with minimum 10% of the allocation to States.
- State specific schemes for housing construction/upgradation with a mix. of subsidy and loan component, sanctioned in a State-level Project Committee with one representative from the Department of UEPA, which is the nodal Department for this scheme in the GOI.

The focus is on community infrastructure, provision of shelter, and empowerment of urban poor women, training, skill upgradation and advocacy and involvement of NGOs, CBOs, Private institutions and other bodies. The scheme is applicable to all the States and Union Territories having urban population.

At the national level, Ministry of Urban Affairs and Employment is the nodal Ministry to monitor this programme. The Planning Commission in the beginning of each financial year allocates funds under this scheme and Department of Expenditure releases Additional Central Assistance to States/UTs.[13]

The Importance of Slum Upgrading

Action taken so far for slum improvement or *in situ* upgrading is inadequate. Re-designing and re-constructing settlements with the participation of residents and assistance from public bodies is a viable option with the least amount of disturbance to the settlers or their livelihood. This method of slum improvement needs to be practised on a much wider scale. The VAMBAY Project permits *in-situ* upgradation, and it is necessary that an early decision is taken regarding land on which slums are situated in order to facilitate upgradation.[14]

Role of Urban Local Government-National Slum Policy prescribes the following role for local self-government:

Planning for Integration

(a) Modify Existing Planning Framework

All existing planning instruments such as Master Plans, Land Use Plans, etc. should be modified to ensure that slums and informal settlements can be properly integrated into the wider urban areas. In order to achieve this objective, it will be necessary to:

(i) Ensure that all Master Plans and Land Use Plans allow for high density; mixed use (for micro-enterprise) land occupation in all slums/informal settlements. This will ensure that every ULB designates sufficient and more appropriate (higher density lower cost) living and working space for the urban poor within the urban area.

(ii) Master Plans and Land Use Plans should also ensure that all new land development schemes make sufficient provision for land to house low income workers as required by such schemes.

(iii) All plans and other regulatory instruments must provide sufficient flexibility to modify layouts and building regulations in line with more realistic density/mixed use requirements.

The powers to implement such changes outlined in (i) to (iii) above should be vested in the ULBs, within parameters laid down by State governments.

(b) Integrated Municipal Development Plan (IMDP)

All ULBs should begin to work towards the formulation of an Integrated Municipal Development Plan. The principle objective of this plan is to ensure that the ULB has an adequate and sustainable level of infrastructure and services for all its residents and that such infrastructure and services are planned and delivered in an equitable manner. In order to achieve this objective it will be necessary to identify the capital and recurrent requirements and costs for the city as a whole (e.g. Bulk water supply) as well as the specific wards and neighbourhood within the city (secondary and tertiary water supply). The plan should prioritize ways and means of narrowing the gap between the better-serviced and less well serviced (slums) areas of the ULB.

(c) Convergence

The IMDP process assumes the implementation of the 74th Amendment and embodies the principle of convergence of activities and funds to achieve more efficient and equitable urban development. The IMDP will incorporate existing plans and reflect schemes and budget allocations as follows:

- Master Plans/Land Use Plans and other statutory instruments.
- Urban Development Plans and Schemes.
- Urban Poverty Alleviation Plans and Schemes.
- Department Plans and Schemes in the ULB area.

(d) Dynamic Multi-Year Planning

The IMDP, outlined in (b) above, should be undertaken as a dynamic process which will be updated and reviewed every three years. The overall plan should then be implemented through Annual Action Plans and budget allocations so that development work can be taken up in a phased manner. These Annual Action Plans should reflect plan priorities based on the level of service deprivation or service gaps pertaining in the wards and neighbourhood.

(e) Bottom-up Planning

Planning should begin at the micro-level with each urban poor area drawing up a list of existing services and identifying gaps and deficiencies. This activity should be undertaken by the community using participatory planning techniques and each plan should include a clear prioritization of needs and an indication of different stakeholder contributions towards costs. ULBs will be required to submit evidence of community participation in planning service provision.

ENVIRONMENTAL IMPROVEMENT

The provision of physical infrastructure components such as water supply, drainage, sanitation, improved access, electricity, etc. should support the ultimate objective of improved quality of life. The evidence from existing slum improvement projects clearly shows that an improved physical environment greatly facilitates the integration of the settlement in the wider urban area and at the same time, contributes to improved livelihoods and health and well-being of the community.

(a) Approach

(i) Community Based Approach

All physical upgrading and improvement in informal settlements should adopt a Community Based Approach with the active involvement of members of the community at every stage of design, implementation, and maintenance of services and assets. Community structures and systems should reflect local conditions and preferences rather than conform to any uniform pattern. Communities have an important role to play at all stages of service delivery in terms of location of the service points, day-to-day functioning of the service and guarding against its misuse. Communities should be encouraged to contribute land and resources to help establish community centres and to promote the collection of user charges to contribute to the operation of certain services.

(ii) Target Women and Children

There is a need to target women and children directly in the design and implementation of physical infrastructure and the delivery of social and economic services. Infrastructure users, especially the urban poor and women are central to the sustainability of any investment decisions related to infrastructure.

(iii) Service Delivery on Individual Household Basis

Wherever possible, the delivery of basic services such as water, sanitation and electricity should be provided on an individual household basis and may even precede the granting of full tenure rights. Individual connections will improve operations, maintenance, and facilitate recovery of user charges and thus improve the overall environment.

(iv) Contracting-out

Wherever possible works should be undertaken by communities/ CBOs under appropriate supervision of ULBs. Such works must be done according to departmental norms and procedures with proper muster rolls maintained and other stipulations to be observed. Services may also be contracted-out, where appropriate, to NGOs and other private companies. Solid waste management has already been successfully contracted-out by many ULBs. Similarly, the maintenance of pay and use toilets has also been contracted-out to NGOs and community-based organisations (CBOs). State enactments/procedures dealing with improvement works should be modified to allow the implementation of such works to be undertaken on a contract basis by the community/CBOs.

(b) Physical Infrastructure Development

The guiding principle and expected outcomes to be kept in focus while planning and implementing the following basic infrastructure and services are outlined as:

(i) Water Supply

Quantum, duration, timing and water quality are the four critical factors in planning water supply delivery. Dual and standby systems, such as piped supply supported by local hand-pumps should be considered as a means of helping to address these four factors.

Even where individual water tap connections are provided, it may be desirable to install hand-pumps or community storage facilities to offset poor frequency of supply and inadequate storage capacity at individual household level.

(ii) Sanitation

ULBs should avoid constructing community latrines within slum/ informal settlements as these quickly degenerate on account of poor operations and maintenance (O&M) thus becoming counter-productive to public health. Where there is insufficient space for individual sanitation options (mostly where on-site disposal systems have to be adopted) groups or cluster latrines with clearly demarcated and agreed household responsibilities for O&M may be a suitable alternative option.

It is vital that any community-wide sanitation programme be preceded by an awareness campaign designed to raise demand for the implementation of specific sanitation options. This would greatly facilitate all subsequent O&M activities as would also assist the process of raising financial contributions. Many members of the community, especially male members, do not perceive sanitation, as a clear priority need. This needs to be addressed before embarking upon the installation of sanitation.

Considering the limitations on improving sanitation in many towns due to absence of underground drainage and sewerage systems, low cost sanitation options, particularly twin pit pour flush latrines may be a more appropriate and cost effective option for slums duly keeping environmental safeguards in mind. Efforts should be made to popularize and facilitate the introduction of such systems wherever appropriate. The tenurial status and likelihood of a settlement getting relocated at some point in the future should not deter promoting such systems since the benefits of such environmental improvement far exceed the initial investment incurred.

(iii) Pedestrian and Vehicular Access Ways

Paved access for pedestrians and/or vehicles will greatly improve overall accessibility. Paved access will encourage investment in the community and promote physical integration with neighbouring areas. It may also help to improve social integration within and between communities. Paved access will also greatly facilitate the introduction of other related infrastructure such as storm water drains, underground drainage water supply, electricity and collection/removal of garbage. Paving would also help in maintaining a clean environment and help reduce flooding and water stagnation. Paved access ways also facilitates the use of such facilities for social activity, extension of household activities and space for economic activity.

(iv) Storm Water Drains

Drains in slums serve the dual purpose of carrying sullage water from individual houses as well as draining storm water. It is crucial to integrate the outfalls of such drains with the city's main drainage system. The planning of slum drainage should be fully integrated into the planning of neighbouring systems as well as the city as a whole.

(v) Electricity

Individual house connections will greatly enhance the comfort and safety of living and working conditions for residents. The mere provision of street lighting without formal household connections leads to illegal tapping and loss of revenue and at the same time causes unplanned loading of the system and fire hazards. Community management systems for collection of user charges will facilitate improved revenue recovery and reduce revenue losses.

(vi) Solid Waste Collection

Sustained awareness campaigns and provision of waste collection receptacles will facilitate a cleaner environment. Urban Local Bodies could organize 'clean slum competitions' and institute prizes to create more awareness and encourage the community groups to maintain a clean environment within their localities. At community level, management systems that employ private sweepers by collecting monthly charges may also be adopted.

9. Improving Access to Social Services

Basic services of health, education and access to credit are crucial for human capital development and reduce the incidence of poverty. Improved access to social services would also help building up the capacities of poor and empowering them to improve their own living conditions and quality of life. Effective delivery of these services would also reduce social inequities and promote integration of people residing in slums into the social and economic networks of the city as a whole, thereby enhancing the overall productivity of the city. Various physical infrastructure components such as water supply and sanitation have a direct bearing on improving health conditions in slums. This section outlines a number of complementary services where ULBs should actively seek to improve access for the urban poor.

SUGGESTIONS

There is a continuous tug-of-war between city level authorities and the slum-dwellers and the battle line is continuously redrawn in the form of regularization of unauthorized colonies. This causes considerable stress on the city administration including law and order problems leading to considerable costs and inconvenience to the city population as a whole. In many cases, such unauthorized colonies are demolished or upgraded incurring huge costs. The city authorities undertake a sort of fire-fighting salvage operation from time to time incurring large expenditure. This cost is estimated to be many times more than the cost involved in habitating them by proper planning, by reserving pre-planned land for this group of population. Past experience indicates that no amount of legal and regulatory mechanisms could stop movement of people in search of economic upliftment. What, therefore, is there to be done? More specifically, what our local governments do? Never in the history have there been such large urban agglomerations. Future emphasis must be on working out ways and means for interdependence between national and local units and between local governments with one another. It is realized that the solutions to slum-dwellers' problems can be found together with them.[15]

It is worthwhile to examine how our governments, specifically the urban local governments are dealing with this situation after five decades. The growth of slum population in these growing cities is so prolific that, our local governments have lost control of the deteriorating urban decay. In other words, the government organisations have generally found themselves largely ineffective to forge authentic partnership with the urban slum people in solving habitat-related issues.[16]

2. Legislative Support

Legislative supports for slum improvement has been provided by the Slum Areas (Improvement and Clearance) Acts adopted by various States. The operation of the improvement schemes is made possible by statutory provisions in the Slum Act in those states, where it has been passed. The Act broadly provides the following powers:

(a) Power to the competent authority to declare an area to be slum area if the buildings in that area are unfit for human inhabitants or are detrimental to the safety of health or morals.
(b) The Act empowers the competent authority to serve notice upon the owner of a building or land in a slum area, to execute the works of improvement.
(c) Power to acquire land in a slum area to execute the improvement work.
(d) Protection to tenants in slum areas from eviction.
(e) Slum Improvement Boards were to be set-up under the Act to organize, supervise the work of slum improvement in the State.

3. Judicial Support

In a major judgment affecting at least 30 lakh people living in the Capital's slums, the Supreme Court has asked the authorities concerned to remove their shelters and stop further growth of unauthorized hutments on public land. It also asked the civic authorities to comply with the 10 directives, which are aimed at providing better hygiene, clean environment and ensuring that "the Capital of the biggest democracy in the world is not branded as being one of the most polluted cities in the World."

Passing strictures on the civic authorities, the court said: "Tolerating filth, while not taking action against the lethargic and inefficient work force for fear of annoying them, is un-understandable and impermissible." "The employees", the judges said, "were perhaps sanguine in their belief that non-performance is not frowned upon by the government or by the head of organisation and no harm will befall them."

On the mushrooming growth of the slums, the court said, "establishment or creating of slums, it seems, appears to be good business and is well organized. Large areas of public land, in this way, are usurped for private use free of cost. It is difficult to believe that this can happen in the Capital without passive or active connivance of the land-owning agencies and/or the municipal authorities."

4. People's Participation

Participatory development is not an attempt to replace the top-down development approach with slum-dwellers/low income participation. Rather, it should stress the need for the government participation in terms of national-level economic planning and coordination of development planning and the demerits of widening disparities and worsening poverty inherent in slum-dwellers. Participatory development attempts to introduce a bottom-up style of development in order to remedy the government approach's shortcomings, specifically by focusing on qualitative improvements in slum-dweller's participation.[17]

5. Taxing the Beneficiaries

Most of the Services in urban slums are free of cost. The slum dwellers can contribute in a small way, which should be tapped. This would add to the resources to make slum life better as well as create interest among slum-dwellers, when they spend their own money.

The environmental improvement scheme is based on total subsidy from the Central Government. The promise of public grants, which is a corollary to the declaration of an area "as slum often encourages the inclusion of settlements belonging to middle income households also. In some cases private land has been illegally sub-divided and sold by owners to circumvent the Urban Land Ceiling Act, they managed to get the area declared as slum. The area was subsequently improved at Government cost. In such cases beneficiaries of government subsidy are certainly not the "Urban Poor." Even in square settlements, there are significant number of households, who can afford and are willing to pay for improvements, which they want. The study of popular settlements in Bhopal confirms this (Risbud, Neelima, 1987).

Resource mobilization from beneficiaries has not at all been explored and Slum Improvement Programme is offered as a welfare action. This has gradually shaped people's attitude of expecting everything free of cost from Government. This is further strengthened, when the politicians condone the recoveries. Credit available for improvement from Housing and Urban Development Corporation (HUDCO) and World Bank requires recovery and minimization of subsidy. In some cities all the three programmes are implemented simultaneously in different settlements (e.g. in Indore, the Environmental Improvement Schemes, the HUDCO aided schemes and World Bank-aided schemes, all are operative).[18]

CONCLUSION

We have to cease presenting slum-dwellers and squatters as a total liability to the city. In most of today's mushrooming cities, the work force living in peripheral areas has become an essential and irreplaceable component of the urban economy.[19]

Urban slums are a slur on the face of the modern civilization. There is a need to help the slum-dwellers to lead a decent life since they are doing a lot for the development of the city.

Notes and References

1. WHO: Dr. Layi Egunjobi, Tackling Africa's Slums, *World Health*, March-April, 1991, p. 14.
2. Puri, K.K., "Urbanization and Slums: A Dimensional Analysis", in "Revamping Urban Governments in India", edited by Dr. Pardeep Sachdeva, New Delhi, Kitab Mahal, p. 43.
3. Sanganal, Ashok, "Participation of Slum-Dwellers in Urban Governance", *Shelter*, Vol. III, No. 1, p. 35.
4. Gurumukhi, K.T., "Slum-Related Policies and Programmes", *Shelter*, Vol. 3, No. 2, April 2000, pp. 57-58.
5. Goel, S.L., "Planning and Administration of Urban Basic Services: A Case Study of Una (H.P.)" in "Development Planning and Administration", Ed. S. Bhatnagar and S.L. Goel, pp. 167-68.
6. Government of India, Planning Commission, "Tenth Five Year Plan (2002-07); Volume II, Sectoral Policies and Programmes, pp. 627-28.
7. *The Hindustan Times*, 24 December, 1999.
8. *Shelter*, Vol. III, No. 1, p. 35.
9. *Ibid.*, p. 42.
10. Risbud, Neelima, "Slum Improvement in India—Some Issues", Delhi Vikas Patra, p. 27.
11. *Shelter*, Vol. VIII, No. 1, pp. 36-37.
12. *Ibid.*, p. 36.
13. Annual Report, 2002-03, Ministry of Urban Affairs and Employment, Government of India.
14. *Shelter*, Vol. VIII, No. 1, pp. 36-37.
15. *Shelter*, Vol. VIII, No. 1, pp. 36-27.
16. *Ibid.* p. 36
17. WHO: Dr. John Clements and Dr. Diana Silimperi, Immunizing the Children of Poverty, *World Health*, March-April, pp. 18-20.
18. *Shelter*, Vol. III, No. 1, p. 43.
19. Risbud, Neelima, Delhi Vikas Patra, p. 28.

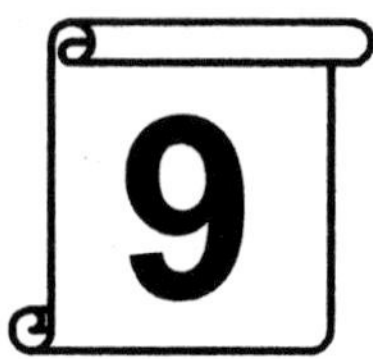

Health Education for Rural Sanitation

It is well known that a direct relationship exists between water and health. Consumption of unsafe drinking water, improper disposal of human excreta and lack of personal and food hygiene are the major causes of many diseases in developing countries. High Infant Mortality Rate (IMR) is also attributed largely to poor sanitation. It was in this context that Centrally Sponsored Rural Sanitation Project (CSRP) was launched in 1986.

To keep the household and village environment clean and to reduce risks, solid waste (refuse) should be disposed of properly. Untreated excreta is unsightly and smelly and degrades both the quality of the environment and the quality of life in the community. It also provides a breeding ground for disease vectors,. such as mosquitoes flies and rats. If waste is not properly disposed of animals can bring it close to the home and children can come into contact with disease vectors and pathogens. To be effective, solid waste disposal programmes require action at both household and community levels-if only a few households dispose of waste properly, the village environment may remain dirty and contaminated. Community members should decide how important solid waste management is and determine the best ways to achieve waste-management goals.[1]

Sanitation has become a yardstick of socio-cultural development of a nation. It is an important health index of any developing country. Since health and sanitation has an important bearing on the productivity, sanitation also has a correlation with economic progress of a country.[2]

In the Johannesburg Earth Summit it has been agreed to halve, by the year 2015 the proportion of people who do not have access to basic sanitation, which would include action at all levels to develop and implement efficient household sanitation systems, improve sanitation in public institutions, especially schools, promote affordable and socially and culturally acceptable technologies and practices, promote safe hygiene practices and integrate sanitation into water resources management strategies.

CHART 9.1

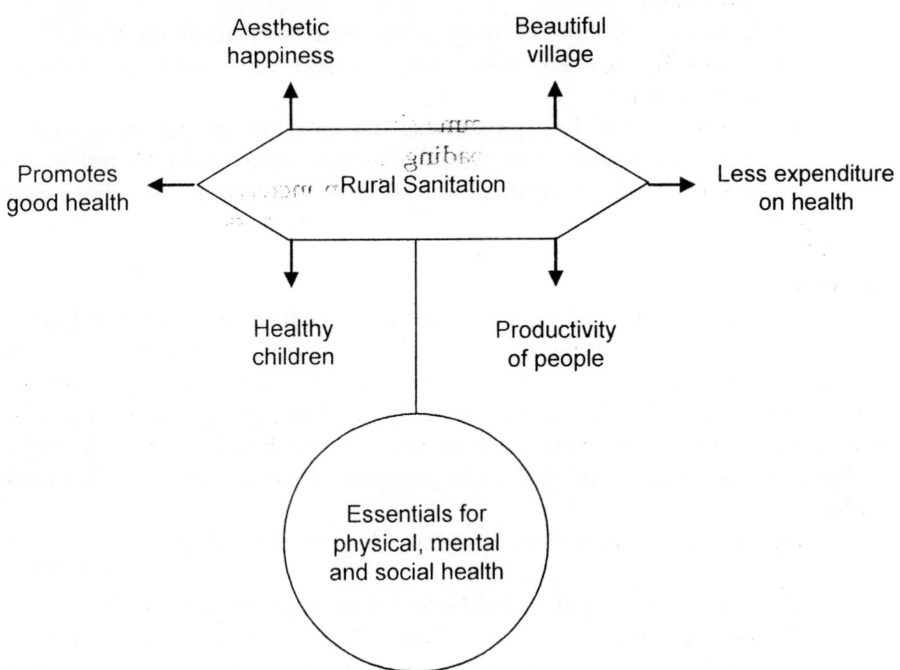

Sanitation is a broad term that includes disposal of human excreta, wastewater, solid wastes, domestic and personal hygiene, etc. Human excreta is the cause of many enteric diseases such as cholera, diarrhoea, dysentery, typhoid, infectious hepatitis, and those based on worm infestation, etc. Studies reveal that over 50 infections can be transmitted from diseased person to healthy ones by various direct/indirect routes from human excreta that cause nearly 80% of sickness in developing countries.

The health implications of this state of affairs as said are appalling. Improved hygiene and sanitation help reduce sickness from diarrohoea considerably. Intestinal worms infect about 10% of the population of developing countries that can be controlled through better sanitation, hygiene and water supply. As per the WHO report globally 200 million people are infected with schistosomiasis, of whom 20 million suffer seriously. Basic sanitation facilities reduce the disease by up to 77%. Sanitation facilities help check transmission of many faecal oral disease by preventing human excreta contamination of water and soil.[3]

Objectives

The objectives of the RCRSP is to bring about an improvement in the general quality of life in the rural areas. The policy changes envisaged shall help achieve the objective by:

(a) Accrelerating coverage of rural population.
(b) Generating felt need through awareness creation and health education.
(c) Covering schools in rural areas with sanitation facilities.
(d) Encouraging suitable cost effective and appropriate technologies.
(e) Consequently bringing about a reduction in the incidence of water and sanitation-related diseases (as evinced by fall in the infant/child mortality rates and incidence of diarrhoeal diseases.)

Strategy

The programme will be implemented as community led and people centred. A demand driven approach will be adopted with increased stress on awareness building and meeting the demand with alternate delivery mechanisms. Subsidy for individual units will be progressively reduced and phased out. Rural school sanitation will be introduced as a major component and entry point for wider acceptance of sanitation by the rural masses.

Some of the major elements of the Programme include:

(i) Shift from a high subsidy to a low subsidy regime.
(ii) Greater household involvement (Demand Driven Approach).
(iii) Technology improvisations according to customer preferences and location specific.
(iv) Development of back-up services—Central Sanitaryware, Production Centres (PCs) at District/Block levels, Rural Sanitary Marts (RSMs) as retail outlets, Trained Masons.
(v) Stress on software-intensive IEC Campaign-closer liaison with Prasar Bharti and other media.
(vi) Emphasis on School Sanitation.
(vii) Seek Institutional Finances for latrine units, production centres and rural sanitary marts.
(viii) Dovetail funds from other Government of India (GOI)/State programmes aimed for rural development (IRDP, IAY, JRY, etc.) to supplement the efforts being made under the TSCs.
(ix) Involve Co-operatives, Women Groups (such as DWCRA, RMK, etc.), Self Help Groups, NGOs, etc.

It has been envisaged that during the 9th Plan, the PHEDs shall be transformed into multi-disciplinary organisations. Their professional capabilities shall have to be enhanced so as to handle the IEC, HRD and MIS activities, etc., as well. Water and Sanitation Missions will be constituted at the State and District levels, to institutionalise community-based water and sanitation programmes. These Missions shall be responsible for implementing the Total Sanitation Campaigns (TSC) as well as implementation of the reforms measures-involving increased community participation, adoption of demand driven approach and capital cost sharing by the stake holders in the Rural Water Supply Sector.[4]

Sanitation Technologies

In developed countries, the standard solution for the sanitary disposal of human waste is sewerage. Due to severe financial constraints and exorbitant maintenance and operational costs, sewerage is not the answer to solve the problem of human waste management in India. Sewerage was first introduced in the world in London in 1850, followed by New York in 1860. Calcutta in India was the next city in the world to have this privilege in 1870, yet only 232 town cities of 4,700 in India have sewerage coverage but too partially.

In developing countries neither the government nor the local authorities or the beneficiaries can bear the capital or the maintenance cost of sewerage system. Moreover, it requires skilled person and good management for operation and maintenance. It consumes a lot of water to clean the human excreta, so with each flush over 10 litres of clean water goes down the drain. We build huge dams and irrigation systems to bring waster, which on the other hand is flushed down, into an expensive sewage system, all to end up polluting our rivers and ponds. Most of our rivers get choked up because of the domestic sewage load from the cities. This has lead to heavy pollution of rivers and urban groundwater aquifers.

Sewerage systems are built to protect public health but badly managed sewers can become a serious health hazard. There can be serious outbreaks of waterborne diseases from:

I. River pollution because of sewage outfalls.
II. Ground water contamination because of leaky sewer lines.
III. Contamination of piped water supply systems because of leaky sewer lines leading to infiltration of pathogens into drinking water pipelines.[5]

Water Supply and Sanitation are very important components of urban infrastructure services for improvement of quality of life and health standard of human habitat. While there has been perceptible improvement in access to drinking water, the provision of sanitation facilities has not received adequate attention. The status of sanitation in urban areas is even worse than the water supply scenario. Sewerage systems are not yet accessible to 54 per cent of the urban population and refuse collection and disposal has yet to reach 28 per cent of the population. Out of the more than 3500 urban areas in India only 200 towns have a sewerage system. However, even these 200 sewerage systems cover only parts of the urban areas they serve. Also the systems are in many cases old and need repairs, up-gradation rehabilitation and replacement. Toilets are not available for close to 26 per cent of the urban population. In many areas open defecation is still prevalent and it is one of the main cause for many diseases. The provision of proper sanitation in rural/urban areas will ensure personal hygiene and community health. While sewerage systems are prohibitively expensive, the twin pit latrine system based on UNDP design has become more popular and acceptable low cost on site disposal system.[6]

Low cost sanitation is rightly seen as a most appropriate solution to the dehumanizing practice of carrying night soil. The problem of manual scavenging is not unidimensional but a multi-dimensional one because it involves social, economical, political, financial, humanitarian and cultural aspects. In order to achieve the goal of eradicating manual scavenging during the 10th Five Year Plan a concerted effort is needed at levels. Awareness campaign at National level for the hygiene and human dignity can change the mindset and help in 11 abolition of dry units and open defecation. The acceptability and adaptability of the technology will not only improve the sanitation situation in the country but also put an end to the social stigma on the nation.[7]

Community management of WES services and the adoption of good hygiene practice are critical to achieving sustainable improvements in people's live. Encouraging health-promoting attitudes and behaviours plays a major role in these efforts. At the community level, for example, people's willingness to take on new responsibility and costs will make it more likely that communities will manage their water systems and not depend solely on outside assistance. Within the household, clean water washing and other practices are not routinely followed, the promised health benefits do not materialize. Likewise, access to latrines does not ensure that people will use and maintain them. Behaviours related to' sanitation are particularly difficult to both understand and change. The private nature of sanitation undoubtedly accounts for some of this difficulty, as does the fact that sanitary control and disposals of excreta may not be viewed as a problem in villages surrounded by substantial open space.

In recent years, UNICEF and its partners have experimented with new ways to engage people in planning for, using and maintaining WES services, which encompass:

- Community participation,
- Gender considerations,
- Intersectoral convergence, such as linking sanitation with broader health and economic concerns.

These three elements merge in new strategies and approaches. For are to participate productively in programmes, they must first understand how gender considerations affect their roles and responsibilities. Likewise, linking sanitation with everyday concerns, such as diarrhoeal disease control, can increase community involvement.[8]

Lessons From India

The WES programme in India yields lessons that other countries may find useful in adapting aspects of the programme to their own conditions and needs:

1. Long-term commitment and partnerships produce results: UNICEF has supported India's WES programme for several decades, coordinating its activities closely with the Government, NGGs and the private sector. The depth of this support contributes to UNICEF's credibility and access in India.
2. An external agency such as UNICEF has greater freedom than a government does to test new approaches: This relative freedom suggests an important role for UNICEF in WES and in other sectors to develop and test new approaches and build capacity among its partners.
3. Partnerships can maximize results, but they must be closely coordinated and mutually advantageous for each participant. Partners should build on each other's capabilities, strengths and comparative advantages to have greatest impact.
4. Local realities must be taken into consideration in implementing policies made by the central government: To be effective, a national policy framework must be shaped by local realties, including behaviours and values.
5. It is crucial to develop technology (pumps and other hardware) suited to local conditions, especially where water is scarce: To ensure access to clean drinking water for all children, it is especially important to create technical solutions that are feasible and sustainable.
6. A balance must be maintained between technology and the social and behavioural aspects of WES services: Technological improvements must be accompanied by changes in behaviours and a focus on how communities use and maintain systems if lasting improvements are to be made in people's lives.
7. Gender and poverty need priority attention when programmes are planned, implemented and monitored: These issues are key to community participation, education, training and other aspects of WES.
8. Cost data are needed for comprehensive and effective analyses: These data help programmes improve decision-making, especially in an era of limited resources and need for greater accountability.
9. Convergence among sectors can maximize impact in a community: Efforts to improve people's lives have greatest impact when they combine health, education, nutrition, water and environmental sanitation. For example, improving sanitation and water facilities in schools will help increase enrolment and retention, especially of girls.

10. Going to scale too quickly has adverse repercussions: It is tempting to expand on pilot projects that seem successful. However, it is better to move slowly to ensure that promising approaches are replicable on a larger scale.[9]

Central Rural Sanitation Programme

Rural Sanitation is a State subject. The efforts of the States are supplemented by the Central Government through technical and financial assistance under the Central Rural Sanitation Programme (CRSP). The programme was launched in 1986 with the objective of improving the quality of life of rural people and provide privacy and dignity of women. The concept of sanitation was expanded in 1993 to include personal hygiene, home sanitation, safe water, garbage and excreta disposal and waste water sanitary toilets for households below the poverty-line (BPL), conversion of dry latrines to water-pour flush toilets, construction of village sanitary complexes for women, setting up of sanitary marts, intensive campaign for awareness creation and health education, etc.

Keeping in view the experiences of the Central Government, State Governments, NGGs and other implementing agencies and the recommendations of the Second National Seminar on Rural Sanitation the strategy for the Ninth Plan was revised and the programme was restructured with effect from 1 April, 1999. The restructured programme moves away from the principle of state-wise allocation of funds primarily based on poverty criteria to a demand-driven approach in a phased manner. Total Sanitation Campaign (TSC) has been introduced and the allocation-based programme was phased out by 31 March, 2002. The TSC is community-led and people centred. There will be a shift from a high-subsidy to a low-subsidy regime. The TSC approach emphasizes the awareness building component and meets the demand through alternate delivery mechanism. School sanitation has been introduced as a major component and as an entry point encouraging wider acceptance of sanitation among rural masses. The States/UTs are required to formulate project proposals under the TSC in order to claim Central Government assistance.

Under the TSC, so far 179 projects in 27 States/UTs have been sanctioned with the total project outlay of about Rs. 1,952 crore. The Central, State and Beneficiary/Panchayat contribution are about Rs. 1,180 crore, Rs. 408 crore and Rs. 364 crore respectively. The components sanctioned in the 179 projects are (a) construction of 165 lakh individual household latrines; (b) 1.64 lakh toilets for schools; (c) 20,000 sanitary complexes for women; (d) 8,024 toilets for Balwadis/Anganwadis, and (e) 1549 rural sanitary marts/production centres. Besides, funds have been earmarked for start up activities, Information, Education and Communication (IEC) and administrative charges.

The total number of household toilets constructed upto 2001-02 are 98,65,980 (provisional).

The Working Group constituted by the Planning Commission has recommended and outlay of Rs. 3,663 crore for Rural Sanitation in the Tenth Five-Year Plan. During 2002-03, Rs. 165 crore have been provided for the Programme, of which Rs. 16.50 crore is earmarked for North-Eastern States.[10]

Rural Santitation

In the rural India, the low levels of household sanitation (only about 22 percent of households are estimated to have toilet facilities as per Census 2001) and the haphazard provision of environmental sanitation infrastructure (e.g. drainage) occasioned by un-coordinated planning and inadequate finances render the settlements in the villages as potential sites for a host of diseases like Schistosomiasis, Dysentry, Japanese Encephalitis, Malaria, Dengue fever and Trachoma. Indirect loss of working days due to repeated episodes of these and other diseases such as asthma, tuberculosis, jaundice, results in huge economic loss. About 1,00,000 usually suffer from morbidity in terms of asthma, tuberculosis, jaundice, and malaria by age and sex in rural India.

The practice of open defecation in India is borne out of a combination of factors—the most prominent of them being the traditional behavioural pattern and lack of awareness of the people about the associated health hazards. In certain cases, lack of access to affordable and appropriate technology is also one of the constraints.

The Central Rural Sanitation Programme (CRSP) was launched in 1986 in the Ministry of Rural Development with the objective of improving the quality of life of rural people and to provide privacy and dignity to the women. The programme provided 100 percent subsidy for construction of sanitary latrines for Scheduled Castes, Scheduled Tribes and landless labourers and subsidy as per the prevailing rates in the States for the general public.

The programme was supply driven. Highly subsidized and gave emphasis for a single construction model. Based on the feedback from various agencies, the programme was revised in March 1991 incorporating some changes in the subsidy pattern and also included village sanitation as one component. Based on the recommendation of the National Seminar on Rural Sanitation in September 1992 the programme was again revised. The revised programme aimed at an integrated approach of rural sanitation. Since its inception and up to the end of the 9th Plan, 94.5 lakh latrines were constructed for rural households under the CRSP as well as corresponding State MNP. The total investment made has been Rs. 621 crore under the CRSP and Rs. 1045 crore under the State sector MNP. This has led to only a marginal increase in the rural sanitation coverage. On an average Annual increase in the rural sanitation coverage has been only 1 percent, which was insignificant.

The CRSP was restructured in 1999 with a provision for allocation based component of CRSP to be phased out by the end of the 9th Plan, i.e.

2001-02. The Total Sanitation Campaign (TSC) under restructured CRSP was launched with effect from 1.4.1999 following a community led and people centered approach. TSC moves away from the principle of state-wise allocation. primarily based on poverty criterion to a "demand-driven" approach. The programme gives emphasis on Information, Education and Communication (IEC) for demand generation for sanitation facilities. It also gives emphasis on school sanitation and hygiene education for changing the behaviour of the people from the younger age itself.

The components of TSC include start-up activities, IEC, Individual house hold latrines, community sanitary complex, school sanitation and hygiene education, Anganwadi toilets, Alternate delivery mechanism in the form of Rural Sanitary Marts and Production centers and administrative charges.

Various Components of TSC

Start-up Activities

The start up activities include the setting up of Water and Sanitation Missions in the States/UTs and the respective districts. Conducting of preliminary surveys (after a phase of me, has been carried out) to assess the demand and thereafter preparation of the District TSC project proposals for seeking Government of India assistance. Upto 5% of the total TSC project cost has been earmarked for the above and shall be 100% funded by the GOI.

IEC Activities

With the setting up of the Missions in the Districts, the NGOs/ Alternative Mechanisms and their volunteers shall start the process of information dissemination related to various aspects of the water and sanitation sector, create awareness to the extent that he/she motivates them to construct their own latrines and soakage pits for solid and liquid waste disposal. The willingness of the people to construct latrines is translated/ interpreted as demand generated. The motivator shall be given his/her incentive from the funds earmarked for IEC. The incentive shall be based on his/her performance, i.e. in terms of motivating the people to the extent that they construct the latrine and soakage pits. At least 15% of the total TSC project cost has been earmarked for the above and the funds in a ratio of 80:20 will be provided by the GOI (80%) and the State (20%), respectively.

Alternate Delivery Mechanism [Central Production Centres (PCs)/RSMs]

The IEC activities shall help generate demand. The preliminary survey thereafter shall reveal the quantity of demand based on which the supply of related goods (squatting; slabs/plates with water seal pans, pipes, etc.) shall be selected and ensured, keeping in view the cost factor (predetermined).

The Central Production Centres at the district/block level (depending upon quantity of demand and the spatial concentration of demand) shall be established. The PCs could be opened and operated by NGOs/ Panchayats. Up to 5% (subject to a maximum of Rs. 35.00 lakh) of the total TSC project cost has been earmarked for establishing PCs with a notional earmarking of Rs. 3.5 lakh per PC/RSM envisaged.

Provision of Hardware

As stated earlier, for the purpose of this scheme, a duly completed household sanitary latrine shall comprise of a Basic Low Cost Unit (BLCU) without the super structure (Cost of superstructure shall be borne by the beneficiary). As per the "Technological Options for Implementation of the Rural Sanitation Programme" Handbook, the simplest and least expensive BLCU on an average is estimated to cost between Rs. 625 and Rs. 1000. Maximum subsidy shall be available for the least expensive sanitary latrine, i.e. costing upto Rs. 625. Units with the higher cost (i.e. between Rs. 625 to Rs. 1000) shall be eligible for a lower subsidy.

The financing pattern (subsidy) for the BLCU's is given in Table below:

S.No.	*BLCU Cost (Rs.)*	*Contribution (as %age) to the cost*		
		GOI	*State*	*Beneficiary*
1.	Upto Rs. 625	Upto 60%	20%	20%
2.	Between Rs. 625 and Rs. 1000	Upto 30%	30%	40%
3.	> Rs. 1000	Nil	—	—

The BLCUs costing upto Rs. 625 shall be open to 80% subsidy, to be shared between the Gal (60%) and the State Government (20%) and shall not exceed Rs. 500 (i.e. Rs. 375 Gal share and Rs. 125 state share in a BLCU costing Rs. 625. The beneficiary is expected to make a minimum contribution of 20% to the BLCU cost.

The BLCUs costing between Rs: 625 and Rs. 1000 shall attract a subsidy of 60% to be shared equally between the Gal (30%) and the State Government (30%), subject to a maximum of Rs. 500 the beneficiary is expected to make a minimum contribution of 40% to the BLCU cost.

No subsidy will be provided to beneficiaries opting for BLCUs costing more than Rs. 1000. The extent of Gal participation will be fixed. However, states are free to generate greater beneficiary participation with a view to reduce their financial liability and ensure greater sustainability. States/UTs wishing to adopt a single flat rate of subsidy, will be free to do so, subject to a maximum of Rs. 500 inclusive of both Gal and State shares.

SUBSIDY DISBURSEMENT

Subsidy disbursement shall be subject to close supervision and monitoring and linked with the construction activity so as to ensure sincere and full involvement of the community, thereby ensuring the sustainability of campaign. The construction (assuming that the beneficiaries opt between the two models viz. (i) single pit brick lined, and (ii) single offset pit (brick lined) with provision for (2nd pit) linked subsidy disbursement shall be effected in the manner as under:

- Once the institutional framework for implementing the TSC in the State/UT has been set-up, the mc activities shall be initiated through the NGOs/Alternative Mechanisms networking. The preliminary survey shall follow wherein a demand (for sanitary latrines) estimation shall be made which shall be the basic input of a TSC project proposal. The demand estimation shall be based on the number of sites of 3×3 metre suitably raised/ developed by the beneficiaries as a part of their contribution in kind. It must also be ensured that the site is Oat least 3 metres away from the Drinking water source. The final beneficiary list shall be drawn by the motivator after physical verification of the sites which will bear countersignatures of the beneficiaries and one villager attesting to each as witness. Based on this list the TSC project proposal shall be prepared. Wherever the beneficiaries are not in a position to provide a 3×3 mtr space, provision for a Community latrine may be considered.
- With the acceptance of the TSC proposal, submitted for the district, the PCs shall be established. Once the PCs are established and production commences (at rates approved by the District Water and Sanitation Committee) the list shall be sent to the PCs in the respective areas for supply of goods and services. The PC shall have its schedule of production, delivery and construction at site (TSC village) by its trained masons. The payment for the goods (bricks, cement, mortar, squatting plate, pit cover, pipe, etc.) and services shall be made to the PC directly from the District Mission. The amount shall exclude that remaining portion of the total contribution of (20% or 40%), which the beneficiary is to make. This amount shall be collected directly from the beneficiary by the skilled mason on behalf of the Pc. The motivator shall oversee, assist and supervise all through. The payment to the PC shall be effected after the motivator physically verifies the construction work. The District Water and Sanitation Committee will take the help of field level Government/PRI functionaries for verification. The duly filled and signed schedule of completion shall be sent to the District Mission by the NGOs/Alternative mechanisms concerned.
- Based on the verified schedule (shall include verification of completion of construction work of soakage pits) the District Mission shall release the NGO motivator's incentive.

- A TSC village shall be rewarded if it completes the works/ activities planned in the scheduled manner/time. The reward amount may be fixed by the District Water and Sanitation Mission and may be given to the village panchayat, preferably, in kind.

School Sanitation (Hardware and Support Services)

Children are more receptive to new ideas and therefore the school is the best suitable institution in changing the conditioned habits of people from open defecation to the use of lavatory through motivation and education. The experience gained by children through use of toilets in school and sanitation education imparted by teachers would definitely be carried home and passed on to parents, in most cases who do not have formal education. This has long been neglected. The Tenth Finance Commission had also drawn attention to this issue and has provided funds for toilet facilities in primary and upper primary schools. This initiative needs to be supported and pushed further.

School sanitation shall form an integral part of every TSC. Accordingly, it is proposed to allow the construction of toilets in schools. The school authorities and Parents Teacher Association (PTA) shall be responsible for mobilising an initial corpus of 5% of the unit cost. The unit cost shall not exceed Rs. 20,000. Once this is in position, the construction of the unit can he taken up. The GOI/State share shall be 60% and 30% respectively with the balance 10% coming from the Panchayats/ beneficiaries.

While drawing up the Action Plan for School Sanitation, it shall be ensured that the total number of schools to be provided with sanitary facilities under TSC have to be estimated taking into account, schools to be taken up under JRY, DPEP, Tenth Finance Commission funds., etc. and OJ ensure that actual break up is clearly mentioned. Construction of the sanitary facilities in the schools shall be done preferably by the construction wing of the DPEP and under close supervision of the Parent Teacher Association. It may also be ensured that approval for the construction of all new schools shall be accorded only if the sanitary and drinking water facilities are integral parts of the plan.[11]

Total sanitation campaign is being implemented in 451 districts of the country. The project outlay for 451 TSC projects sanctioned so far is Rs. 4413.19 crore. The Central, state and beneficiary contribution are Rs. 2620.89 crore, Rs. 979.90 crore and Rs. 812.40 crore respectively. During the current year, 53 projects have been sanctioned. The physical and financial progress of the TSC projects is available on the Departmental web site at www.ddws.nic.in.

Progress

During the current year, the TSC programme has taken off in the right direction and the implementation has been improved tremendously. The monitoring mechanism was strengthened while the hand holding exercises including Capacity development activity has been improved substantially. Some of the key areas of improvement made are as below:

Monitoring Mechanism

Progress is monitored through review meetings taken up by Secretary (DWS). In addition, review Missions are sent to various TSC projects to assess the extent of implementation as well as support the project authorities in implementing the project in an effective manner. In addition to the above, a Mid-term evaluation study of the TSC programme has been initiated. Over and above, the On-line monitoring of TSC programme has been launched and many States are now feeding their performance On-line on the Departmental web.site at www.ddws.nic.in

Ninnal Gram Puraskar, an award scheme for achieving 100% open defecation free environment has been launched on 2/10/2003 to the Panchayati Raj institutions (PRIs). The individuals and Organisations other than PRIs who playa key role in achieving this feat will also be rewarded. This has generated sufficient enthusiasm amongst the PRIs. Large number of applications were received. The scrutiny process has been completed and the award will be granted in February, 2005.

- HRD training modules for Capacity Development of grass-root level, district and state level officials involved in TSC implementation has been finalized. Training of TSC implementation officials is structured through 4 National Resource Centres at ESI, Ahmedabad, RKNLSM, Kolkata, GRI, Dindigul and SIPRD, Kalyani, WHO.
- Booklets on Community participation in water supply and sanitation has been finalized through NIRD, Hyderabad.
- During the current year special thrust was given on School sanitation and hygiene education. Modules on Food hygiene to environmental sanitation has ocean prepared and printed in two technical notes called "School Sanitation and Hygiene Education and Angwanwadi toilet designs." These technical notes have been circulated to all the states. Decision has been taken to cover all Government schools in the country with safe sanitation facilities by 2005-06. Accordingly, an Action Plan for school water and sanitation has been initiated and all the states have been requested to comply for the same.
- Realizing the facts that poor rural men population who do not have adequate land for construction of individual latrines, the earlier Women complex has been expanded to a Community complex. Further, hygiene education in schools has been highlighted. Featuring these changes which also include provisions for coverage of all Anganwadi toilets and Ninnal Gram Puraskar, the revised TSC guidelines has been made in

January 2004. One of the most important features of these revised guidelines is emphasis of coverage of Individual latrines for APL households without subsidy incentive through proper change of mind set. These are hosted in the web site and the guidelines are being distributed to all the states and district implementing agencies. Further, all the states have been asked to translate. the revised TSC guidelines and SSHE technical notes into their regional languages so as facilitate the grass-root level workers also in effective TSC implementation.

- Inter-sectoral Co-ordination meetings with other Ministries! departments at the Secretary level was held with DWCD, Health and Elementary Education. Co-ordination with external agencies for enhanced facilitation for TSC implementation through UNICEF, WSP-SA has been taken up.
- National Communication strategy has been worked out for the National and District levels utilizing the services of UNICEF and Ogilveyand Mather. The TV spots have been developed.
- As a result of the above initiatives taken up, 24.68 lakh individual household latrines, 32364 school latrines, 1190 women community complex, 6068 Anganwadi toilets have been constructed during the current year along with establishment of 904 Rural sanitary marts and production centers.

Gender Budgeting Under CRSP

Central Rural Sanitation Programme (CRSP) administered by this Department is meant for providing sanitation facilities in the rural habitation. All the inhabitants of the rural areas irrespective of cast, creed and sex benefit of this programme.

Physical and Financial Progress

Plan Period	*CRSP (GOI) releases (Rs. Crore)*	*Latrines constructed (Units)*
Eighth Plan period, 1992-93 to 1996-97	260.33	4337609
Ninth Plan	—	—
1997-98	96.66	1387080
1998-99	64.90	1631272
1999-2000	92.00	1087604
2000-01	130.86	734514
2001-02	130.46	—
Tenth Plan	—	—
2002-03	141.10	2471945
2003-04	205.30	4513884
2004-05 (as on 3.2.2005)	294.10	2841053

Under Rural sanitation programme there is a special provision for construction of Community Sanitary Complexes for women in order to ensure better hygience conditions and support dignity of women. Separate toilet blocks for girl student in each co-education rural Government schools is being provided under TSC. However, since the bifurcation cannot be made on gender lines in respect of rural sanitation sector, it is not possible to earmark separate budget provision and fix separate physical targets in respect of this programme.[12]

Other Related Matters

Maintenance

It is essential to train the community, particularly all the members of the family in the proper upkeep and maintenance of the sanitation facilities. The maintenance expenses of individual household sanitary latrines should be met by the beneficiaries where as that of sanitary complexes for women may be at the cost of the panchayats/voluntary organisations/charitable trusts.

(i) The State shall prepare an Annual Action Plan one month before the commencement of the year on the basis of the shelf of schemes and taking into account the size of the allocation as well as carryover funds. Annual Action Plan should indicate clearly targets under each component for each quarter. A copy of the,Action Plan should be sent to Government of India by 30th April.

(ii) While preparing the Action Plan, the completion of the incomplete works should be given priority over new works. It should be ensured that the works taken up are completed as per schedule to avoid cost escalation.

Cost Escalation of the Schemes not Allowed

There is no need or scope for delay in implementation resulting in cost overrun. Hence no additional funds shall be allowed under the TSC as well as the "allocation-based" Sanitation Programme towards cost overrun.

Schedule of Inspections

Monitoring through regular field inspections by officers from State level and district level in essential for the effective implementation of the programme. The inspection should be to check and to ensure that construction work has been done in accordance with the norms, that the community has been involved in construction, that the latrines are not polluting the water sources and also to check whether there has been correct selection of beneficiaries and proper use of latrines after construction. Such inspection should ensure that the sanitary latrines are not used for any other purpose, as has happened some times in the past.

Reports and Returns

The following reports and returns will be sent by the States/UTs:

- An Annual Action Plan for the schemes to be taken up during the year shall be furnished by 30th April of the year to which it relates.
- Monthly progress report will be furnished by the 20th of the succeeding month.
- Quarterly progress report shall be furnished by the 20th of the succeeding month.
- Annual Report of achievements under the programme during the year shall be furnished by 30th April of the succeeding year.

These reports shall enable authorities both at Centre and the State level to monitor the progress of the performance and to take appropriate collective measures.

Evaluation of the Programme

The implementation of the programme, results achieved and its impact will be evaluated at the end of each year by the Government of India through reputed Organisations. The States/UTs may also undertake the Evaluation of the programme through the reputed agencies in the States. Follow-up action taken by the States/UTs should be intimated to GOI front time to time. Any further modifications in the programme could be formulated based on the results of such evaluation.

Audit

The funds released under the Restructured Rural Sanitation Programme will be subject to audit by the Comptroller and Auditor General of India.

Introduction

Allocation-based Sanitation Programme

In order to allow time for proper grounding of the new approach, the existing "allocation-based" programme will also be continued and will be progressively phased out. While the third year of the 9th Plan period will have 50% funds earmarked for the existing scheme, only. 30% will be allocated for the fourth year, followed by 10% during the fifth year of the Plan period, mainly to handle spillover costs and small pending commitments.[13]

Programme Components

The components of the programme are as under:

- Construction of individual sanitary latrines for households below poverty line with subsidy (80%) where demand exists.

- Construction of exclusive village sanitary complexes for women, where adequate land/space within the premises of the houses do not exist and where village panchayats are willing to maintain.
- Setting up of sanitary marts and production centres.
- Construction of toilets in schools.
- Total sanitation of village through the construction of drains, soakage pits solid and liquid waste disposal.
- Intensive campaign for awareness generation and health education for creating felt need for personal, household and environmental sanitation facilities.

(a) Construction of Individual Latrines

The pattern of subsidy prescribed under TSCs will be followed.

(b) Conversion of Dry Latrines

As regards conversion of dry latrines, as per records, there are no such latrines in the rural areas. However, the Baseline survey does point to the existence of such latrines. A sum of Rs. 50 lakh shall be earmarked for this purpose for the third and fourth years of the 9th Plan. Unutilized balances shall be merged into the general pool of the resources of the Programme.

(c) Village Sanitation Complexes for Women

Though public latrines have not proved to be very successful in the past in view of the difficulties experienced by rural women in some areas, where individual household latrines are not feasible, village sanitary complexes exclusively for women could be attempted on a pilot basis. Upto 10% of the annual funds can be utilized to provide public latrines in selected villages during the plan period, where the panchayats/charitable trusts/NGOs offer to construct and maintain village complexes exclusively for the use by women.

(d) Rural Sanitary Marts (RSMs)/Production Centres (PCs)

Upto 5% of the allocation, subject to a maximum of Rs. 35 lakh/ district @ Rs. 3.5 lakh per unit can be used to set-up RSM/PCs.

(e) Total Sanitation of Village

Other Sanitation facilities such as drains, soakpits, solid and liquid waste disposals, etc. should be taken up as far as possible under Jawahar Rozgar Yojana GRY) or any other programme for providing civic amenities in the Panchayat. Where this is not feasible due to other priorities and non-availability of adequate financial resources, the facilities can be taken up under allocation-based sanitation programme. For village that achieve more than 50% sanitation coverage in the below poverty line (BPL) segment, total sanitation packages can be taken up with 50% GOI assistance. No project will be sanctioned by the GOI, duration of which exceeds beyond the 9th Plan period. The facilities may include provision for construction of cattle troughs, sanitation of cattle sheds including provision of drinking water facilities, disposal of solid and liquid waste and Insecticide sprays for mosquitoes! flies.

(f) Campaign for Creation of Felt Need

This is a very important aspect of the programme. While government machinery for publicity may be useful to some extent, a well-orchestrated programme of publicity, health, education and creation of required facilities only can make any change in the attitude of the people. Support of the reputed local voluntary organisations, autonomous institutions, social, political and religious organisations who carry conviction with the people can be enlisted in creating the felt need. These organisations should be selected for their reputation for good and adequate infrastructure already available with them. These details should be collected at the field level. These organisations should be selected for environment creation and generation of felt need-based on clear norms such as number of years of good work, extent of good work, availability of infrastructure, extent of geographical coverage, etc.

These voluntary organisations should be encouraged to prepare projects covering various components of the programme but with focus on generation of felt need and construction of individual sanitary latrines. The incentive scheme provided under TSC for the NGOs/volunateers will be applicable for this also.[14]

CONCLUSION

There is a need of integrated approaches for water, waste disposal and health. In areas where drainage and sanitation are poor, water runs over the ground during rainstorms, picks up faeces and contaminates water sources. This contributes significantly to the spread of diseases such as typhold and cholera, and may increase the likelihood of contracting worm infections from soil contaminated by faeces. Flooding itself may displace populations and lead to further health problems.

It is often essential that community members participate in maintaining drains. In Indonesia, for example, residents agreed to clean the drains in front of their houses every day and this was inspected twice a week. Community members responded well to friendly inspectors who provided support for clearing the drains. Maintaining the drains soon became part of the daily routine for responsible community members.[15]

Responsibility of Panchayati Raj System

1. Provide health education to people outlining the importance of sanitation to individuals and community.

2. Provide health education through demonstration of the impact of insanitation on the health of the people.
3. Encourage people's participation in making their house and village clean and beautiful.
4. Provide essential items for keeping the village clean.
5. One day a month may be celebrated as cleanliness day.
6. Encourage school children to keep their village clean.
7. Remove the weeds harmful to health.
8. Do plantation to make the environment of the village good.
9. Provide health education as not to throw things any where except in the space provided.
10. Encourage co-operative effort to promote sanitation.

Notes and References

1. Healthy Villages-A guide for communities and community health workers, WHO, p. 52.
2. Building Materials and Technology Promotion Council India, BMTPC, "Water and Sanitation for Cities", *World Habitat Day*, 6 Oct. 2003, p. 22.
3. *Ibid.*, p. 4.
4. Rajiv Gandhi National Drinking Water Mission, Ministry of Rural Development, GOI, New Delhi, pp. 2-3.
5. Building Materials and Technology Promotion Council India, BMTPC, "Water and Sanitation for Cities", *World Habitat Day*,
6. 6 Oct., 2003, p. 22.
7. *Ibid.*, p. 4.
8. K.Subramanian: Shelter, Vol. 6, No. 3, October 2003, p. 48, *Ibid.*, p. 52.
9. UNICF: Learning from Experience, Water and Environment Sanitation in India, p. 9.
10. *Ibid.*, p. 15.
11. India 2004, Ministry of Information and Broadcasting, GOI, New Delhi, pp. 579-80.
12. Rajiv Gandhi National Drinking Water Mission, Ministry of Rural Development, GOI, New Delhi, pp. 10-13.
13. Rural Development, Book, pp. 1332-35.
14. Rajiv Gandhi National Drinking Water Mission, Ministry of Rural Development, GOI, New Delhi, pp. 18-19.
15. Healthy Villges: A guide for Communities and Community Health Workers—WHO, p. 50.

10

Health Education for Rural Drinking Water Supply

"For most people, it is not a problem to obtain the minimum amount of water necessary to sustain life. Rather, problems relate to the quantities of water required for different activities (resource allocation) and the quality of the water available (source suitability). Many places with water shortages actually receive abundant rainfall and community-based initiatives could alleviate water scarcity. Such initiatives may incorporate traditional approaches and include water management and conservation measures; sustainable rates of extraction; sustainable crop production; catchment protection; rainwater harvesting; and soil conservation."

—*WHO*

Dr. Able Wolman's Charter is one of the "father-figures" of environmental health in today's world. Professor emeritus of sanitary engineering at the Johns Hopkins School of Engineering, Baltimore, USA, he is also a former President of the American Public Health Association, and has spent the greater part of a long lifetime engaged in research into the control of the environment for the reduction of disease and the welfare of man. Here he contributes his own 20-point "Charter" for improving the world's health:

(1) Life is impossible without water. The statement is accurate. It always leads great conferences to pass resolutions to do something about providing water to impoverished people. Resolutions become opiates, because they are gratifying substitutes for action.

CHART 10.1

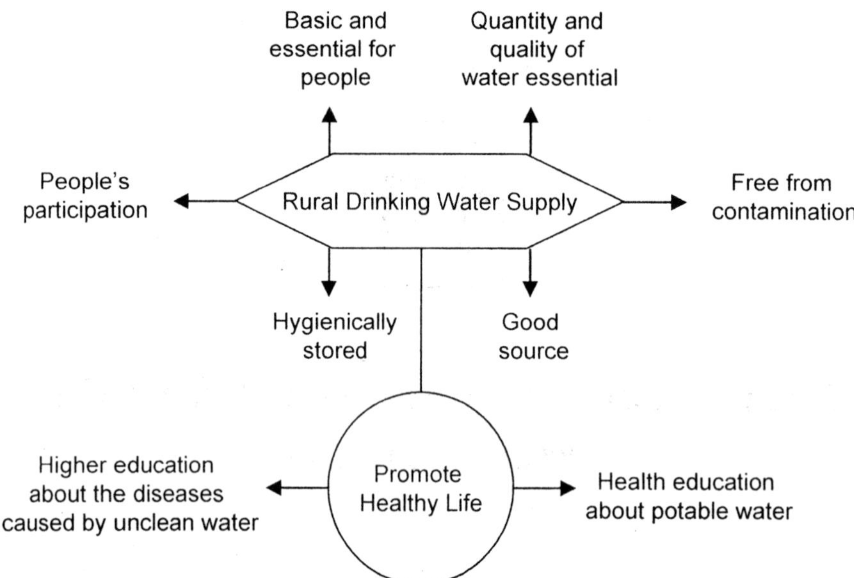

(2) Statistics are necessary, but they do not stir the emotions! One sick child, if it is yours, makes the world weep.

(3) How much drama is there is repeating, time and again, that more than 1,000 million people in developing countries cannot conveniently and safely drink, cook or wash with water? Astronomical numbers, of anything, are so often unintelligible. One should see people *en masse*, without these amenities, in villages or in slums, bidonvilles or favelas!

(4) Progress, of course, has been made in the last 30 years. WHO reports, in its recent survey of some 90 developing countries, that 69 per cent of urban dwellers had adequate community water supply and excreta disposal services.

(5) The situation for the rural or urban fringe dweller is dismal. For them, only 20 per cent have even reasonable access to safe water. Less than 10 per cent of these individuals have any real form of sanitary excreta disposal facilities.

(6) Viewed on a global basis, we have little to be sanguine about. The disease consequences of poor and insufficient water, of living with human excreta, and of unhygienic personal habits, are disastrous; they have been familiar for so long a time that they no longer excite even the statistician or epidemiologist. People accept their devastation, as they so often abjectly bear their real and spiritual poverty. We speak of the toll of deaths, due to environmental deficiencies, in a casual way, even though the figures mount to hundreds of millions. The communicable

diseases, often the sequels of poor sanitation, are maiming and killing men, women, and children—not computer data.

(7) No "health house" can or should be built on an in-sanitary foundation. Healthcare and hospitalization, important as they are, will always be in default when structured upon a sanitary environmental quicksand.

(8) Why are hundreds of millions of people still without even minimum sanitary facilities—and, at the present rate, unlikely to get them for another half a century? Some say religion, custom, money, education, economics stand in the way.

(9) As in all social diagnoses, no single cause and non-single therapy account for all environmental disabilities. No two countries are alike and no two regions within the same country are the same. Let us look at some of the blocks to progress.

(10) It has been abundantly demonstrated that no one likes to be sick or die. Everyone (whether Moslem, Hindu, Christian, or any chosen religion) likes to wash so as to sleep at night, free from wake fullness infighting hordes of body vermin. Regardless of history or culture, people learn to protect themselves when given the opportunity and understanding.

(11) Too often, the slow pace has been blamed upon the people. The major cause for delinquent action lies in the motivation of governments. Do they really mean what their resolutions say—militantly enough to go into action? Is only lip service the main response of presidents, prime ministers, kings, and ministers?

(12) Unfortunately, the exceptions are still too few. What lessons stem from their successes? Motivation and intention, diligently and persistently pursued, remain in first place.

(13) Equally important are the desires of the people themselves, which can be met through education, understanding and participation. Much of the time these factors are missing and must be created and stimulated.

(14) This is not easy, but must be deliberately undertaken, preferably village by village, by the local "barefoot" somebody.

(15) To do this well requires the machinery and personnel of a permanent and sympathetic government, operating through regional and local units. Their nature and number will vary from country to country.

(16) Movement toward broad sanitary reform should go forward jointly or in parallel with other social and economic undertakings in the same areas. Room for exceptions must be available.

(17) It should be clear by now that maneuvering on this complex stage demands manpower, unfortunately in scarce supply in too many countries. The spectrum of manpower required runs from the highly skilled supervisor to the equally important, earthy village worker. Almost always, training on the spot is essential

(18) What about money? Strangely enough, this is not the dominant constraint. Some is needed, of course, but often, with local self-help (material, physical, and monetary), money can be found.

(19) Technology likewise is at hand. Failures lie in its abuse rather than in its unavailability. Certainly, innovation, simplicity, lower cost will all help, but progress is not retarded greatly by the inadequacy of present tools, materials or equipment.

(20) The task for the future is difficult, but possible. People should not be consigned to premature death, simply because we are less than courageous and diligent. The pace must be accelerated.[1]

Government of India in its document, "Guidelines for Implementation of Rural Water Supply Programme" observes that since independence, India has been making earnest efforts for achieving social and economic development. India has been implementing national strategies and plans through various multi-pronged development schemes and programmes. To relieve the women and young girls from the drudgery of fetching water from long distances and, to combat the scourge of water-borne diseases, the Government of India and States/Union Territories have been implementing water supply programme in the rural areas.

The importance of a country attaches to the provision of adequate and safe water supply is an index of its concern for socio-economic development of its people. The ever-increasing population in the country inevitably brings in its wake complex problems of potable water supply systems and environmental concerns in the implementation of the rural water supply programme.

India's rural water supply programme is the biggest in the world and has been remarkably successful. Around 95% of the rural habitations have access to one or more sources of drinking water. However, there are still a number of challenges to be faced in providing potable water to the remaining uncovered rural habituations. Depleting ground water, pollution, problems of quality of drinking water add to this. Developing hygiene awareness, helping people to become conscious of the relationship between safe water, sanitation, health and development and bringing about a change in the attitude and behaviour appear to be some of the difficult tasks to be carried out in the coming years.·

M.M.N. Saxena in his article, "Initiatives in Promoting Water Resources in India", in *Yojna,* June 2003 clearly mentions that water being precious, finite and in view of growing demand, ultimately is a scarce natural endowment. Our main strategy is to optimize its availability for different purposes, and accordingly National Water Policy has defined water allocation priorities broadly for supply of water for drinking, irrigation, hydropower, ecology, agro-industries and non-agricultural industries, navigation and various other uses. Of equal importance are the objectives of achievements of efficiency, equity, and sustainability in the use of water.

With the existing water resources of the country, per capita availability of water varies in the range of 2000 to 13745 cubic meters (cu. m.) per year with the national annual average of per capita availability about 1829 cu. m. in 2001. By 2015 AD the country will be facing water stress conditions with annual per capita availability of water at about 1557 cu. m. The conditions will be further worsening due to continued population growth and by 2050 AD the projected annual per capita availability of 1168 cu. m. would take the country to the threshold of water scarce conditions. It is estimated that by 2050 AD 22% of the geographical areas and 17% of population of the country will be under absolute scarcity conditions having access of water availability of less than 500 cu. m. per year and 70% of the area and 76% of population will be on the verge of affected health and economic activities with access to water available of less than 100 cu. m. per year, which is identified as stress or scarcity level.

Water is life. This colourless, odourless and tasteless liquid is essential for all forms of growth and development—human, animal and plant. Water is a fundamental basic need for sustaining human economic activities. Not only does water support a wide range of activities, it also plays a central symbolic role in rituals throughout the world and is considered a divine gift by many religions.

Dr. Halfdan Mahler, WHO, former Director-General mentioned that: I am utterly convinced that the number of water taps per 1,000 population will be an infinitely more meaningful health indicator than the number of hospital beds per 1,000 population

Providing water in the desired quantity and quality; and at the right time and place, has been a constant endeavour of all civilizations. No other natural resource has had such an overwhelming influence on human history. As the human population increases, as people express their desire for a better standard of living, and as economic activities continue to expand in scale and diversity, the demands on fresh water resources will continue to grow.

While water is a renewable resource, its availability in space (at a specific location) and time (at different periods of the year) is limited, being largely determined by climatic, geographical and physical conditions, by affordable technological solutions which permit its exploitation, and by the efficiency with which water is conserved and used.

Much of the world's fresh water is consumed by the agricultural, industrial and domestic sectors. Increasing water demands and the inadequacy of these sectors to effectively manage this resource, has meant that crises situations have arisen in many parts of the world, crises over the availability of adequate, quality water.[2]

WATER FOR ALL: A HUMAN RIGHT

Water is a basic human need for health—indeed, for survival—and therefore it is not an exaggeration to call it one of the basic human rights.

Without safe water and sanitation, there is no real development. A community ravaged by diarrhoeal diseases, dracunculiasis or schistorsomiasis cannot look beyond its immediate problems towards social and economic welfare. Safe water is the doorway to health and health is the prerequisite for progress, social equity and human dignity.

Despite the achievements of the 1980s—an additional 1600 million people were served with safe water supplies—an estimated 1200 million people in developing countries still do not have proper access to safe water. They are at constant risk of contracting water and sanitation-related diseases. The upsurge of cholera since 1990 has underlined the need for clean water to protect health, particularly in the expanding shanties and slums in and around the cities of developing countries.

An adequate quantity of water, by itself, is not enough to safeguard health. Unsafe water supplies lead directly to diseases that affect hundreds of millions of people, mainly living in the tropics. This issue of *World Health* describes some of the problems and what is being done about them.

An accessible and safe water supply, improved personal and domestic hygiene, and stronger community participation are the main ways to avoid water-borne diseases. But to be really effective they must be accompanied by other measures such as pollution control and proper drainage of surface waters. Since environmental protection of fresh water source is the basic step to ensure a sustainable clean water supply, this must always be an integral component of both environment and health programmes.[3]

Water is essential to life on earth. Plant and animal life are vitally dependent on water, which is an essential ingredient and a lubricant of nature. Human existence is affected if there is too little or too much water and, if it becomes polluted, it becomes a health threat and a hindrance to economic prosperity. There is hardly any current issue that more conclusively demonstrates the integrated nature of environment and development than that of fresh water. The challenge of securing for all people the basic human need of a reliable supply of fresh water, adequate in quantity and quality, is perhaps the most fundamental development issue.[4]

IMPROVEMENTS IN WATER AND SANITATION CAN SAVE LIVES

Drinking water and sanitation improvements could reduce the overall incidence of infant and child diarrhoea by one quarter and cut total infant and child mortality by more than one-half. Country programmes are increasingly taking measures to improve water supply and sanitation within their primary healthcare programmes. Guinea-worm disease can be effectively prevented by providing safe drinking water and its global eradication is clearly possible within the next few years. As for schistosomiasis, some 60% reduction could be achieved by improving water supplies. Building latrines, giving health education and introducing selected drug therapy could reduce the prevalence even more.[5]

Water is part of a large constantly moving cycle. Simply explained, it evaporates from the surface of the earth, and turns into clouds that produce rain and snow, which fall on the earth's surface. Then through rivers and underground water tables it passes to the oceans and lakes, and thus the cycle continues.

Climatic changes caused by human activity—like cutting down forests—have reduced the water supply in many parts of the world. As temperature and rain and snow precipitation patterns change, many rivers carry less water. At times they carry too much water, resulting in floods. Trees and other vegetation help to retain water in the solid and prevent landslides. Chemical substances from industry sometimes pass into the air. One of the results is acid rain, which kills fish and vegetation in many lakes and rivers. Sometimes dangerous products from industry, agriculture and other human activities enter the rivers, lakes, oceans and underground water, and can contaminate our drinking water.

At the same time, the demand for water from villages and towns, and from industry and agriculture, is steadily increasing. Water can therefore no longer be considered an unlimited resource, which costs nothing and which can be wasted. In the next century water supplies will certainly be considered a very valued service, and each one of us will have to pay what it costs to have clean water.[6]

Safe water and improved sanitations are a necessary condition for better health, and there can be no lasting improvement of public health without them.

We all know that determined government action is needed to change the prevailing situation. We also know that clean water and sanitation will remain an unattainable objective in poor countries without development assistance.

Many countries are making efforts towards implementing the objectives of the International Drinking Water Supply and Sanitation Decade. But much still needs to be done-and can be done.[7]

The Americas: Attainable Goals—Governments in the Americas are increasingly aware that providing water and sanitation services is the single most important activity they can undertake to improve people's health and raise productivity.

Hours of personal drudgery are devoted to obtaining safe water and disposing of human wastes in a sanitary manner. When water must be carried from a source, which is five kilometers from the house, someone must spend about three hours a day in making the two trips that will be needed to carry the 30 to 40 litres of water the family will use. And this amount, which is often of dubious quality, will barely serve to quench their thirst, meet their cooking needs, and leave a little over for basic hygienic needs. Unless even this limited amount of water is properly disposed of, it can serve as the focus of a long of diseases.[8]

Millions in Need

Drinking water and sanitation are health programmes, not disease programmes. They are the essential precondition for the promotion of health, where health is under threat from communicable diseases.

A good drinking water supply is good for health. This simple fact was recognized more than a hundred years ago during one of the great cholera epidemics in London. John Snow stopped the pump on Board Street that supplied parts of the city with water from the River Thames and, by doing so, not only demonstrated that the disease was caused by infected river water but also showed that diseases like cholera cannot be permanently resisted unless people are provided with safe drinking water.

Why then are researchers today spending time and money yet again to disprove what has already been proven? Because of a misconception. They start from the premise that drinking water and environmental sanitation are interventions designed to control the diarrhoeal diseases. This is wrong. Drinking water supply and sanitation are the only permanent solutions that can prevent infant deaths from diarrhoea (and remember there are more than five million such deaths a year in the developing world). But it is wrong to assume that they should be provided merely to fight the diarrhoeal diseases. Drinking water and sanitation are health programmes; they are the essential precondition for the promotion of health, where health is threatened by a vast array of communicable diseases, and often the only permanent solution.

Moreover, drinking water and sanitation are an essential precondition for community development, and ultimately for social and economic development. Since we know this, we may ask why economists like the researchers referred to above continue to ask questions about these essential services? Is it because they prefer to invest the money in projects, which seem to offer a higher financial rate of return? Is it because they shy away from putting money down for water supply and sanitation since-admittedly-to build and maintain these services will call for more ingenuity and hard work than putting money into a bank where it will earn interest?

When delegates to the 39th World Health Assembly last May reviewed the progress made so far in the International Drinking Water Supply and Sanitation Decade, they started by saying that the case for adequate water supply and sanitation did not need to be restated. However, they noted the disparities in progress made between urban and rural areas, and between water supply and sanitation. They insisted that more should be done for water supply and sanitation in the future, and not less.

Children and women are suffering most in the present situation and they felt it was important to promote local technologies for water supply and sanitation, and to develop health education strategies aimed at increasing the awareness of communities of their role, especially in planning and maintaining their own water supply and sanitation facilities.

The delegates also stressed that improving water supply and sanitation means meeting the basic needs of millions of people; it followed, therefore, that financial resources should be made available in the light of a new and more equitable international economic order and as a contribution to the quest for peace. Everybody had to get involved, not only the health sector; the delegates concluded that inter-sectoral cooperation would be of prime importance to the attainment of the objectives during the second half of the decade.[9]

There is today just as much fresh water on the earth as there was millions of a year ago: about 40,000 cubic kilometers. But whereas there were 1,000 million people on the planet in 1820, there are 6,000 million today. Obviously this means that there is less water to go round. In addition, since the advent of the industrial era, there has been a dramatic increase in demand for water, commensurate with population growth and improved living standards. Each individual is using more fresh water every day for domestic, agricultural and industrial use, so it is all the more urgent to protect the water that is available to make the most of it and share it equally.

The International Drinking Water Supply and Sanitation Decade, is striving to bring safe water to everyone's doorstep. All too often, women and children spend hours in the drudgery of collecting water from remote and possibly polluted streams and wells. Having safe water means better health and nutrition, more time for education; it also means a better chance of a style of life that opens the way to social and economic growth. The technologies exist to bring water into every household. People must now work together to make this a reality and prove that "Happy are those who build their development on water."

Health plays a crucial role in any effort for development, and good health is closely related to the status of water supply and sanitation. Our graph on the opposite page shows the direct and indirect effects of water supply and sanitation on health. It indicates how water and health, in common with many other sectors, form a basis for development.[10]

Fresh water from inland sources can be broadly classified into, (i) Surface Water comprising rivers, lakes and ponds, and (ii) Ground Water comprising of wells and springs. A portion of the water falling on land soaks into the ground. This is stored in underground tunnels as groundwater. Groundwater is pure as it has already percolated through the solid and purified by a natural process of filtration. This is increasingly being preferred for use by people. But finding adequate groundwater sources for supplying large urban populations is difficult. Cities that do have good groundwater supplies benefit, because the cost of treatment is minimal. The treatment basically removing excessive minerals. Often the water is pure enough so that chlorine or other chemicals are not needed to make it usable, even for drinking.

Of all the water available on earth, potable or water fit for human consumption can be found only in the rainwater, inland surface water bodies like rivers, lakes, ponds and underground water from wells and handpumps.[11]

Until very recent times, most people took water for granted—as free, on nearly so, and certainly inexhaustible. But a long with the rapidly increasing population and greed of people have led to severe water shortages. And because people are spread widely over the world, water must be transported long distances to supply their needs.

Since water resources are limited, this trend of increasing use creates considerable pressure on declining water supplies. Further quality of water is also deteriorating because on increased levels of pollution and increases in salinity.[12]

The ground water is exploited by tube wells causing its level go down and hence potable water is becoming a problem. In villages and cities, water is obtained through wells, which may be shallow—(water above the first impervious layer), Deep wells (Below the first imperious layer) and tube wells run mechanically or electrically.

The order to avoid the wells or surface water from contamination, we should make wells on an elevated area at least 15-20 meters away from source of contamination and we should not urinate or put night soils near the well. The environment of wells and tube well need to protect scientifically to obtain potable water supply. There is also need of disinfecting wells frequently through chlorination and in the days of epidemics, it must be done on every night. Even chlorine tablets of 05 gram are available to make 20 litres of water clean.

Water purification is done through sedimentation, filtration, chlorination ozonation, ultraviolet irradiation, etc. The water is not completely purified because of less use of material or material of sub-standard quality.

The standards for drinking water take into account the following constituents in determining the quality and make water free of them through treatments.

- Microbiological pollutants: bacteria, viruses, etc.;
- Toxic substances: arsenic, cadmium, cyanide, lead, mercury, selenium, etc.;
- Specific substances affecting health: fluorides, nitrates, poly-nuclear aromatic hydrocarbons;
- Acceptability of water colour, odour, hardness and taste or water; and
- Radio-active substances.

No matter how it is accomplished, keeping water pure enough to be usable has become expensive. Clean water in the future will undoubtedly account for a large percentage of money, but the investment in clean water contributes greatly to public health. Clean water is a people's issue. Because of corrupt practices, clean water even in beautiful city like Chandigarh has become a remote possibility.[13]

WATER QUALITY ASSESSMENT AUTHORITY

The problem of pollution of national water resources has become a matter of serious concern in India. To circumvent the situation on the advice of Ministry of Water Resources (MoWR), the Ministry of Environment and Forests (MOEF), Constituted the "Water Quality Assessment Authority (WQAA)" with effect from 29 May 2001 for the purpose of performing the powers and functions enumerated therein to protect the quality of National Water Resources. The 12-member Authority is headed by the Secretary, Ministry of Environment and Forests as the Chairman and the Commissioner (Water Management), MoWR as the Member Secretary.[14]

Drinking water supply and Sanitation are State subjects, included in the Eleventh Schedule of the constitution among the subjects that may be entrusted to Panchayats by the States. The Government of India supplement efforts made by the States by providing financial and technical assistance under the two centrally sponsored programmes, namely, the Accelerated Rural Water Supply Programme (ARWSP) and the Central Rural Sanitation Programme (CRSP).

Substantial investment to the tune of about Rs. 50,000 crore has been made in the rural water supply sector alone by the Central and State Governments since 1st Five Year Plan in approx. 37 lakh hand Jumps and 1.45 lakh piped water supply schemes, crediting the country with one of the largest rural drinking water supply networks in the world. While significant achievement has been made in terms of providing access to potable drinking water with 5.34% rural habitations fully covered and another 28% partially covered, the sanitation coverage in rural areas continues to be a challenge, with only 22% of the rural population having access to basic sanitation, as per the 200I Census.

A national water supply and sanitation programme was introduced in the social sector in country in 1954. The Government of India provided assistance to the States to establish special investigation divisions in the Fourth Five Year Plan to many out identification of problem villages. Taking into account the magnitude of the problem, and to accelerate the pace of coverage of problem villages, the Government of India introduced the Accelerated Rural Water Supply Programme (ARWSP) in 1972-73 to assist States and Union Territories with 100% grants-in-aid to implement drinking water supply schemes in such villages. The entire programme was given a Mission approach when the Technology Mission on Drinking Water Management, called the National Drinking Water Mission (NDWM), was Introduced as one of the five Missions in social sector in 1986. NDWM was renamed as Rajiv Gandhi National Drinking Water Mission (RGNDWM) in 1991. During the International Water and Sanitation Decade in 1980s, Central Rural Sanitation Programme (CRSP) was launched in 1986 in the Ministry of Rural Development to accelerate sanitation coverage in rural areas with the objective of improving quality of life of the rural people and also to provide privacy and dignity to women.

Presently Rajiv Gandhi National Drinking Water Mission (RGNDWM), Department of Drinking Water Supply, Ministry of Rural Development administers the Centrally Sponsored programmes in Rural Drinking Water Supply and Rural Sanitation sectors.

The Xth Plan accords the highest priority to providing the Not Covered (NC) habitations with sustainable and stipulated supply of drinking water.

It is envisaged to cover all the rural habitations including those which might have been slipped back to NC/PC category by the end of Xth Plan. The Tenth Plan emphasizes the participatory approach where PRIs should be the key institutions for convergence of drinking water supply programmes at the ground level. Considerable success has been achieved in meeting drinking water needs of the rural population and 95.34% rural habitations are Fully Covered with stipulated level drinking water facilities. The Partially covered habitations are 4.28%. The Not Covered habitations are about 0.38%. As per the latest report from the States/UTs, the coverage status as on 1.11.2004 based on comprehensive Action Plan, 1999 and coverage reported by States/UTs.

Thereafter is as under:

Type of coverage	*No. of habitations*	*Percentage of total*
Not Covered (NC)	5368	0.38
Partially Covered (PC)	60884	4.28
Fully Covered (FC)	1356031	95.34
Uninhabitated migrated	381	
Total	1422664	

Statement showing State-wise coverage position is given at Annexure XL/II.

The strategy to achieve the Tenth Plan objectives can be briefly summarized as Accelerating coverage of the remaining Not Covered and Partially Covered habitations, including those slipped back from Fully Covered to Partially and Not Covered categories, with safe drinking water systems.

- To tackle problems of water quality in affected habitations and to institutionalize water quality monitoring and surveillance systems.
- To promote sustainability, both of systems and sources, to ensure continued supply of safe drinking water in covered habitations.

The quality problems of drinking water both due to geogenic factors leading to chemical contamination like excess fluoride, arsenic, iron, salinity, nitrate, etc. and anthropogenic factors resulting in bacteriological contamination, pose serious public health problems. Water Quality survey data has revealed 2,16,968 quality affected habitations, with the following break-up: excess Fluoride—31,306, excess Arsenic—5,029 excess Salinity—23,495, excess iron—1,18,088, excess Nitrate—13,958 and Multiple reasons—25,092. Water quality has to be ensured through a comprehensive surveillance process, incorporating monitoring data processing, evaluation sanitary surveys, public health assessment and remedial and reventive action throughout the length and breadth of the country. Separate Sub-Mission programmes have been part of the ARWSP to address specific quality problems. The Department has finalized a Water Quality Monitoring and surveillance programme on Catchment Area approach by Utilizing the available district and sub-district level rater-testing infrastructure in educational institution and private and suitable capacity development PRIs and other villages level functionaries.

Despite respectable coverage in terms of access to drinking water proper upkeep of water supply themes has been a problem. Many factors like sources going dry increase in quality problems systems becoming defunct due to poor maintenance demand from other competing sectors like culture industry, etc. pose threat to sustainability of drinking water supply schemes. Putting in place an effective operation and maintenance system calls for huge investments. The total estimated cost of operation and maintenance of the water supply networks created so far is estimated at Rs. 6750 crore per annum whereas the total funds being utilized for O&M purposes under ARWSP are approx. 5.450 crore only. As such, as a part of the strategy to ensure sustainability of systems, reforms were introduced in 1999 with approval of the Cabinet which meant a paradigm shift from supply driven, norms based, centralized form of funding to one based on the principles of demand responsiveness, community leadership and decentralized mode of management.

Initially, the reforms were introduced in 67 pilot districts as Sector Reform Projects. Based on the experience gained, the reforms initiative was scaled throughout the country by launching Swajaldhara December 2002.

Unlike Sector Reform Projects, which had district as the unit for implementation. Swajaldhard themes can be implemented by the Beneficiary group, Gram Panchayat, Block Panchayat or District Panchayat. All the States across the country are implementing Swajaldhara schemes now. Under the Sector Reform and Swajaldhara, the individual water supply schemes are planned, designed, implemented, operated and maintained by the community through the village level committees. A major thrust of the reforms initiative in the rural water supply sector is on empowerment of Panchayati Raj system, for not only operating and maintaining drinking water schemes but also managing the entire rural water supply sector.

During the Ninth Plan period special initiative was taken to cover rural habitations with proper sanitation. The CRSP was restructured in

1999 with a provision for phasing out the allocation-based component by the end of the IXth Plan, i.e. 2001-02. The total Sanitation Campaign (TSC) under the restructured CRSP was launched with effect from 1.4.1999 following a community led and people centered approach. TSC moves away from the principle of state-wise allocation to a "demand-driven" approach. The programme gives emphasis on Information, Education and Communication (IEC) for demand generation of sanitation facilities and offering a wide range of technological choices of sanitation hardware through an effective delivery mechanism of Rural Sanitary Mart and Production Centre to meet the demand for sanitation facilities so generated. It also lays emphasis on school sanitation and hygiene education for bringing about attitudinal and behavioural changes for relevant sanitation and hygiene practices from young age.

SCHEMES OF RURAL WATER SUPPLY

I. Accelerated Rural Water Supply Programme (ARWSP)

Objectives

- To ensure coverage of all rural habitations with access to safe drinking water;
- To ensure sustainability of drinking water systems and sources;
- To tackle the problem of water quality in affected habitations; and
- To institutionalise the reform initiative in rural drinking water supply sector.

Rural water supply is a State subject. States have been taking up projects and schemes for the provision of safe drinking water from their own resources. However, recognising the importance of providing safe drinking water in rural habitations, Government of India has been providing financial assistance to State Governments under the Centrally Sponsored Scheme, "Accelerated Rural Water Supply Programme (ARWSP)."

Coverage Norms

- Ipcd of drinking water for human beings;
- 30 Ipcd of additional water for cattle in areas under the DDP;
- One handpump or standpost for every 250 persons; and
- Availability of water source in the habitation or within 1.6 km in the plains and 100 metres elevation in hilly areas.

Funding Pattern

(i) Under ARWSP, funds are provided to States for making provision of safe drinking water in rural habitations. 15% of these funds can be spent on operation and maintenance (O&M) of the existing drinking water systems and sources. State Governments should match funds released by this Department on 1: 1 basis.

(ii) Upto 20 per cent of the funds can be utilized by the State Governments: (a) to take up projects under the Sub-Mission programme to tackle water quality problems like fluorosis, arsenic, brackishness, etc., and (b) to ensure source sustainability by conserving water, recharging aquifers, etc.

Out of this, 15% should be utilised for projects for quality and 5% for projects for sustainability of sources. Funding is done in the ratio of 3: 1 between Central and State Governments.

(iii) 20 per cent of the annual outlay of ARWSP have been earmarked for implementation of reforms-oriented Swajaldhara and Sector Reform projects. The funding pattern for these projects is 90% from Government of India and 10% by way of community contribution.

(iv) About 5 per cent of the annual allocation is also earmarked to States covered by Desert Development Programme (DDP) under ARWSP. This is funded as 100% Central grant to the States.

(v) Further, to meet the contingencies arising due to natural calamities and emergent situation, 5% of the ARWSP allocation is earmarked. This is funded at 100% grant from the Central Government.

(vi) In pursuance of the announcement made by the then Prime Minister on 15.8.2002 three programmes viz. Installation of one lakh Hand Pumps providing drinking water facilities to one lakh rural Primary Schools and revival of one lakh traditional sources of water. The programmes will be completed in two years, 2003-04 and 2004-05.

Implementing Agencies

State Governments side the implementing agencies for the programme. The agencies may be the Public Health and Engineering Department (PHED), Rural Development Department or the Panchayati Raj Department. Implementation is also taken up by the Government Boards/ Nigams/Agencies in a few States, for example, the Gujarat Water Supply and Sewerage Board is the implementing agency in Gujarat, Uttar Pradesh Jal Nigam is the agency in Uttar Pradesh and Tamil Nadu Water and Drainage Board in Tamil Nadu.

Financial Progress

Government of India and State Governments have so far invested about Rs. 50,000 crore on rural drinking water supply schemes. The Central outlay for the Rural Water Supply Sector for 2004-05 is Rs. 2900.00 crore, which is likely to increase to Rs. 3148.00 crores through supplementary grant.

State-wise allocation of funds and releases made under ARWSP (Normal), ARWSP (DDP), Swajaldhara and three programmes of Prime Minister (as on 31.1.05) may be seen at Annexures XLIV, XLV, XLVI and XLVII respectively.

Delegation of Power

Keeping in view the concept of decentralisation of power, Government of India has delegated powers to States. All projects and schemes proposed under ARWSP are approved by the State Level Scheme Sanctioning Committee. Under Sector Reforms Pilot Projects, powers to plan and implement projects and schemes have been delegated to the community, who will also own, operate and maintain the systems. The community also has the power to choose the systems of their preferences. As per the Guidelines issued in June 2003 the District Water and Sanitation Committees are empowered to sanction projects under Swajaldhara.

Role of Panchayats

As per the 73rd Amendment to the Constitution of India, the subject of rural water supply vests with the Panchayati Raj Institutions (PRIs). The Panchayats are to play major role in providing safe drinking water and managing the systems and sources in their respective areas. They can be involved in the implementation of schemes, particularly in selecting the location of hand pumps, standposts and spot sources; in Operation and Maintenance (O&M), etc. Moreover, Government of India emphasis on empowering and capacity building of the PRIs to enable them for discharging their responsibilities in drinking water supply.

North-Eastern States: The States of the North-East have been facing problems to meet State matching share against central releases in the past.

As a result arrears of matching share has been accumulated. The Department of Drinking Water Supply has given maximum financial flexibility in the guidelines for implementation of Rural Water Supply Programme in respect of North-Eastern States in view of the fact that 10% of the total Central outlay for the programme is earmarked for the NE States. To ensure that the unutilized funds released to North-Eastern States are not lapsed, a Non-lapsable control Pool of Resources has been created. Any unutilised funds of Government of India share are credited in to this Pool under which the State Governments can take up various projects.

Sub-Mission programmes of the Government of India were launched with the objective to provide safe drinking water facilities in rural habitations affected by water quality problems like fluorosis, arsenic, brackishness, excess iron, nitrate, etc. The States undertakes these projects. For ensuring source sustainability through rainwater harvesting, artificial recharge, etc. State Governments also use funds under Sub-Mission. Quality problems in groundwater are of two types, viz. chemical and biological. It is inherent in the form of contamination caused by the nature of the geological formation.

Excess fluoride, arsenic, iron or brackishness fall under this category. Groundwater pollution is also caused by human intervention (biological contamination).

It has been noticed that groundwater depletion has aggravated water quality problems due to excess fluoride arsenic and brackishness in certain areas. This gets manifested in the form of various diseases like floozies and arsenical dermatitis. This has forced the State Governments to abandon low-cost handpumps preferring costly piped water supply schemes.

Central Assistance under Sub-Mission Programme

Control assistance is extended to States for the following:

- Approved capital cost of treatment plants desalination, defluoridation, arsenic; and Iron removal;
- O&M cost of desalination plants;
- Cost of water conservation measures;
- Cost of holding awareness camps epidemiological surveys and water quality testing;
- Water testing laboratories non-recurring cost of equipment and recurring cost on technical staff, chemicals, etc., and
- Mobile water quality testing laboratories.

20 per cent of ARWSP funds are earmarked and utilized new projects under the Sub-Mission activities. However, if the States/UTs have achieved full coverage of habitations as per the national norms, they may utilise more funds to tackle quality problems subject to Government of India concurrence. Priority is given to the NC and PC habitations which are also affected by quality problems. In order to assess the ground position with regard to quality problems. water quality survey was conducted. As per the information furnished by the State Governments, the following number of habitations were affected with quality problems of drinking water shown on next page.

The Department has prepared a concept paper on tackling the water quality problem. It is estimated that Rs. 10,000 crore as the Central share are required to tackle water quality problem. The project has been posed for World Bank funding.

Even though the coverage has been impressive over the last decade, various studies indicate that there is no institutionalized quality monitoring and surveillance system in the country. This is going to be critical to the entire water supply sector in the future owing to increase in pollution and depletion of water sources. The National Workshop held on 7-9 August, 1997 recommended that there is a need to institutionalise water quality monitoring and surveillance systems in the country. Establishing of water quality labs could be only one of the components of the programme. A "Catchment Area Approach" would be adopted by involving various grass-root level educational and technical institutions by utilising existing resources and strengthening them by providing additional financial resources to these institutions. This may be implemented at three levels consisting of a Nodal Unit at the top level catchment like a premier technical institution, university, etc., intermediary level units like district laboratories, polytechnics, etc. and grass-root level units like (+2) level education institutions, labs., etc. Activities relating to preliminary water testing, etc. could be carried out at the grass-root level itself and more complicated cases could be referred to higher levels in such a way that only focussed cases of complex nature and of value and utility at State level reach the nodal unit. The nodal units will be networked with the State headquarters (PHED). 100% funding, as per the approved norms, would be provided to the States for strengthening water quality monitoring facilities, based on projects received from the State Governments. Restructuring the State PHEDs with the required grant-in-aid support, as indicated in para 3.7, to bring in the much missed link up with the Health authorities will also be attempted as a part of institutionalising the monitoring system. Health Department officials will be increasingly involved in the surveillance activity.

Nature or Quality problem habitations	*No. or affected*
Excess Fluoride	31306
Excess Arsenic	5029
Excess Salinity	23495
Excess Iron	118088
Excess Nitrate	13958
Multiple	25092
Total	216968

A programme for water quality monitoring and surveillance system has been finalized in consultation with Ministry of Health and Family Welfare. The system will be implemented through a National Level, and State Level Referral Institutions. National Institute of Communicable Diseases (NICD) has given consent to act as National Level Water Quality Referral Institution. Manual on Catchment Area Approach has been finalised. Information on district level WQ Testing Laboratories, listing problems in their functioning and listing of alternative facilities is under compilation. Many States have already identified State Referral Institutes and matter is being pursued with the remaining.

Sustainability

This is an important Sub-Mission for the success of water supply schemes on a long-term basis. Central Ground Water Board (CGWB) and National Geophysical Research Institute (NGRI) have been engaged in the programme since the inception of the Mission. Further State Governments have been advised that up to 5 per cent of the funds released under ARWSP should be used for Sub-Mission—

- Reasons for taking up sustainability in drinking water sector:
- Fast depletion of groundwater level leading to quality problems like arsenic and fluorosis;
- Sources go dry due to deforestation, leading to reduced recharge of aquifers;
- Poor maintenance of the existing water supply systems;
- Non-participation of people in the operations and maintenance of the systems; and
- Neglect of traditional water management practices and systems.

In order to overcome these problems, Government of India aims to concentrate on: (a) control on over extraction of groundwater; (b) funds for repairs and rehabilitation; (c) emphasis on community participation; (d) promotion of water as a socio-economic good; and (e) stronger links with watershed development programmes.

Further, the following action has also been taken by the Department of Drinking Water Supply for source sustainability:

- Ministry of Urban Development has been requested to make rainwater-harvesting structures mandatory for urban constructions;
- Ministry of Water Resources has been requested to promote water-harvesting measures;
- All MPs have been requested to encourage/take up water harvesting schemes from their Local Area Development Fund;
- Technical Manual on Water Harvesting and Artificial Recharge has been finalized;
- A CD indicating different models of rainwater harvesting has been prepared and circulated to the States for wider dissemination;
- A model bill for Legislation by States to promote rainwater harvesting is being finalized in consultation with Ministry of Law; and
- For finding household, community and institution level rainwater harvesting structure, bankable schemes have been worked and are being finalised in consultation with the States.

Sector Reform

It has been realised that to strengthen the socio-economic conditions of rural India, mere administrative decentralisation or increased investment is not enough. The power of people's participation has been recognised and brought to therefore. Despite good investments, and improvement in the rural water supply and increased outlay by the Government, particularly in the last one decade, general satisfaction is rather limited at the community level. Earlier emphasis was laid on hand-pumps fitted to tube-wells and bore-wells had resulted in an impressive increase in the total rural water supply coverage. However, the availability of potable drinking water in rural areas, especially during the summer months is still not satisfactory. Though about lakh habitations are covered every year, the number of problem habitations has not declined proportionately. Hence, Government of India realized that sustainability of sources and system is key to people's satisfaction. Systems are falling idle and into disrepair. This is due to the perception of the rural people that water is a social right to be provided by the Government, free of cost.

The Government tried to drive home the principles that water is an economic and social good and should be treated as such. It should be managed at the lowest appropriate with users involved in the planning and implementation of projects. With this aim in view, Government of India has brought about policy changes by introducing reforms in the rural drinking water supply sector. ARWSP was improved in April 1999 to include proposals to mobilize community participation in rural water supply programmes, and 20 per cent of the annual outlay has been earmarked for providing funds for such projects.

This shift envisages demand-responsive approach, community participation and decentralisation of powers for implementing and operating drinking water supply schemes. To ensure people's participation, the Central Government is following three basic principles:

- Adoption of a demand-responsive and adaptable approach based on empowerment of villagers to ensure their full participation in the project through a decision-making role in the choice of scheme design control of finances and management arrangements;
- Shifting role of government from direct service delivery to that of planning policy formulation monitoring and evaluation and partial financial support; and
- Partial capital cost sharing either in cash or kind or both and 100 per cent responsibility of O&M by the users.

Accordingly, on a pilot basis, Sector Reform projects were sanctioned in 67 pilot districts across the country for implementation. Based on the demand-generated the total estimated project outlay of Sector Reform Pilot Projects was only Rs. 1328.38 crore. These pilot projects will enable the community to plan sanction partially fund, and implement, operate, maintain and replace Rural Water Supply Schemes of their choice. In order to instill a sense of ownership in the project, the community has to contribute at least 10% of the capital cost either in cash or kind (labour, land or material). The community will also shoulder the entire O&M cost.

In this new approach the government plays the role of a facilitator. Efforts are being made to create awareness through Information Education and Communication (IEC) amongst the people about the need for their effective participation in this programme. The community should be willing to be involved in the implementation of the water supply schemes for which they should have a feeling of ownership of the assets created. With the experience gained from Sector Reform pilot projects the reform process has now been extended to the entire country by launching Swajaldhara programme on 25.12.2002.

COMMUNITY PARTICIPATION

Background

Water is today perceived by the rural public as a social right to be provided free by the Government, rather than as a scarce resource which must be managed locally as a socio-economic good in order to ensure its effective use. This perception has been grown out of the fact that the present rural water supply systems are designed and executed by the Department/ Boards and, imposed on end-users. Demand preferences of the people are not taken into account while executing the schemes. In other words, rural water supply programme till now has been adopting a supply driven approach. Experience has shown that the present approach has led to the failure of a large number of water supply systems/schemes due to poor operation and maintenance.

Now that substantial investment has been made in the sector and huge infrastructure and systems built up, it is paramount that they are made functional to a great degree to achieve sustainability. There is a general recognition that a transformation from a target-based, supply-driven approach which pays little attention to the actual practices and/or preferences of the end users, to a demand-based approach where users get the service they want and are willing to pay for is urgently required. Implementation of a participatory demand-driven approach will ensure that the public obtain the level of service they desire and can afford to pay. Further, full cost recovery of operations and maintenance and replacement costs will ensure the financial viability and sustainability of the schemes. The conditions under which people would be willing to maintain and operate water supply schemes are:

- If they own the assets,
- If they have themselves installed the handpump, or being actively involved throughout,

- If they have been trained to do simple repairs,
- If they know the government will not maintain the asset,
- If they have sufficient funds for maintenance, and
- If they have to pay for O&M.

Hence, it is possible to institutionalise community-based rural drinking water supply programme if the Panchayati Raj Institutions/local communities are empowered to generate resources and are trained and equipped to plan, implement, use, maintain and replace water supply schemes themselves in coordination with the Government agencies/Private Sector/NGOs.

Swajaldhara

The Government of India has been emphasizing the need for taking up community-based rural water supply programmes and with this end in view a beginning was made in 1999 by sanctioning Sector Reform Pilot Projects on experimental basis. With the experience gained, the reforms initiatives in the rural drinking water supply sector has now been opened up throughout the country by launching the Swajaldhara programme on 25.12.2002. The key Principles of the programme are:

Principles of Swajaldhara

- adoption of demand responsive, adaptable approach along with community participation based on empowerment of villages to ensure their full participation in the project through a decision-making role in the choice of the drinking water scheme, planning, design, implementation, control of finances and management arrangements;
- full ownership of drinking water assets with appropriate level of panchayats;
- panchayats/communities to have the powers to plan, implement, operate, maintain and manage all Water Supply and Sanitation schemes;
- partial capital cost sharing either in cash or kind including labour or both, 100% responsibility of operation and maintenance by the users;
- an integrated service delivery mechanism;
- taking up conservation measures through rain water harvesting and ground water recharge systems for sustained drinking water supply; and
- shifting the role of Government from direct service delivery to that of planning, policy formulation, monitoring and evaluation, and partial financial support.

As per the guidelines issued in June 2003, Swajaldhara will have two Dharas. First Dhara (Swajaldhara I) will be for a Gram Panchayat (GP) or a group of GPs or an intermediate panchayat (at Block/Tehsil level) and the second Dhara (Swajaldhara-II) will have a district as the project area.

Funds under Swajaldhara are now allocated to the States/UTs and the allocated amount is intimated to the States/UTs. The States/UTs make district-wise allocation and furnish the details to the Department of Drinking Water Supply. On receipt of such information, the funds are released directly to SWSM/DP/DWSM by Department of Drinking Water Supply.

Three Programmes of the Prime Minister

The Honourable Prime Minister in his Independence Day Address (15.8.2002) announced three programmes viz. Installation of one lakh hand pumps, providing drinking water facilities to one lakh Primary Schools and revival of one lakh traditional sources of water. Thereafter EFC memo for the programmes was prepared and the case was processed for Cabinet Approval. CCEA gave the approval in June 2003. The guidelines for implementation of the programmes have since been prepared and circulated to all the states. The programme is to be completed in two years, i.e. 2003-05. The total cost involved is Rs. 800 crore have been made.[15]

Providing Community Water Supplies

To promote community health an easily accessible water supply should be available that provides sufficient safe water to meet community needs. Household water needs can be estimated by questioning community member about their daily water use. If this is not possible, a minimum water need can be circulated by assuming that the average person uses 25 litres per day for drinking, cooking and personal hygiene. More water will be needed for laundry, but this may be available from other sources such as rivers or ponds.

To ensure that the water is potable, either the water supply should be protected the water should be treated before use. Low-risk water supplies for drinking and other domestic uses can be provided to communities in many ways. Often, unprotected water sources, such as springs, traditional wells and ponds, can be improved and this may be preferable to constructing completely supplies. However, unprotected sources are open to contamination and pose a potential health risk. Community hygiene programmes should therefore promote the use of protected drinking-water sources.

Characteristics of Low-risk Water Sources

- The water source is fully enclosed or protected (capped) and no surface water can run directly into it.
- People do not step into the water while collecting it.
- Latrines are located as far away as possible from the water source

and preferably not on higher ground. If there are community concerns about this, expert advice should be sought.

- Solid waste pits, animal excreta and other pollution sources are located as far as possible from the water source.
- There is no stagnant water within 5 metres of the water source.
- If wells are used, the collection buckets are kept clean and off the ground or a handpump is used.

When resources are limited, it may be necessary to decide whether greater emphasis should be placed on the quality of the water, or on its availability. Where sufficient safe water for all is not immediately available, intermediate steps should target the provision of larger quantities of lower-quality water. Deciding on an acceptable level of contamination is difficult and depends on the willingness of community members to pay increased costs for better water, as well as on their willingness to treat water within the home. If payment is required for water use, it must be affordable to the whole community. In only case, water with high levels of contamination, particularly with faces, should never be used. Local health officials should be consulted about the quality of water provided and the level of health risk.

Many rural water supply programmes aim to develop water sources that can be fully managed by users, with only limited additional support from local government. While this can make a sense of community ownership more achievable, it also require communities to make long-term commitments, such as maintenance of improved water sources, and even to contribute financial towards their construction This means that it is important to involve communities during all stages of development of the improved water sources, from initial planning and implementation to long-term management. Community members should be actively involved in selecting the type of water supply they receive and have access to information that allows them to make informed decisions. However, discussions must be balanced and should also consider what the supporting agency considers feasible, not simply what the community desires. On the other hand, solutions chosen solely by outside agencies are more likely to fail.

From the outset it is also essential that community members are fully aware of the short and long-term implications of their choices, for while it is relatively easy to build an improved water supply sustaining, it is often a major problem. For example, boreholes with hand pumps are often recommended to communities, but this technology requires relatively expensive maintenance, and access to spare parts and tools is essential. In one country, spares for handpumps were available only in the capital city, a two- or three-day journey for remote communities. As a result, the hand pumps were likely to fail in a very short time and the investment would have been wasted.[16]

K. Pandimurga Chinnan in his article, "No Fresh Water—No Future" in *Yojana*, Vol. 48, Feb. 2004 clearly indicated the essential steps for tackling water crises.

The main constraints that are faced in the water sector are inadequate trained personnel, inability to mobilise internal and external resources, inadequate project preparation, uncoordinated development approach, institutional weakness, technological shortcomings, poor quality of water resources itself, water losses through leakage intermittent services, haphazard garbage collection and disposal systems, inadequate drainage of surface run off, non-involvement of community in project planning development, operation and maintenance activities, etc. The following suggestions for solving the water crisis are given below:

- A large share of water to meet new demands must come by saving water from existing uses through comprehensive reform of water policy.
- New strategies for water development and management are urgently needed to avert severe national, regional and local water scarcities that will depress agricultural production, damage the environment and escalate water-related health problems.
- Major institutional policy and technological initiatives are required to ensure efficient socially equitable and environmentally suitable management of water resources.
- In facing the enormous challenge of meeting the requirements of water supply for domestic irrigation and industrial uses it is natural to expect that the R&D sector should play an important rule.
- Since a major portion of water resources are used in agriculture the farmer's co-operation is a must in the process of water management at all levels. An efficient irrigated cropping system also can sustain India's large and expanding population. During the years of poor monsoon, the farmer can go in for crops demanding less irrigation such as gram, barley and mustard during the rabi system.
- Attention should be paid by researchers and extension personnel in increasing the production per unit area/per unit of water in agriculture.
- Water management programmes should be implemented in a systematic way with integrated coordination of all relevant government departments at State and Central level. There is a need for revision of water legislation/ground water control regulation acts to maintain water table at a reasonable depth for sustainability.
- Clearcut water rights system is indispensable for the sustainability of our agriculture.

- Integrated watershed development actions have to be taken to use rainwater, soil water, ground water and run off water to increase production in rainfed areas.
- A data base should be created among all water boards and corporations for effective transfer of best practices.
- Immediate steps should be taken for drastic reduction of wastage of water in all sectors and protection of water sources from industrial pollution.
- The beneficiaries role should be modified from passive recipients to active participants in water conservation activities. As woman know better all the matters related to water, participation even from the selection of the site for water projects to the maintenance is important.
- Above all, a strong political will of government to frame appropriate water policy and equally important indomitable conscience of water users to utilize water judiciously are absolutely necessary for sustainable utilization of water.

CRITICAL APPRAISAL

I. Need of Sectoral Reforms

Provisions of high quality and sustainable drinking water services for all the citizens, particularly the rural poor, is critical to enhance the economic productivity of any nation. Supply of safe and quality drinking water to the rural community remains a significant issue in the governance in India. The traditional approach for implementing programmes for supply of drinking water in rural areas was top-driven, the result being that the community involvement was minimal and the problems of providing drinking water in all villages could not be addressed fully. What were needed, therefore, were reforms in this sector and a new programme, namely, Sector Reforms Project (SRP), was introduced by the Government of India.

The Rajiv Gandhi National Drinking Water Mission introduced the Sector Reforms Project in selected districts of the country in 1999. The Project envisaged community participation in creating and maintaining drinking water sources and sanitation facilities. It redefined the role of the government from being a "provider" to that of a "facilitation." The Project was to be driven by demand originating from within the community in contrast to the erstwhile practice of thrusting a source on the community without involving them.

Reforms Objectives

The Sector Reforms Project envisaged mission approach and emphasized creation of institutions that are relatively more independent and focused. The basic approach was "decentralized governance." Some of the objectives of Mission were:

(a) Increasing community participation and creating awareness the water is a resource, which has to be paid for.

(b) The operational and maintenance aspects of the source created would be the responsibility of the community.

(c) The community needs to consider imposition of user charges for maintenance of the source.

(d) Full freedom to the villagers in the selection of a water source and its implementation.

(e) Gender sensitive approach towards drinking water problems.

(f) Emphasis on quality of drinking water and reliability of the reforms.[17]

2. Sustainability

The Government has accorded the highest priority to rural drinking water for ensuring universal access as a part of policy framework to achieve the goal of reaching the unreached. Despite installation of more than 3.5 million hand-pumps and over 116 thousand piped water supply schemes, in many parts of the country, the people face water scarcity almost every year thereby meaning that our water supply systems are failing to sustain, despite huge investments. The examination of sustainability issues of drinking water supply as well as systems has, therefore, become imperative.

World Bank, in its Review Report (1998), has made the following findings of much interest on India's Water Resources Management Sector:

(i) Water is becoming an increasingly scarce resource in India, its finite and fragile water resources are depleting, yet it continues to be used inefficiently on a daily basis in all sectors, while various sectoral demands are growing rapidly.

(ii) The Current approach emphasizes development of water resources and construction of new infrastructure under a top-down, supply-oriented and fragmentary framework.

(iii) The present institutional arrangement in India, including central, state and local institutions, and both formal and informal structures, do not enable comprehensive water allocation, planning and management.

(iv) Existing organisations, furthermore, lack capacity in key management areas as well as effective mechanisms for implementation.

(v) Appropriate economic incentives for efficient water use and conservation are lacking on various levels, thereby impacting negatively on water provision and usage in these sub-sectors.

(vi) The absence of appropriate direct water pricing, and lack of adequate application of other economic and financial incentives at the sub-sector level has also served as an obstacle to the smooth transfer of water between sectors and states.

(vii) Supporting technological and informational systems, to enable effective planning and management of water are also weak.

(viii) The current situation in water service delivery in India is, in general, characterized by a vicious circle of inadequate financial allocations to the sector (particularly for O&M) and inefficient and bloated service institutions, which have led to poor quality and unreliable services, user dissatisfaction with their services, and an unwillingness of users to pay for those services. The inadequate resources generated by the sector due to low prices and user unwillingness to pay for services further undermine sector financial resources contributing to a perpetuation of the circle. The end result is a sector that has become unsustainable.

(ix) The vicious cycle of the drinking water sectors (both rural and urban) varies due to the varied and desegregated institutional structures that make up the RWSS and UWSS sub-sectors within the states in India.

Further, GWSS, Assessment Report—2000 identified similar sector constraints viz. (i) financial difficulties, (ii) institutional problems, (iii) inadequate human resources, (iv) lack of sector coordinating, (v) lack of political commitment, (vi) insufficient community involvement, (vii) inadequate O&M, (viii) poor water quality, (ix) insufficient information and communication and lack of hygiene education are equally applicable to India.

Acknowledging the necessity to involve local community or community-based organisation for sustainability of the systems, the following necessary elements are identified:

- Community mobilization and capacity building.
- Community share in the capital investment.
- Community ownership and control.
- O&M and management by the community.
- Dependable water source to meet community needs.

Having achieved appreciable physical coverage of habitations with water supply system through the normal "supply-driven" and "cent per cent Government funded" programme, it is now, high time to reorient the programme-approach. The present water resources scenario is critical, especially the status of ground water exploration and availability is causing a lot of concern. Apart from the severe threat to sustainability of the sources due to indiscriminate ground water use, water quality problem has emerged as a major issue adding a new dimension. Taking into account all the constraints relating to proper management and conservation and protection of ground water source *vis-a-vis* the action needed to be taken at different levels, a multi-pronged integrated approach with a well conceived mix of professional, technical, administrative and legal aspects with a focus on "community-based-demand-responsive approach would pave the way for making sustainable rural drinking water supply in the country.

Providing safe and adequate water to the people is one of the several challenges that our country is encountering. The problem is particularly severe in rural areas. Government has been addressing this as a priority issue since the commencement of the first five year plan. An overview of the rural water sector indicates that still a lot needs to be done. The problem is multi-dimensional and area specific in nature. Several factors like increased urbanization, negligence of traditional water sources, poor water management, resource depletion due to over exploitation of existing resources, lack of co-ordination between departments and poor institutional set-up in addressing the problem have led to the severity of the problem over the years. It is important to understand the existing situation and the complexities in order to address the problem in the context of project design and implementation and factors affecting sustainability of Rural Water Supply (RWS) programmes. Sustainability through water conservation and water management is seen as the best option.[18]

3. Poor Availability

The annual per capita availability of freshwater in 1951 was 5,177 cubic meters, that declined to 1,869 cubic meters in 2001. It is likely to fall further to 1,341 cubic meters in 2025, and in 2050, it will be 1,140 cubic meters. It is generally presumed that if per capita level falls to 1,000 cubic meters, it could seriously affect the health and economic activity of the entire country. At this level, water crisis will be seen in 25 percent of India's geographical area, affecting 21 percent of the total population. Already, 5.5 percent of the country's geographical area and 7.6 percent of the population are facing acute water shortage, with availability less than 500 cubic meters.[19]

4. Poor Quality of Water

"Lack of reliable data, however, makes it difficult to appreciate the magnitude and impact of the crippling and incurable diseases like fluorosis and arsenical dermatitis. Fluoride contamination affects districts in 15 states and excess arsenic affects 8 districts of West Bengal. Fluoride levels are high in Andhra Pradesh, Gujarat, Haryana, Karnataka, Punjab, Rajasthan, Tamil Nadu and U.P. and iron levels are high in the north-eastern and eastern part of the country. Similarly, salinity is high in Gujarat, Haryana, Karnataka, Punjab, Rajasthan and Tamil Nadu. The number of quality affected habitations with excess fluoride/arsenic/salinity/iron, etc. is about 1.54 lakh.

Towards following up the quality problems as outlined, a large number of district water testing laboratories have been established in Panchayat Raj Engineering Department in different States under an elaborate action plan of the RGNDWM. In the present socio-economic condition, reaching the vast rural areas of the country with decentralized water quality-monitoring programme is an almost impossible task and the formidable problem is to bring water samples from the remote parts of the districts to the labs. Although samples may be collected and brought to the labs for examination, pooling them at one place for subsequent transportation is extremely difficult. Also, to collect and bring samples regularly for chemical/bacteriological quality assessment has also been not easy because of storage problems.

Therefore, there is need for introducing simple bacteriological quality assessment tests such as the H2S Strip test, which can be done by people themselves. Routine quality assessment (both chemical and bacteriological) can be done in the local field labs that may be established in schools or PHCs.

Research studies in 144 countries by Esrey and Nookes (1992-93) show that interventions like Safe Disposal of Excreta; Household and personal hygiene, Quantity and quality of water can make significant difference in the overall health and quality of life of people, especially that of children.

A Status of Water Quality

Providing safe water has been one the major focuses in the recent years with the increasing levels of contamination observed in the ground water sources. Under the National Drinking Water Mission by the Government of India, a submission on water quality monitoring is integrated as a part of drinking water supply programme. Water quality testing has been conducted in all the rural areas of the state. Major contaminants found are excess fluoride, iron, nitrate and hard water problems. 66 million people in India are estimated to be consuming groundwater with unsafe levels of flouride. Nearly 30 million people in the eastern states are estimated to be at risk of consuming water with higher than acceptable arsenic levels (Kolavalli and K.V. Raju, 2003).

Reasons for Quality Decline

Degradation in water quality has been observed due to various reasons. Contamination of ground water sources due to disposal of untreated sewage, disposal of industrial effluents without treatment, disuse of wells, extensive usage of chemical fertilizers. over exploitation of ground water and poor sanitation and hygiene.[20]

5. PRIs must be made Responsible for Water Supply

Lack of safe drinking water was been identified as major causes of sickness and death, especially of the children. Therefore, rigorous efforts need to be made by all to sustain, safeguard and provide drinking water to the people. Community has to be mobilized and sensitized to save India from a water scarce country to a water resource country. This is possible if we learn from our traditional water resource management and harvest the knowledge and transfer to the modern local self-governments—the Panchayati Raj Institutions (PRIs).

The three-tier Panchayati Raj Institutions (PRIs) are increasingly being recognized as the cornerstones of people-centered and self-reliant village development programmes. Therefore, PRIs can play a major role in managing and maintaining drinking water supply in the villages.

6. Harvesting Rain Water

Rain is the first form of water in the hydrological cycle. Rainwater offers advantages in water quality both for irrigation and domestic use. Rainwater is naturally soft (unlike well water), contains almost to dissolved minerals or salts, is free of chemical treatment and is relatively a reliable source of water for households. Rainwater collected and used on site can supplement or replace other modern sources of household water. Generally, the conservation/harvesting of water refers to collection and storage of rainwater and other allied activities aimed at prevention of losses through drain off, evaporation and seepage, etc. Rainwater conservation makes droughts less severe, rivers will have water throughout the year and soil holds greater level of moisture and consequently, there is increase in agricultural yield and thus economic conditions of rural poor is appreciably improved. All this leads to regeneration of vegetation and forests and thus overall environment of the region is positively impacted.[21]

In a document of Rajiv Gandhi National Drinking Water Mission, Deptt. of Rural Development, Ministry of Rural Areas and Employment, GOI, 1999, "Guidelines for Implementation of Rural Water Supply Programme."

HUMAN RESOURCE DEVELOPMENT

A National Human Resource Development Programme (NHRDP) has been launched by the Mission from 1994 based on the Human Resource Development Policy Document evolved jointly by the central and state governments. The NHRDP, *inter alia,* aims at training at least one grassroots level trainee through district level trainers who in turn may be trained at selected institutions forming the Indian Training Network (ITN). Under the NHRDP the States and UTs should set-up state level HRD cells for planning, designing, implementing, monitoring and evaluating an appropriate and need-based HRD programme. The HRD programme should aim at empowerment of Panchayati Raj Institutions/Local Bodies with the objective of enabling them to take up operation and maintenance activities related to rural water supply systems. It should also aim at capacity building of local communities by giving requisite training to mechanics/ health motivators/masons, etc. especially women to operate and maintain handpumps and the components of other water supply systems as well as to generate demand for adequate sanitation facilities. To train the grass-root trainees, the States/UTs may build be a pool of district level trainers who could be sent for training to the participating and key institutions. The States/UTs should establish state level HRD cells. The suggested staffing pattern, norm for equipment alongwith delineating of major functions already communicated vide D.O. Letter No. W.II038/1/94-HRD dated 15.9.94 and D.O. letter No. W-II043/1/95(Media) dated 31-12-1997.

INFORMATION EDUCATION AND COMMUNICATION

The emphasis of IEC programme should not be on hardware aspects but should be aimed at front loading software with the objective of generating a felt need which would result in an increased demand for safe drinking water and better sanitation facilities. Awareness on matters related to water borne diseases manifestations and symptoms should be created. The services of the State Publicity/Public Relations Department should be utilised to provide publicity to the rural water supply programme through mass media to disseminate information about the programme, highlighting the achievements, emphasis on use of safe water to overcome water borne diseases, etc. The importance of using safe water, using water as a socio-economic goods and the problems related to water quality in any specific area should be highlighted. This could be done by bringing to the public knowledge through appropriate methods like folk songs, folk drama, documentary films, pamphlets, brochures and other local means suited to the area. Publicity should also be given in the local newspapers about the action plan for coverage of habitations actually covered on year to year basis with other details like the type of schemes provided, the service level, delivery system, agency responsible for operation and maintenance, etc. 100%.

MONITORING AND INVESTIGATION UNITS

The Government of India has been providing assistance to the States to establish and continue special investigation divisions from the Fourth Five Year Plan to carry out investigation, planning and feasibility study of the schemes. The special monitoring cell and investigation unit at the State headquarters should be headed by an officer suitably qualified and of suitable level for monitoring and investigation with necessary supporting staff. Monitoring unit shall be responsible for collecting information from the executing agencies through prescribed reports and returns (Progress Monitoring System), maintenance of the data and timely submission of the prescribed reports and returns to the Central Government by due dates. The unit shall also be responsible for monitoring at field level of aspects of quality of water, adequacy of service and other related qualitative aspects of the programme. The Unit shall also maintain water quality data in coordination with the concerned Department, Central/State Ground Water Board, details of different technologies developed by institutions for tackling different problems and to provide the same to the field level executing agencies. The Monitoring and Investigation Units should also have technical posts of hydrologists, geophysicist, computer specialists with data entry operators, etc. A Quality Control Unit should be an integral part of M&I Units and should work in coordination with the R&D Cell. This unit will be responsible for controlling/regulating the quality of construction works in water supply schemes and will ensure practical application of latest technologies in the field. The expenditure will be borne by the Central Government and the State Governments on a 50:50 basis.

MONITORING AND EVALUATION

Central Government takes up monitoring and evaluation studies through reputed organisations/institutions from time to time. The State Governments may also take up similar monitoring and evaluation studies on the implementation of the rural water supply programme. 100% financial assistance will be provided by the Centre to the States for taking up such evaluation studies with prior approval of the Mission. The reports of these studies should be made available to the Mission and immediate collective action should be initiated as a follow up to improve the quality of programme implementation.

MANAGEMENT INFORMATION SYSTEM

For effective planning, monitoring and implementation of various schemes under different programme, Information Technology (IT) based Management Information System provides for the following:

(i) Maintenance of micro-level status of water supply to ensure planning and monitoring based on micro-level data,
(ii) Assistance for computer facilities up to division level in phases to ensure latest technology for processing and storing data and its communication from one office to another through NICNET,
(iii) Assistance for conducting training programmes; and
(iv) Development of customised software for enabling States/UTs to fully utilise for power of computer systems for planning, monitoring and implementation of various activities in the sector. 100% Central assistance will be provided for all MIS activities including training during the plan period.

RESEARCH AND DEVELOPMENT

To strengthen the R&D facilities in the concerned Departments in various States, State Governments are encouraged to establish R&D cells with adequate manpower and infrastructure. R&D Cells are required to remain in touch with premier technical institutions within the State. The network of technical institutions may follow the guidelines issued by the Mission from time to time for effective implementation of the rural water supply programme. R&D Cells are also required to be in constant touch with the Monitoring and Investigation Divisions and the Monitoring and Evaluation Study Reports for initiating appropriate follow up action. The R&D Cell should keep in constant touch with the documentation and information centre of the Mission and visit at the Mission's web site. The Mission will provide necessary assistance to the States.

PROVISION OF DRINKING WATER IN RURAL SCHOOLS

All the States are required to compile data regarding district-wise rural schools in existence and number of them having drinking water facilities. The remaining rural schools and Anganwadis are to be provided with drinking water facilities. A part of this work will be accomplished through the funds provided by Tenth Finance Commission and the rest would have to be covered under the rural water supply programme, in addition to the work of covering NC and PC habitations. Expenditure for this purpose would also be shared by the Central and State Governments on 50:50 basis from the funds allocated for ARWSP. States would be required to fix target for coverage of rural schools on an yearly basis and intimate its achievement to the Mission on monthly basis along with the progress reports being submitted to intimate coverage of NC and PC habitations. This activity is to be carried out in coordination with NEP, DPEP, DWCRA, Anganwadis, Department of Social Welfare and Department of Education. All the rural schools should be covered with drinking water facilities by the end of the 9th Plan.

CONCLUSION

Organizing IEC Campaign in a Village Panchayat

The Information, Education and Communication (IEC) campaign is aimed at creating awareness in the community about safe drinking water and its relationship with their health, with a view to changing their behaviour to use, maintain, protect and sustain the assets created for safe water supply. Therefore, the PRIs can play a key role in changing the attitude of the users of water supply and sanitation programme being implemented by Village water and sanitation committee/District water and sanitation Mission. The Village Panchayat should be concerned more with the village level activities. Hence, the members should be familiar with the objectives of the campaign with a focus on:

- To put an end to indiscriminate open defecation by creating a felt need among households for construction of individual latrines.
- To create awareness about the need for safe disposal of children's excreta.
- To create awareness about the collection, storage, handling and consumption of safe drinking water.

- To create awareness in the community about sanitary aspects of water supply, including keeping water source pollution free, safe disposal of waste water and solid waste.
- To create a sense of participation in the community so that the people are involved in the water and sanitation programme from the pre-planning stage to execution of and evaluation.
- To create a sense of competitiveness among individuals and families on sanitation through social marketing.
- To create a sense of willingness to pay for the creation of common and household assets and their operation and maintenance.
- To promote low-cost location specific appropriate technologies.
- To facilitate participatory planning and development through PRIs.

After the formation of the VWSC, the Village Panchayat must take initiative to organise campaigns to create awareness about the importance of safe water supply and sanitation. Since a VWSC member is link person between the village community and DWSM/DWSC/CBOs/NGOs it has an important role to play as an initiator and facilitator. The PAI/VWSC can organize following activities to create demand from the people for better water supply and sanitation facilities.

- The PRIs are expected to organise or to help community to organize the following with the active participation of the panchayat members.
- Organize Jathas/prabhat pheris in the village.
- Contact local folk artists to include messages of hygiene practices.
- Contact schoolteachers to promote school sanitation.
- Actively participate in the WATSAN Committee meetings.
- Provide feedback to the Gram Sabha and the Panchayat Samiti.[22]

The strategies of Rural Water Supply Programme hitherto adopted revolve around the basic premise that provision of safe drinking water is the responsibility of the Government. Increased outlay by the Government, particularly in the last one decade and, a change in technology focus to handpumps fitted on the tube wells and bore wells, had resulted in an impressive increase in the total rural water supply coverage. However, the availability of potable drinking water in rural areas, especially during the summer months, is still not satisfactory. Eventhough about 1 lakh habitations are covered every year, the number of problem habitations has not declined proportionately.

To focus in future would be:

- To ensure coverage of all rural habitations especially to reach the unreached with access to safe drinking water.

- To ensure sustainability of the systems and sources.
- To preserve quality of water by institutionalising water quality monitoring and surveillance through a Catchment Area approach.

Notes and References

1. WHO: Abel Wolman's Charter, *World Health*, January 1977, p. 17.
2. WWF, UNICEF: Fresh Water for India's Children and Nature, April 1998, pp. 1-2.
3. WHO: Nikolai P. Napalkov, Editorial, *World Health*, July-August 1992, p. 3.
4. WHO: Richard Helmér, News from the Waterfront, *World Health*, July-August 1992, p. 4.
5. WHO: Dennis B. Warner and Louis Laugeri, The Legacy of Water Decade, *World Health*, July-August 1992, p. 7.
6. WHO: Bruce M.W. Fisher, We must not lose hope, *World Health*, July-August 1992, p. 17.
7. WHO: Willy Brandt, *World Health*, August-September 1982, p. 3.
8. WHO: David Donaldson, Frank A. Butrico and Guillermo Davila, The Americans Attainable Goals, *World Health*, August-Sept. 1980, p. 25.
9. WHO: "Million in Need", *World Health*, December 1986, p. 4.
10. WHO: *World Health*, Water is Development, December 1986, p. 16.
11. IGNOU: "Public Health and Hygiene", Environmental Sanitation and Safety, p. 27.
12. IGNOU: "Public Health and Hygiene", Environmental Sanitation and Safety, p. 30.
13. IGNOU: "Public Health and Hygiene", Environmental Sanitation and Safety, p. 36.
14. India 2004, Ministry of Information and Broadcasting, GOI, New Delhi, p. 673.
15. GOI, Ministry of Rural Development, Annual Report, 2004-05, New Delhi, pp. 121-30.
16. Healthy Village—A Guide for Communities and Community Health Workers, WHO, pp. 19-21.
17. Ashutosh Jindal, "Community Participation in Drinking Water supply", *Kurukshetra*, March 2004, pp. 36-37.
18. Dinesh Chand, Towards Sustainable Rural Water Supply, *Kurukshetra*, March 2004, p. 3.
19. *Kurukshetra*, October 2003, p. 10.
20. K.V. Raju and S. Manasi, "Water For Rural Areas", *Kurukshetra*, October 2003, p. 33.
21. V.P. Rajvedi, "Rainwater Harvesting", *Kurukshetra*, October 2003, p. 63.
22. Dr. S. Ponnuraj, "Role of Panchayati Raj Institutions in Drinking Water Supply", *Kurukeshtra*, Oct. 2003, pp. 21-22.

11

Health Education for Rural Housing

EXISTING SITUATION

Housing is not a luxury but a basic necessity, as all activities depend upon the quality of housing because good housing energies the inmates leading to productivity and happiness. As per the provisional estimates made available by 2001 census, the housing shortage in the rural areas is about 149 lakhs as compared to 137 lakh housing shortage per year 1991 census. Under the IAY, for the last three years, on an average, about 14-15 lakh houses are being constructed every year whereas the annual requirement is about 30 lakh houses per annum as per the 2001 census. In addition to this, it is estimated that about 10 lakh shelterlessness are added every year. Thus, the total requirement is about 40 lakh houses are constructed leaving the gap of about 25 lakh houses every year in the rural areas. In addition to the number of houses, the quality of houses and facilities in them are very poor causing many diseases and a dull life.

Housing Constitutes not only a basic necessity but also a crucial economic activity in view of its contribution to the construction industry. The banks, of late have been alive to the potential of this industry since the demand for housing remains insatiable even as the supply is constrained by various structural deficiencies and institutional obstacles.

G. Srinivasan in his article, "The Big Push in the Housing Sector" in *Yojana*, January 2004 clearly states that the Government's thrust on housing in the form of facilitating steps such as the Reserve Bank of India (RBI) regulations pertaining to priority sector lending, fiscal concessions and budgetary support has started yielding handsome returns through construction of dwelling units to lakhs and lakhs of people over the years. This is also corroborated by the latest Report on Trend and Progress of Banking in India 2002-03 of RBI. Assistance to the housing sector in the form of gross bank credit flows had gone up from Rs. 6203 crore (38.4 per

CHART 11.1

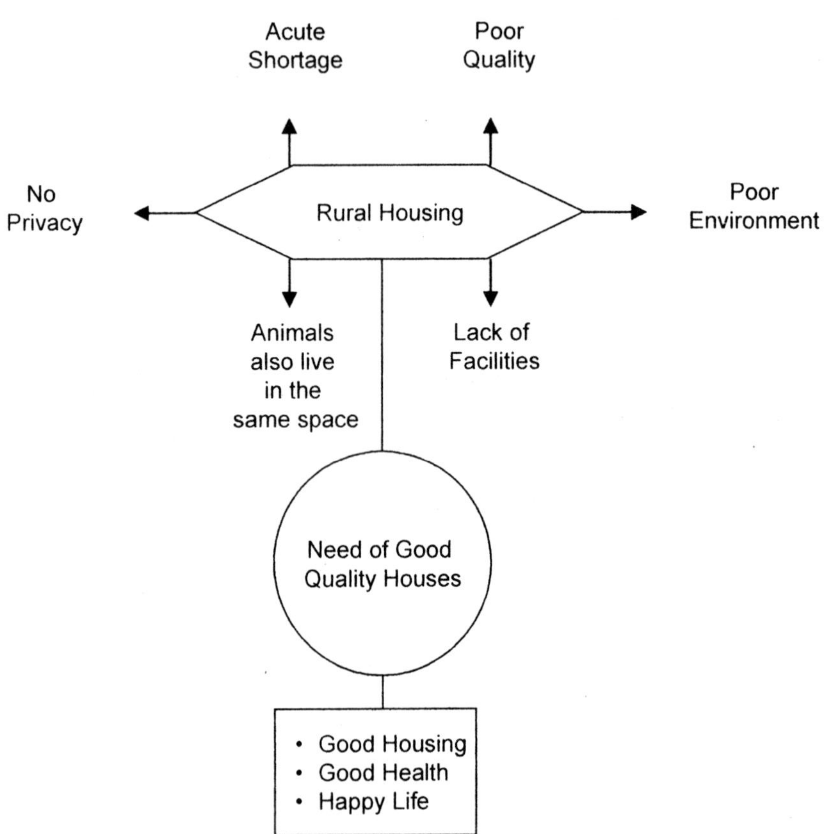

cent of the gross bank credit) in 2001-02 to Rs. 12,308 crore (55.11 per cent) during 2002-03. In order to increase further credit flow to the housing sector, the limit of housing loans for repairing damaged houses was raised from Rs. 50,000 to one lakh in rural and semi-urban areas. Because of the escalating demand for housing in rural and semi-urban areas as also the compulsive need to improve financing to housing sector here, the banks are being directed to extend direct finance to the housing sector upto Rs. 10 lakh per individual as part of priority sector lending with the approval of their Boards.

On its part, the Central government has come out with a series of well-meaning policy ballast to the housing sector in order to augment investment in housing. These include fiscal sops. Lowering of interest rate on housing loans, enhancement of bank finance for housing to the extent of 3 per cent of their annual incremental deposits, support to HUDCO and other housing finance institutions in the public sector.

THE NEW POLICY SHIFT

The long-range objective of the NHP was to stamp out houselessness to ameliorate the housing conditions of the inadequately housed and to accord a minimum level of basic services and amenities to all. It deservedly recognised that the magnitude of housing stock demands the involvement of various agencies including government at different levels, the cooperative sector the community at large and the private corporate sector. The NHP of 1994 envisaged a tectonic shift in the Government's role which would henceforth be only a facilitator than as a provider in tune with the changed economic realities of the reformist path the Indian economy had traversed since July, 1991.

As the NHP provided for review and modification in the light of changing scenario in the housing domain the National Housing and Habitat Policy was unveiled in 1998 to address the issue of sustainable development infrastructure development and for wholesome public-private partnership for delivery of shelter. This policy, laid in Parliament on July 29, 1998 was to foster surpluses in housing stock and facilitate construction of two million dwelling units each year in pursuance of National Agenda for Governance. It also sought to ensure that housing along with supporting services is treated as a priority sector at par with infrastructure. The focus of the policy is robust public-private a partnership for dealing with housing and Infrastructure impediments. Accordingly, the Government is providing fiscal fillips carrying out regulatory and legal reforms and bringing about an enabling milieu. The private and cooperative sector the other vital pillars in the partnership, would come forward to undertake actual construction activities and invest and run infrastructure services.

Efforts are well under way to prop up institutional mechanism for housing finance so that they do not get saddled with non-performing assets. One such proposal is the Mortgage Credit Guarantee Scheme of the National Housing Bank. This would cover housing loans extended by nationalised banks thereby protecting lenders (banks) against potential default. The NHB had begun securitisation of housing loans and has been making operational foreclosure of mortgage (rights of creditors to acquire the property). This would preclude borrowers from wilfully defaulting on repayments now. It is also praiseworthy that the prudence of lending bodies has kept the non-performing assets to the barest in this significant segment of the economy. With foreclosure laws in place lending institutions will become freer and flexible in loan disbursals. These measures are salutary in that they minimise the cost of funds to the banks and housing finance companies while simultaneously enhancing the effective yield. This would also help bolster the profitability of the lending banks which are flush with funds but could not find savvy borrowers.

SCHEMES

Indra Awaas Yojana

The Ministry of Rural Development is implementing Indira Awaas Yojana (IAY) with a view to providing financial assistance for shelter to the rural poor living below poverty line. The details of the Scheme alongwith its performance are given below:

(a) The Government of India is implementing Indira Awaas Yojana (IAY) since the year 1985-86 to provide assistance for construction/up gradation of dwelling units to the below poverty line (BPL) rural households belonging to the Scheduled Castes. Scheduled Tribes and freed bonded labourers categories. From the year 1993-94, the scope of the Scheme was extended to cover non-Scheduled Castes and Scheduled Tribes rural BPL poor subject to the condition that the benefits to non-SC/ST would not be more than 40% of tile total IAY allocation. The benefits of the Scheme have also been extended to the families of Ex-servicemen of the armed and paramilitary forces killed in action. 3% of the houses are reserved for the rural Below the Poverty. Line physically and mentally challenged persons. The IAY became an independent Scheme with effect from 1.1.1996.

(b) The funding pattern of the IAY is shared between the Centre and State in the ratio of 75:25. From 1999-2000, the allocation of funds under the Indira Awaas Yojana to the States/UTs is being made on the basis of the poverty ratio, as approved by the Planning Commission, and rural housing shortage, as specified in the Census. Both parameters have been accorded equal weightage. Similarly. allocation to Districts in the States/UTs is made on the basis of proportion of SC/ST population of the District to the total SC/ST population of the State and housing shortage. The ceiling on construction assistance under the IAY currently is Rs. 25,000 per unit for the plain areas and Rs. 27,500 for the hilly/difficult areas. The ceiling on upgradation of unserviceable kutcha house to pucca/semi pucca house is Rs. 12,500 for all areas. This ceiling came into effect from 1.4.2004.

(c) On the basis of allocations made and targets fixed. District Rural Development Agencies (DRDAs)/Zilla Parishads (ZPs) decide Panchayat-wise number of houses to be constructed under IAY and intimate the same to the concerned Gram Panchayat. Thereafter the Gram Sabha selects the beneficiaries, restricting its number to the target allotted from the list of eligible households. No approval of other authorities is required. The Panchayat Samities/Zilla Parishads IDRDAs should, however, be sent a list of selected beneficiaries for their information.

(d) As the need for upgradation of unserviceable kutcha houses in the rural areas is acutely felt, therefore, with effect from 1.4.2004, upto 20% the total funds can be utilized for conversion of unserviceable kutcha houses into pucca/semi- pucca houses and for providing subsidy to the beneficiary availing loan under the credit-cum-subsidy scheme of Rural Housing (RH). Amaximum assistance of Rs. 12,500 per unit is provided for conversion of unserviceable kutcha houses into pucca/semi-pucca houses.

(e) Further, the dwelling units should invariably be allotted in the name of a female member of the beneficiary household. Alternatively, it can be allotted in the name of both husband and wife. The Sanitary latrine and smokeless chullah and proper drainage are required for each IAY house latrine could be constructed separate from the IAY house on the site of beneficiary. The construction of the houses is the sole responsibility of the beneficiary. Engagement of contractors strictly prohibited. No specific type design has been stipulated for an IAY house. Choice of design, technology and materials for construction of an IAY house is the sole discretion of the beneficiaries.

PROVISION OF ADDITIONAL FUNDS FOR NATURAL CALAMITIES

5% of allocation is kept at central share to meet the exigencies arising out of natural calamities and other emergent situations like riot, arson, fire, rehabilitation. The State Government should make necessary recommendation for additional funds in this regard which are to be shared by the Centre and State on 75:25 basis. The maximum limit for such assistance is Rs. 50.00 lakh per district. The relief will be as per the norms of IAY.

During the year 2004-05, the country is affected by various natural calamities. Majority of the victims are from rural areas, their dwelling units get partially or fully damaged apart from other losses. An amount of Rs. 400 crore has been sanctioned for the 20 flood-affected districts of Bihar as Additional Central Assistance under the Indira Awaas Yojana II (IAY). Similarly, on 26.12.2004, a large number of houses were damaged due to Tsunami tidel waves in the region of South-East coast and in some parts of South-West coastal areas of India and for this purpose an amount of Rs. 200 crore are likely to be released under the Indira Awaas Yojana (IAY) in order to provide immediate financial assistance for reconstruction of houses in the rural areas.

PERFORMANCE UNDER IAY

About 121 lakh houses have been constructed under IAY since inception of the Scheme with an expenditure of Rs. 21419.64 crores (upto

31st December, 2004). During the Tenth Five Year Plan, i.e. last two years, the progress of IAY is as under:

Year	*Funds Utilized Centre + State share) (Rs. in crores)*	*Targets Houses constructed/upgraded*	
		(No. in lakhs)	*(No. in Lakhs)*
2002-03	2795	13.14	15.48
2003-04	2580	14.84	13.61
2004-05*	1377	17.76	5.75

* As reported by the State Governments (upto 31st December, 2004).

During the current financial year 2004-05, the central allocation under IAY is Rs. 2900 crore with a target of 17.76 lakh houses. Out of this allocation, Rs. 2422.86 crore have been released under the scheme (upto 31st December, 2004).

Discontinuation of the Schemes such as Innovative Stream for Rural Housing, Samagra Awaas Yojana and Rural Building Centres

The small schemes under Rural Housing namely Innovative Stream for Rural Housing and Habitat Development, Samagra Awaas Yojana and Rural Building Centres (RBCs) have been discontinued and merged with the main scheme, i.e. Indira Awaas Yojana (IAY) with effect from 1.4.2004.

NEW INITIATIVES

Unit Cost of the Indira Awaas Yojana Houses

The ceiling on construction assistance under the IAY has been enhanced from Rs. 20,000 to Rs. 25,000 per unit for the plain areas and from Rs. 22,000 to Rs. 27,500 for the hilly/difficult areas. The ceiling on upgradation of unserviceable kutcha house to pucca/semi pucca house has also been enhanced from 10,000 to Rs. 12,500 for all areas. This ceiling came into effect from 1.4.2004.

Construction of Sanitary Latrines and Smokeless Chulhas

Sanitary latrine and smokeless chulha will be provided with each IAY house. In case, the beneficiary is unable to construct sanitary latrines due to some reasons, an amount of Rs. 600 would be deducted from the assistance to be provided for construction of the new IAY house or for upgradation of an unserviceable kutcha house. Similarly, where smokeless chulha is not possible, deduction will be Rs. 10.

Loan for IAY Beneficiaries

In addition to the assistance provided under the IAY, loan for construction of IAY houses or for upgradation of unserviceable kutcha houses can be obtained from the banks/other financial institutions if the concerned State Governments/DRDAs take the responsibility in order to coordinate with the financial institutions to make available the credit facilities to those beneficiaries who are interested.

Ownership of IAY House

Under IAY, the houses can be allotted in the name of male member of a deserving BPL family if there is no eligible female member in that family is available.

Equity Support to HUDCO

To meet the housing requirement of economically weaker sections in rural areas and to improve the outreach of housing finance in rural areas, equity support to HUDCO is being provided. During the first two years of the Tenth Five Year Plan, the equity support to HUDCO by the Ministry of Rural Development was as under:

Year	*Equity Support To HUDCO (Rs. in crores)*
2002-03	50.00
2003-04	10.00
2004-05.	5.00

Not yet released.

Provision of Houses for Physically and Mentally Challenged Persons

Under the IAY Guidelines, 3% of the IAY funds are reserved for construction of houses for the rural. Below the Poverty Line (BPL) physically and mentally challenged persons belonging to SCs/STs. As per the information received from the various States/UTs, about 45,083 houses have so far been concerned for the physically and mentally challenged persons under the Scheme.

North-Eastern Region

From the financial year 2000-01, a separate non-lapsable provision working out to 10% of the total budget of Rural Housing was earmarked for North-Eastern States. During the current financial year 2004-05, an amount of Rs. 250 crore has been earmarked for the North-Eastern Region for with a target of 150301 houses. Of this, an amount of Rs. 190.83 crore has already been released and about 69,380 houses have been constructed under the Indira Awaas Yojana (IAY).

Success Stories in Rural Housing and Habitat Development

Smt. Bhagyamma w/o Late Chikkaraju of Alkere village in Mandya Taluk is from BPL family. She is wage labourer and a widow belongs to Scheduled Caste having two female school going children, one is 7th and second one is 5th standard. She is the only wage earner in the family. Before she was staying in a thatched hut. Grama Sabha decided her name for house grant under the Indira Awaas Yojana (IAY) and to construct house herself without involving contractor she came forward and constructed house to her own satisfaction along with smokeless chulha and sanitary latrine as per guidelines. Now she feels much better having own pucca house to live.

Gender Budgeting under IAY

In order to provide social security to women, it is provided in the Indira Awaas Yojana (IAY) guidelines that the houses constructed is to be allotted in the name of female member of the beneficiary household Alternatively, it can be allotted in the name of both husband and wife under the Programme. When there is no eligible female member in the family, available/alive, IAY house can also be allotted to the male member of a deserving BPL family.

However, IAY guidelines do not provide separate earmarking of provisions and physical targets benefiting women. During 2003-04, 5.22 lakh houses were allotted exclusively in the name of women members, while 4.15 lakh houses were allotted in the name of both husband/wife. During 2004-05 (upto 31st January, 2005), 4.49 lakh house were allotted exclusively in the name of women members and 2.26 lakh houses allotted in the name of both husband/wife.

Congested

In small houses there are many things stores—grains, garments, utensils, animals, feet, etc. which allow little space for people living in the house.

Hence there is a need of health education to people to provide them guidance as to how they should live and enjoy a life free from disease.

PROBLEMS

1. Lack of knowledge

People in the villages are ignorant and they are not provided all the benefits under various schemes resulting in low quality housing. There is a lot of corruption in these schemes sponsored by Governments.

2. Lack of Health Education

The villagers do not give much importance to hygiene, hand washing and other facilities resulting into many diseases caused by poor house environment.

3. High Population as Compared to House Capacity

Many people live in a house which has been constructed for 4-5 members. How can they enjoy while sitting, sleeping and existing care should to taken about the size of the house *vis-a-vis* renders.

A visit to villages in Hungary by the authors revealed that villages are heaven possessing all the facilities of the city—good quality housing, lighting, ventilation, decorative as well as pure air of nature with good plantations. While a visit to an Indian village in despressing as the houses are unplanned, insufficient and unclean from where the outsiders want to run away. That is why government officials visit the villages and come back to the city on the same day. Housing is a basic necessity but it must of good quality so that the residents can enjoy the quality of life.

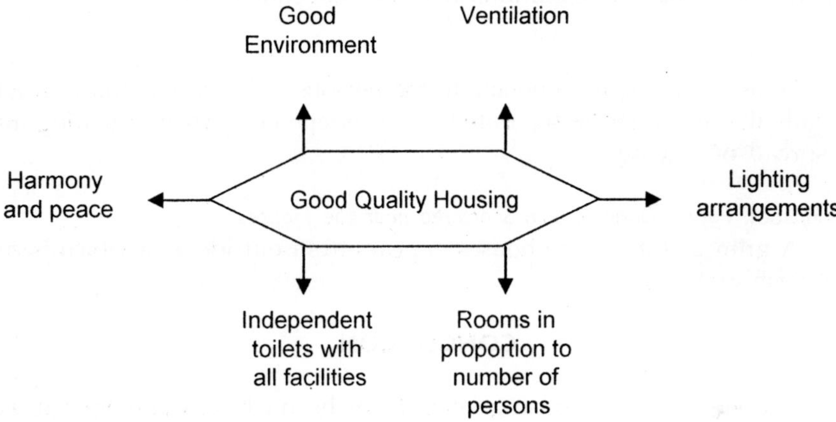

Improvement: Health Education

Panchayati Raj Institutions, i.e. gram Panchayat's must take the initiative to provide health education to the people to help three houses clean. This can avoid them from many diseases and make the villages healthy and beautiful.

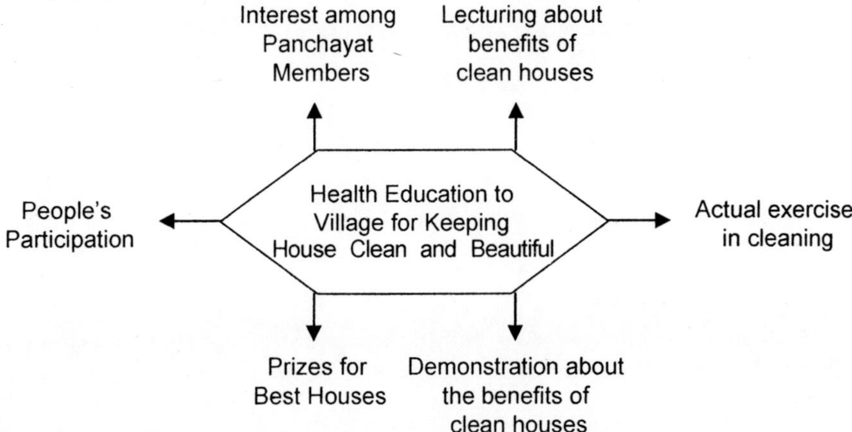

Problems of Housing in Indian Villages

1. Unplanned

Since the villages have expanded without any planning, the houses are congested causing unhealthy environment.

2. Approach Unhealthy

The roads outside the houses is unclean, dirty and insufficient. Children ease in the street resulting into garbage outside the houses.

3. Foul Smell during Rainy Seasons

During rainy seasons, water collect in the locality as there is no drainage resulting into communicable and infectious diseases.

4. Small Houses

Houses are disproportionate to the persons living in the house. If any one falls ill, he cannot be separated to an independent room resulting into the spread of disease.

5. Plastics, Paper, Dung remain Scattered near the Houses

A grim picture of the houses appears from outside area which is full of rubbish material.

CONCLUSION

The emphasis of housing should not be on bricks and mortar but comforts. The houses should be simple with all facilities. There is a need of research to ensure good housing at a minimum cost.

Appendix

Ventilation

Adequate home ventilation is particularly important where wood, charcoal and dung are used for cooking or heating, since these fuels give off smoke that contains harmful chemicals and particulate matter. This can lead to respiratory problems, such as bronchitis and asthma, and make tuberculosis transmission easier. Women and small children are particularly at risk from poor ventilation if they spend long periods within the home or in cooking areas. Where cooking is done indoors, it is essential that smoke and fumes be removed from the house quickly and efficiently. Ventilation may be improved by constructing houses with a sufficient number of windows, particularly in cooking areas. Alternatively, houses can be constructed using bricks with holes drilled through them ("air-bricks"), which allow fresh air to circulate within the house.

Lighting

Poor indoor lighting can have many harmful effects on health and well-being. A poorly lit working environment in the home can lead to eyesight problems, for example. This is a particular concern for women working in indoor cooking areas. Poor lighting within the home can also make people feel more depressed. These problems can be remedied by adding windows to the house to increase the amount of natural light, which is much stronger than light from candles or lamps. In communities where it is important that privacy within the home is maintained, windows can be located where it is difficult for people to see into the house, or constructed with a mesh or lattice work which allows light to enter while guarding privacy. Increasing natural light is also important for home cleanliness: if a house is dark, it is more difficult to see dust and dirt and thus more difficult to clean properly.

Disease Vectors in the Home

Unless homes are kept clean and steps taken to prevent insects from entering, the homes can become infested with disease vectors. In eastern Mediterranean areas, for example, sand flies thrive in the dirt inside houses and transmit leishmaniasis; and in Central and South America, triatomid bugs live in the cracks of walls and in thatched roofs and transmit American trypanosomiasis (Chagas disease). Insect disease vectors can be reduced by keeping food covered and properly disposing of waste. If mosquitoes or flies are a problems windows and doors should be covered with mesh screens and kept shut at night, and mosquito nets placed over beds. Cleanliness within and around home areas significantly reduces the risk of disease transmission.

Overcrowding in Homes

Overcrowding in homes causes ill-health because it makes disease transmission easier and because the lack of private space causes stress. Overcrowding is related to socio-economic level, and the poor often have little choice but to live in cramped conditions. In principle, increasing the number of rooms to live in should improve the health of the people who live there, but increasing house size is often difficult. Careful planning of family size can also help to reduce overcrowding. If community members feel that overcrowding is a problem, they can take the initiative and press landlords to provide more space for tenants at affordable prices. This may necessitate working with local government and pressure groups to ensure that the housing laws and tenancy agreements are revised, and that everyone has access to houses adequate for their family size.

Source: WHO: Healthy Villages, Geneva, 2002, pp. 61-64.

12

Problems of Health Education

The role of education in health development, including family planning, cannot be overemphasized. The literacy rate, in particular the functional literacy rate of women, is of cardinal important to health development. Health is so much in the hands of women that female literacy rate becomes crucial. Likewise, the education of children is important. As with growth, so with education, it is the length of time that improved rates of literacy have prevailed that makes a difference. There is much variation in this regard amongst the countries of the Region. The horizontal spread of primary education seems more critical for health development than the vertical spread of higher education to selected population segments. For example, the success of clean water and environmental sanitation is critically dependent upon education in the hygiene use of water and appropriate disposal of wastes.[1]

Health Education is not being accorded the priority it deserves.

Whatever little priority is accorded, Health Education is not imparted seriously and with full devotion and dedication. Health Education is the last priority among health professionals. They are so busy in curative health, they find no time for health education which is stressed in every five year plans, Health policy and other documents.

Akbar Moarefi has nicely put as: Despite the sporadic but ample evidence on the success of systematic health education in reducing accidents, morbidity and mortality, there must be something drastically wrong with our attempts in health education, otherwise results would have been more encouraging. Granted that health education of some sort is receiving priority, at least verbally and in reports, but a sound, systematic, well-conceived, correctly implemented, well-evaluated health education activity is seriously lacking.

Let us enumerate the problems:

1. Dichotomy between Health and Disease

Health professionals look at health and disease independently causing poor role of health education. Health and Diseases co-exist as no body can be either totally healthy or disease ridden. He must be somewhere in between meaning thereby that health education must act on both disease and health, i.e. minimizing disease and maximizing health. To quote:

People have been taught to feel that health and disease are two separate states similar to light and darkness. This Aristotelian way of thinking in a non-Aristotelian world of various shades of grey has created psychologically and arbitrarily two distinct phases rather than a continuum. A totally healthy or a totally sick individual is a rare phenomenon indeed if physical, mental and social well-being are carefully observed. Any individual at any given time rests on a particular point in this continuum. Whether he moves to the negative or positive side of this continuum is mainly the outcome of his own decision and efforts, or the decision and efforts of his parents if he is a child.[2]

This continuum of well-being, like an algebraic quantity, could be positive or negative but not two separate entities. Neglect of the positive side will undoubtedly lead to the negative and conversely negative may, unless irrevocable harm has been done, with an effort in the right direction be turned into positive. Thus, the role of the individual effort becomes obvious. Health should not be considered a gift, or disease a curse, but in general an outcome of human effort or a lack of it.[3]

Too often, the training of health personnel follows a pattern of yesterday's view of health care, or even of only the clinical care, and falls seriously short of meeting today's and tomorrow's requirement for personnel who can lead or participate in effective health services responding to people's needs.

Population-based education and training of both governmental and non-governmental sectors for health system development and implementation is of paramount importance. That all in a population will be cared for, and not simply. those who knock on the door of the health facility, raises the issues of coverage, quality, effectiveness, efficiency and equity. That all in the population must be of concern requires teams of health workers, functioning at different levels of the health system, each level with its purpose and methods, interacting with communities in support and referral, guided by information systems appropriate for each level.[4]

2. Lack of Inter-Sectoral Co-operation between Health and Total Development: Need of Intersectoral Action

More than ever before, the experts responsible for planning national economies are recognizing that a country's health forms part of an integrated process of development.

The experience of the world's industrialized countries showed that diseases associated with poor sanitation, illiteracy and poverty were eventually controlled, not by spectacular- medical breakthroughs, but by improvements in urban services, housing and the environment, higher levels of education, and better diets.

The moral for all the world today is that the health sector cannot do it alone! Many other ministries, services, institutions, official and unofficial bodies, and all levels of administration down to the community and the family must become involved in health.

So the drive towards the goal of Health for all by the year 2000 and now 2025 can only be inspired and fuelled by concerted intersectoral action. Our graphic model suggests only the eight elements included in WHO's definition of Primary Health Care: education about health, proper nutrition, safe water and basic sanitation, maternal and child care including family planning, immunization, prevention and control of locally endemic diseases, appropriate treatment of common diseases and injuries, and provision of essential drugs.

But these symbolize a huge range of factors to which other sectors besides health must contribute if all people are indeed to attain a level of health that will permit them to lead a socially and economically productive life.[5]

Improvements in the health status of a population cannot be achieved simply by. expanding and developing the health services. The prevention and control of disease and the promotion of health require a concerned effort for the improvement of human well-being as a whole. In this task, what has been defined as "health care" has to be supported by improvements in the social and economic infrastructure, and contributions from various sectors other than health.[6]

Intersectoral linkages which combine increased family income, education, and effective health services targeted to the most high-risk groups can yield positive improvements in health conditions. At the same time, there is a growing awareness that the failure to take account of the implications of macra-economic policies and projects on the environment and on health can have serious negative consequences for national health goals. What Latin America and the Caribbean have learnt from the economic and adjustment crisis is that understanding the nature of intersectoral cooperation are not merely desirable; they are essential to the achievement of both Health for all and economic development objectives?

A health related development, which involves a community, is seldom separated from other developments. Water, for example, is used for irrigation, industry, gardening, domestic purposes and, obviously, drinking. Drinking, in terms of quantity, has a very low requirement in comparison with the others. But its standards are much more exacting. Whilst these exacting standards must be met, the installation of a water supply also needs to take into account several other needs of the people, at the present time and for the immediate future, thus, involving the collaboration of a number of different agencies. Little can be accomplished in continuous utilization and adequate maintenance of this supply by the consumer if no attention is given, from the planning state, to the cooperative efforts of all agencies and the public in meeting all man's basic needs for water. Many unused, or poorly utilized but expensively constructed, water supplies stand idle as monuments to this unwise planning.

Cultivation of food and preparation of adequate nutrition similarly involve a cooperative effort of health, agriculture, economy and several other departments. Irrespective of the hierarchical social form, the function at the field level should be a cooperative one in order to succeed. Health is a very significant factor and a major contributor to what is nowadays called socia-economic development. In order to contribute to this development, health efforts must be integrated with other efforts, and must complement other efforts rather than compete with them. After all, any development is for man and his welfare.[8]

It is now increasingly evident that more and more diseases stem from the degradation caused by man to his own environment. The potential harmful effects of industrial development on our global ecosystem are now better known. Ozone layer depletion, acid rain, climate change, chemical pollution are some examples of the man-made wounds to our planet.

We are at a turning point; warnings of the damage to our health and quality of life are growing louder. An increasing number of people are acting to stop the degradation of our environment.[9]

In our report on Our Common Future, the World Commission on Environment and Development (sometimes called the Brundtland Commission) pointed out that the situation is getting increasingly critical. At the present rate of development, we are rapidly depleting the natural resource base on which man's existence depending. The evidence is growing of a strong relationship between health and the environment. We are filling our environment and our food products with chemicals. Certain infectious diseases show signs of new gains as a result of increasing poverty and an inability to meet people's basic needs. Malnutrition remains a serious obstacle to health and to the development of human resources.[10]

How can we make environmental health a more potent force to serve people faced with growing threats to their health? How can our improving environmental health technology be better used to foster positive health? I know of no country-developing or industrialized-in which this issue is not urgent and important. I know of many countries in which it is critical.

The remarkably wide range of environmental concerns includes the international problems of acid rain, the greenhouse effect, and depletion I of the planet's ozone layer. It includes national concerns with medical wastes disposal, radioactive and toxic wastes control, transportation accidents, health aspects of urbanization and traffic, occupational health and safety, and air and water pollution. It also includes local concerns over inadequate water supplies and sanitation facilities, water quality, clean air, solid wastes management, and finding a balance between the economic incentives of development and a decent quality of life.[11]

3. Health Education must Attend to Essential Information Services and not Waste Time on Hypothetical Situations

Health Education should not operate in isolation. Health Education must be related to the actual health issues, e.g. where to go in case of disease? Where is it located? What are the services available?, etc. Health Education may not talk of Heart Transplant or sophisticated issues for which services are not available near by.

4. Health Education Emphasize Theory and not Practice Resulting into Inefficiency

Health Education should be result-oriented for example, a lecture on Yoga should not merely attempt at understanding the theory of Yoga but also the methods of its implementation to make health better and provide integrated health services. Words, written or spoken are of no use unless put to action.

Emphasis should be on Implementation through hard work rather than being engaged merely in Paper Planning. Words, "Written or spoken", are of no use unless put into action. The emphasis should be more on performance rather than paper planning. Khalil Gibran has rightly said that "Believing is a fine thing, but placing those beliefs into execution is a test of strength. Many are those who talk like the roar of the sea, but their lives are shallow and stagnant, like the rotting. marshes. Many are those who lift their heads above the mountain tops, but their spirit remain dormant to the obscurity of the caverns."[12]

Let us discuss some golden rules about Nutrition education which can help in control of many diseases if implemented carefully—

The first of the TEN GOLDEN RULES FOR SAFE FOOD PREPARATION in the home (or restaurant) is to eat the food as soon as it has been cooked. Since many raw foods are contaminated with foodborne pathogens, it is important to make sure that food is thoroughly cooked, particularly poultry, meats and milk. Thorough cooking means that the temperature of all parts of the food reaches at least 70°C.

In many societies the consumer can choose between foods which, for safety reasons, have been processed and those which have not. So the third of the ten golden rules is to choose foods processed for safety. For instance, choose pasteurized milk instead of raw, milk, and irradiated fresh or frozen poultry instead of non-irradiated.

It is not always possible to eat food immediately it has been cooked, especially when it has to be served on several occasions. If it needs to be kept for more than four or five hours, it must be stored either in hot (near or above 60°C) or cool (near or below 10°C) conditions. A common error, responsible for countless cases of food borne illness, is putting too large a quantity of warm food in the refrigerator. Microbial proliferation, reaching disease-producing proportions, will occur in the centre of food, which remains at a high temperature (above 10°C) for too long. Food for infants should preferably not be stored at all.

The next rule is to make sure that food already cooked is reheated thoroughly (reaching 70°C throughout) prior to eating. In this way microbes which might have developed during the storage period will be killed, thus preventing infection or intoxication.

A void contact between raw foods and cooked foods is another important measure to prevent food borne disease. This contact could be direct (raw poultry meat coming into contact with cooked foods) or indirect (preparing an uncooked chicken and then using the same, unwashed cutting board and knife to dissect the cooked bird). In this way the cooked food is recontaminated with all the potential risks for microbial growth and subsequent illness.

Keep all kitchen surfaces meticulously clean; this is the seventh golden rule of food safety. Utensils, plates, cutlery and so on should be wiped with a clean cloth, which should not, as a rule, be used for more than one day. The cloth should then be boiled for re-use. Separate cloths for cleaning the floor also need frequent washing.

Wash hands before handling food is another vital prerequisite for food safety. This commandment applies in particular after using the toilet and after changing a baby's nappy. Hand infections are frequently pus-filled and the microbes responsible for the infection may cause food borne illness. So it is important to prevent contact or to bandage injuries.

Protect foods from insects, rodents and other animals is the next rule. Animals frequently carry pathogenic micro-organisms, which cause food-borne disease.

The last of the ten golden rules of food safety, but by no means the least important, concerns the purity of the water supply used for drinking and food preparation. If any doubt exists, the water should be boiled or chlorinated. And, as for travellers, slow-release disinfectant tablets in water or filter attachments to domestic taps may be used, if proved to be safe and reliable.

By following this advice, the risk of food borne illness will be reduced significantly. In this way, good food will continue to be one of the greatest pleasures in life.[13]

Lack of people's participation in Health Education—Health Education is imparted by professionals without taking into account as to what people require. Health Education does not attend to those health problems, which affect the community. In addition, there are no practical exercise or demonstration to prove the rationale of Health programmes by health education professionals.

5. Lack Effective Involvement of the Public in the Affairs of the Health Organisation

Merle Fainsod remarks: "The most favourable setting for progress in development administration exists where a polemically influential and dynamic modernizing elite strongly desires development and can successfully project this attitude into both the bureaucracy and the population at large."[14]

Many well-intentioned and technically sound programmes aimed at solving problems have been frustrated by lack of popular acceptance and community participation. It has been observed that such programmes are either not actively associated or passively ignored because they do not 'belong' to the population they are designed to help; they are rather seen by the population as imposed external programmes that belong to the government and consequently deserve and require little, if any, of the population's attention, action, or other response.[15]

6. Lack of Adequate Materials in the Context of the Targeted Group

Health Education is facing a challenge, as they have no material, which can be of direct relevance to the target group. Union Government and State Governments bring out some material but this is of a general nature. Primary Health Centres must prepare the health education material to suit the people of the area. For this work, the teachers in local colleges, schools in the area can be involved. This would make the teaching material specific, interesting and simple.

One of the greatest handicaps under which training programmes are being undertaken today, especially in developing countries, is the grave shortage of relevant teaching and learning materials for use by health workers during their training. Such materials are also needed for reference during their service in the field. Where the materials exist, they are often out of date, of poor quality, in an inappropriate language, or have been translated from material prepared for a country with different needs.

The situation is serious enough for potential leaders of the health team-medical students and physicians but they at least can refer to professional journals. Moreover, they rarely work in isolation, so that they have an opportunity to improve their knowledge through discussion with colleagues.

For auxiliary health workers, however, especially those who work at the periphery, and on whom fall the greatest load of PHC delivery, the materials situation is catastrophic. In most developing countries, auxiliary health training schools have no libraries and their students have no books or manuals. When they finish their training and begin their service to communities, they have no reliable materials to which they can refer. They are often stationed in remote areas where there can be little or no supervision of their work. Little wonder that their competence gradually declines, to the detriment of their patients. And yet the eventual achievement of Health for All depends on the efficacy of this first line of health workers.

Over the past ten years, WHO has been contributing towards the solution of this universal problem of acute shortage of relevant teaching and learning materials for the health team. The development of manuals to serve as models for adaptation, the provision of libraries for teachers of health auxiliaries in different major languages, a large-scale textbook programme in the Americas—these and many other efforts have helped partly to remedy the situation.

The recent emphasis on PHC, however, has created an even greater demand for training, especially at auxiliary level. Surveys in selected countries have confirmed the grave lack of relevant materials for use by health workers in training and in service, and by their teachers. Much of the material required by peripheral level workers must be developed at individual country level because of the variations in culture, language, educational status of staff, and tasks to be performed. It was evident that if all health workers were to have available appropriate materials for teaching, learning, reference and continuing education—national capabilities would need to be created to produce illustrated texts and teaching aids. Such country self-reliance would require heavy funding, and would take several years to build. It would involve an intensive programme of training, so as to produce a permanent structure able to function effectively after the phasing out of external aid.

The educational sector has clearly shown that properly developed teaching and learning materials, readily available to all for training and reference, can accelerate training and thereby improve service performance. A World Bank study (World Bank Staff Working Paper No. 398 (1980) affirmed that "textbooks, teacher editions, and allied materials are the most consistent factors in upgrading academic achievement, especially for poorer schools with less qualified teachers, and ... are cost effective tools which greatly enhance the efficiency of an educational system."

WHO accordingly launched in 1981 a programme to ensure that appropriate teaching and learning materials could be available to all health workers. The approach adopted—since an immediate worldwide project is impracticable—has been to tackle the situation in a selected number of countries, and to use the experience gained to reach out gradually to others. The extension will be brought about through the development of regional networks, by the sharing between countries of newly gained experience and expertise, and by assistance in adapting the materials.[16]

Teaching materials are of obvious importance to health personnel in any programme aimed at promoting health personnel education and community health. Health Teaching Learning Materials (HTLM) is the name that WHO gives to written and audio-visual aids used in the education of health personnel and in health promotion.

In most countries of EMRO, good quality and appropriate health teaching and learning materials are scarce—whether they are needed to train health workers and help them to acquire new skills, or as aids to health workers who will work as health educators of the community.

Efforts to provide health-teaching aids have been made in almost all countries, but they are far from meeting the pressing needs. An exchange of information and expertise is therefore of vital importance. To help promote such an exchange, EMRO, in January 1986, set-up the Health Teaching and Learning Material Clearing House, an information bank which serves to support the development and sharing of good materials. There is often too little exchange of materials among countries and even among institutions within the same country, so the Clearing House facilitates the distribution and use of materials, particularly in health programmes based on primary health care.

7. Lack of Audio-Visual Aids Programmes

Since Audio-Visual aids are more comprehensive and interesting, health education experts must make use of them to make health education interesting and absorbing.

Let us explain with an example: The love of music and the appreciation of drama lie deep in the culture of Jamaicans. This fact has more than once been exploited by the medical students as a vehicle for conveying health concepts.

On one occasion, a medical student who plays the guitar led a group of patients in a song on "how to treat a fever," set to a reggae heat—the strongly accented rhythm of West Indian music. The words were in large type and were held up for all to see. The audience joined in with cheerful gusto. On another occasion, two medical students planned Christmas party and concert for children at the local school. One student was deeply interested in drama while the other was a good pianist. They chose a "knowledge, attitude and practices" study in oral hygiene as their project. The supervisor from Social and Preventive Medicine suggested combining their project report with the Christmas party.

A group of children from the school answered a questionnaire on care of the teeth. The same children then put on a concert, which included not only a nativity play but also a dance about brushing the teeth, with appropriate musical accompaniment. One set of children kneeling represented the lower row of teeth, and children standing behind them represented the upper teeth. One little girl used a large broom to brush the teeth across. Then out from between the children crept a very small boy who declared he was a germ untouched by the broom. As the broom was now used correctly, with an up-and-down movement, he uttered a yell and "died" as he slipped back out of view. The audience cheered, laughed and clapped their hands in appreciation.

Another dance had children bearing letters on sticks spelling HYPERTENSION. A song about the value of taking pills every day for hypertension was danced to a mento rhythm—a catchy tune and dance peculiar to Jamaica. The sticks were turned round and DIABETES came in for its share of management in the form of a dance.

After the concert, the children were asked the same questions .they had been asked before, plus an additional one: "What else should have been done to make the concert better?" They all replied, "You should have asked some of the parents to join us in putting on the concert, since they were the ones who had hypertension and diabetes."

We at the Department of Social and Preventive Medicine are now convinced of the value of music and drama in conveying health messages. The "message of the day" is now frequently conveyed by a group consisting of medical students, the clinic staff and some lay people. The little dramas are kept short and the message is kept simple. In this way we hope to change very gradually the lifestyle of rural communities so that they will in future take better care of themselves. We can follow the same thing in India.

8. Lack of Adequate Training to Personnel Engaged in Health Education

Health Education is a challenging task involving social, psychological and technical components. The most important quality of health educator is communication which most of them lack. Health activities involve multi-dimensional aspects carried out by different functionaries. Therefore, it is essential to make all of them appreciate the intentions of the health programme. Let us take the case of malaria control programme. It involves doctors, paramedical, people, spray men, etc. To make the programme successful, all must communicate among themselves.

Communication is an integral part· of every function of health administration "and that is why it is said to be the bloodstream of an organisation." It is a two-way process between people. In communication a message is transmitted and received..

Communication can be transmitted through audial, visual and audio-visual means. Communication plays the same role as the nervous system in a body. Norbert Wiener has rightly observed that "communication is the cement that makes an organisation." Communication is central to the exercise of authority in an organisation. In the words of Ordway Tead, "Communication is the touching of mind by mind, of person with person, whether it be one man, or a thousand .... It can include conversation, interview, dialogue, visual technique carefully used."[18]

Essentials of Communication

The essentials of communication are:

(a) Clarity of Thought

The first *sine qua non* of good communication is that the idea to be transmitted must be absolutely clear in the mind of the communicator. It must spring out from a 'clear' head. It should be understood by the personnel so that it may be fully appreciated and acted upon.

(b) Importance of Action Rather than Words

In all communication, actions are more significant than words. Example is better than precept. An .officer who is not punctual cannot succeed in enforcing the time-rules on the subordinates.

(c) Participation

In this connection it is essential that both the parties (the communicator and the recipient) should participate in the communication. It is the only way to make the communication effective.

(d) Transmission

The communicator must plan carefully what to communicate, with whom to communicate and how to communicate. How can the top personnel communicate with the workers when they themselves do not know or cannot understand all the facts about the new plans? Further, delegation of authority without responsibility breaks down the spirit of communication.

(e) Keep the System Always Alive

The system of communication should be kept open and alive all the year round. It is only by honest attempts that good communicative relations can be developed.

(f) Cordial Employer-Employee Relations

Effective communication requires good employer-employee relations, which enable mutual appreciation of different viewpoints.

According to Terry, eight factors are essential in making communication effective:

(a) Inform yourself fully;
(b) Establish a mutual trust in others;
(c) Find a common ground of experience;
(d) Use mutually known words;
(e) Have regard for context;
(f) Secure and hold the receiver's attention;
(g) Employ examples and visual aids; and
(h) Practice delaying relations.

According to Millet, seven factors make communication effective it should be clear, consistent with the expectation of the recipient, adequate, timely, uniform, flexible and acceptable.

Difficulties and Barriers to Communication

These can be classified into three categories:

(a) Social and psychological;
(b) Organisational; and
(c) Mechanical.

Social and Psychological

People in an organisation come from different social background. The same problem may be looked differently by different people. The messages are thus interpreted differently by different people. Information is distorted through adding and subtracting one's own ideas. Besides, the connotations of words are not properly understood. We can improve upon this through management by objectives (MHO), which can generate understanding about the true goals of the organisation. Besides, the members of the organisation may be encouraged to meet frequently to sort out differences.

Organisational

Organisation consists of many layers. Communication transmitted reaches the lower levels through all the levels in between and *vice versa.* There is a danger of the information reaching the lower levels in a different context leading to friction, misunderstandings and distortion. It is suggested that the top personnel in the organisation must creates an environment of trust and confidence. There is also a need of constant personal contacts of the top personnel with the subordinates to remove misunderstandings. Organisations generally transmit more information than required (overloading) which needs to be discouraged to ensure compliance.

Mechanical

These emanate from defective system of dispatch and communication within the organisation resulting in delays, etc. These may also result from the wrong use of media. It is suggested that a set procedure must be in vogue for smooth communication from upward downward, and *vice versa,* as well as horizontal. This would avoid overloading and ensure timeiy receipt of communication.[19]

Let us take as example of Family Health.

Viewed from this standpoint, the health of the family might appear to be simply the sum of the health of all the individuals making up the family. In fact, it represents much more than this, since it takes into consideration the interpersonal relationships within the family group and the biological and social environment in which the group functions and lives. In this light, the most important indices of family health are probably the composition of the family, the patterns of its growth until it is complete, and the physical and psychological development of the children. The quality of life or of happiness is difficult to quantify, and there are such negative factors as the effect of morbidity and mortality on the family structure, or crises, both transitory and lasting, which may tend to break up the group.

Family health and community health are distinct entities, even though closely linked with each other. A community cannot be healthy if the families of which it is composed are themselves in a poor shape. One of the afflictions of many modern societies is the existence of underprivileged, excluded or marginal families cut-off from the benefits of expansion and socio-economic progress. These constitute what has been very vividly described as the "Fourth World." Coping with the problems they face simultaneously promotes the health of the community. To go one stage further, it may be asserted that every family should be induced, by means of education rather than coercion, to assume responsibility not only for its own health problems but also for the well-being of the community of which it is a part. Through reliance on such families, public health will be able to make its objectives and activities acceptable.

In our era of rapid change, it is fundamental to have a proper grasp of the concept of the family within the context of its everyday life in order to plan judiciously the services, which are required to meet health needs. The family represents an essential element in the functioning of society; in return, it is entitled to expect society to provide a certain number of services, notably access to education, to welfare and to progress in all fields-not least, in that of health.[20]

10. Lack of Infrastructure for Health Education

A large number of health training Institutions have been set-up but they lack infrastructure for health education like literature, well trained trainers, Audio-Visual aids, demonstration exercises, etc. Health education is given only a lip service. Even in the field health education is given last priority by health workers. In this advanced age, people know very little about positive health. All the family members have forgotten the old preventive practices, which kept the individual and the family healthy. The need is to strengthen infrastructure for health education. All schools, colleges, universities should include health education in different subjects.

WHO also helps countries to assess their need, so that they can derive the best advantage from the resources that the Clearing House offers. Countries are encouraged to develop self-reliance in designing tnaterials produced in Arabic and appropriate to their health training programmes.[21]

11. Not Effective Teaching of Health Education as Part of Under-graduate and Post-graduate Curriculum

Traditionally, the primary role of medical schools has been the training of medical practitioners to deliver service to all persons either as individuals or in groups. In recent years, more attention is being given to health promotion, health education of the community and preventive measures in relation to health and disease. It follows that medical schools can play an important role in community health development through appropriate education of the health professionals.

Let us explains with an example:

Teaching in the hospital setting before students go to the countryside is heavily slanted towards clinical curative or therapeutic medicine in the third or penultimate year prepares the students to deal with the problems of groups of people. The five-week Community Medicine programme in the rural areas in the final year provides a testing ground for the efficacy of the previous year's teaching. It also gives the students a chance to gain confidence in their own ability to function 12 to 14 miles (20 to 25 kilometers) away from the nearest hospital without the instant back-up services of the University teaching hospital.

These realities have thrown into sharp focus the fundamental importance of "sharing the knowledge" with lay people.

How is this accent on education implemented? Firstly, the co-coordinator introduces the importance of this on the first day of the course at the University Campus, not far from Kingston, the Jamaican capital. On the second or third day the students who are now in the field have another orientation exercise arranged by the local health team, when the value of communication is again reinforced. Next, the government's Health Educator for the parish holds a formal session during the first week on how to impart knowledge to rural folk. Finally, the students are warned by the coordinator that "when two or three are gathered together, for whatever reason, the opportunity to 'share the knowledge' must be seized." Thus, from the very first day the rudiments of communication are taught. This session is of vital importance. The target population is the one in the waiting room. The people may have come together for curative medicine, as in the general clinic or the hypertension clinic; or they may have come for "preventive" reasons, as in the baby clinic where mothers are instructed in nutrition or immunization, or are counseled in general child care.

The students decide on the topic for discussion. This they do in consultation with the other members of the health team, including the porter, the elderly and the housekeeper. Once the team decides on the topic only one fundamental concept will be shared with the target group.[22]

A challenging and a slow process—Health Education is a challenging task, as it is very difficult to change habits immediately. Let us explain with an example.

Over the last two decades the government and health agencies in the United Kingdom have placed great emphasis on equipping individuals with the right knowledge and skills to make decisions about their health. There have been valuable success; for example, a large number of people have given up smoking—more than three million in the last decade—to the point where only about one-third of adults now smoke. But there have also been notable failures; there are increasing numbers who are overweight and obese, and who do not take sufficient exercise to gain health benefits-now more than half the adult population.

Our "Heartbeat Award" scheme sought to encourage a healthier eating environment. Developed on a pilot basis early in 1986, it has not only spread to the whole of Wales but also to the rest of the United Kingdom. The scheme is administered by the environmental health department of local authorities during their routine inspection of establishments that sell meals. To qualify for an award, at least one-third of the seating area must be clearly designated as no smoking, a range of healthy foods must be provided on the menu (fresh fruit, non-fried dishes and so on), and the premises must have high standards of food hygiene. A successful proprietor is given a sticker to go on the door and a certificate to display inside. The scheme has a double attraction: each establishment benefits through publicity and endorsement, while the environmental health officer carries out a positive, rewarding action rather than a punitive one. Hundreds of premises, including "pubs" (drinking bars), now display the Heartbeat Award.

Can we draw any wider conclusions from the progress that has occurred in just this one area of Heartbeat Wales' activities? We think so. The underlying principles of the nutrition programme could well apply to other health issues in other parts of the world:

- Emphasizing that it is the people's programme not the authorities.
- Working with people, not against them.
- Building self-confidence, not destroying it.
- Supporting and helping, not coercing people.
- Concentrating on positive, not negative approaches.
- Working with all sectors, not just a few.
- Cooperating with organisations, not "taking them on."
- Drawing on community resources, not funding everything.
- Acting through people, not posters.
- Encouraging participation, not passivity.

Two years after the programme was launched, we carried out a follow-up questionnaire survey among 1,000 adults. This showed that hundreds of thousands of Welsh people were reporting important behavioural changes. For example, 29 per cent of all smokers had made a serious attempt to stop smoking in the past year, more than half of them succeeding for longer than a month. Over a third (35 per cent) of all adults reported having consciously changed their diet to a healthier one; 28 per cent had successfully lost more than five pounds in weight in the last year and a similar number said they were taking more regular exercise; 54 per cent had their blood pressure checked in the past year. The changes were observed in both sexes, all ages and all social groups throughout the whole of Wales.[23]

We should not base our health education on our own principles but should develop them as per the needs of people. We must base our campaign on the scientific views of sociologists, economists, law enforcement organs and, most important of all, on the views of the people themselves. Only this approach will give us a realistic and effective strategy. I have met hundreds and hundreds of people and not one has spoken against this drive for temperance on which the country has embarked. All were in favour-even the chronic alcoholics and hardened drinkers. But how to go about it consciously and in a spirit of patriotism, so that it produces results without giving offence, without humiliating people, nobody knows but the people themselves. We should all join forces to meet this challenge.[24]

12. Health Education does not take into Consideration Cultural Values Causing Misunderstandings and Non-acceptance

To communicate is also to persuade. And a key to effective persuasion may lie in discovering how a situation affects a family or community in such a way that it becomes a part of them personally. Since messages must be interpreted within the cultural framework, the greater the cultural disparity between the communicators and their receivers, I the less likely the communicator will be able to define and interpret.[25]

Successful campaigns against breast cancer, tobacco and AIDS in' California have relied more than health prpgrammes in the past upon dialogue between health professionals, volunteer organisations and the public at large. To I do this, original techniques had to be tailored and adapted to their audiences or, better still, had to involve the public as partners in health.[26]

13. Health Educators do not Understand the Role of Mass Media—Need of Understanding

Health promoters and educators need to be convinced that the mass media can operate in the public interest and should play a critical role in social affairs, including health issues. The health concerns of readers, listeners and viewers are very much the concerns of the print and broadcast journalists. The basis of the relationship between the health and media sectors should therefore be one of partnership, not one of user-helper.

Health and media are not naturally inclined to work in unison. Historically, medical scientists trained in the methodical and meticulous search for knowledge have been somewhat skeptical of any effort at popularizing their work. Some doctors even view the media with suspicion and ambivalence. Media people, on the other hand, need to have their source material in language understandable to the layman; they have no time to dwell on technical details, and often lose patience with lengthy scientific papers.

Yet media and health in a close partnership have much to contribute to the public's welfare. Without the involvement of the media, the health sector cannot hope to inform the public on health issues or to help stimulate a community's involvement, which is critical to the success of any health effort. Without the technical input of the health sector, the media cannot fulfil their obligations to serve the interest of the public and these public interests certainly include health.

The complexity of the media, with their obsession for meeting deadlines and their own technical constraints, is little appreciated or understood by health professionals. Those in health who most work in partnership with the media need to acquire a rudimentary knowledge of how media work not in order to become media specialists but to be more empathetic in their dealings with the journalists and broadcasters. This in turn will call for a good hard look at the core curriculum of the training of health promoters and educators.

Whether the health professionals can play their rightful role in battling successfully against lifestyle-related illness—including AIDS—and whether health education and promotion practitioners will enter the 21st century adequately prepared for the communication challenges, will depend on the actions that health authorities take now.

CONCLUSION

Health Education possess the potentiality and can optimize health action provided it is well planned, designed audience specific, practical in approach and interesting. Health education can play an important role in providing decent health care.[27]

We should following the following to make health education a reality:

- Promote actions which are realistic and feasible within the constraints faced by the community;
- Build on ideas, concepts and practices that people already have;
- Repeat and reinforce information over time, using different methods;
- Use existing channels of communication such as songs, drama and storytelling, and be adaptable;
- Entertain and attract the attention of the community;
- Use clear, simple language with local expressions and emphasize short-term benefits of action;
- Provide opportunities for dialogue and discussion to allow learner participation and feedback on understanding and implementation.
- Use demonstrations to show the benefits of adopting practices.[28]

Notes and References

1. Declaration on Health Development in the South-East Asia Region in the 21st Century, *World Health*, New Delhi, 1997, pp. 24-25.
2. WHO: Akbar Moarefi, 'The Corner-Stone', *World Health*, August-September 1975, p. 32.
3. *Ibid.*
4. Declaration on Health Development in the South-East Asia Region in the,21st Century, World Health, New Delhi, 1997, pp. 33-34.
5. WHO: Intersectoral Action, 2000, World Health, March 1986, p. 16.
6. WHO: Intersectoral Cooperation in primary health care, *World Health*, March, 1986, p. 3.
7. WHO: Mark L. Schneider, Rhetoric and reality, *World Health*, March 1986, p. 13.
8. WHO: Akbar Moarefi, 'The Corner-Stone', *World Health*, August-September 1975, pp. 32-33.
9. WHO: Dr. Hiroshi Nakajima, "A wounded planet", *World Health*, January-February 1990, p. 3.
10. WHO: Dr. Mrs. Gro Harlem Brundtland,. "In tune with Nature, *World Health*, January-February 1990, p. 4.
11. WHO: Dr. Wilfried Kreisel, "Environmental health in the 1990's", *World Health*, January-February 1990, p. 5.
12. Khalil Gibran: Between Night and Morn, the Philosophical Library, New York, 1972, pp. 8-9.
13. WHO: Fritz K. Kaferstein, Pleasure and pitfalls of eating, *World Health*, November 1988, p. 7.

14. Merle Fainsod: "The Structure of Development Administration" in Irving Swerdlow, ed. 'Development Administration: Concepts and Problems' (Syracuse, N.Y., Syracuse University Press, 1963), p. 1.
15. WHO Chronicle, 30, (1976), pp. 177-78.
16. WHO: M.A.C. Dowling, Health Learning Materials, *World Health*, April-May 1983, p. 21.
17. WHO: Kenneth L. Standard and Owen D. Minott, A song and a dance, *World Health*, April-May 1983, p. 7.
18. Ordway Tead, The Art of Administration, New York, McGraw-Hill, 1951, p. 45.
19. Dr.S.L.Goel, Advanced Public Administration, "Communication-Coordination and Control", pp. 188-90.
20. WHO: Michel Manciaus, "The Health of The Family", *World Health*, August-September 1975, p. 9.
21. WHO: Abdulmoneim Aly, "Health education through religion", *World Health*, July 1989, p. 28.
22. WHO: Kenneth L. Standard and Owen D. Minott, *World Health*, April-May 1983, pp. 5-6.
23. WHO: John Catford, "Heartbeat Wales", *World Health*, June 1988, pp. 24-25.
24. WHO: Anatolij Martynov, "Battles won-but not yet the war!", *World Health*, June 1988, p. 27.
25. WHO: Gloria Gordon, Let's Communication, *World Health*, January-February, 1989, p. 13.
26. WHO: Nedd Willard, *World Health*, January-February, 1989, p. 20.
27. WHO: Jack C.S. Ling, "The Media's Role", *World Health*, January-February, 1989, p. 25.
28. WHO: Gloria Gordon, "Let's Communicate", *World Health*, January-February 1989, p. 12.

APPENDIX I

COMMUNITY HEALTH CARE MANAGEMENT INITIATIVE (CHCMI)

(A presentation:25th March, 2008)

"**Community**'s health in **community**'s hand"—central motto of the initiative:

- Promoting **commnity** involvement in health care management through awareness generation, programme and capacity building exercises, while ensuring delivery of services at the **community** level.
- To develop a sense of responsibility among common people towards their own health care management under the leadership of Panchayati Raj Institutions.
- to motivate, enlighten, enthuse and involve individuals and institutions to **community** action for achieving good health and well being of the **community**.

OBJECTIVES OF COMMUNITY HEALTH CARE MANAGEMENT INITIATIVE

- To develop appropriate attitude and knowledge of all concerned Government functionaries, PRI functionaries, self help groups and functionaries of related institutions in order for them to act as change agents.
- To institutionalize the system of public health monitoring by the Panchayats.
- To sensitize communities on the issues of public health.
- To build capacity of the communities to plan, implement and manage health care interventions by developing among them a strong sense of ownership of the system.
- To work out plans at the different levels for improving outreach, particularly in unserved and under-served areas through regular monitoring and facilitation so as to improve access of the communities to basic health services.
- To improve coordination among the various units of service providers, Panchayati Raj Institutions and **community** members.

CHCMI-Programme to build up the capacity of the Panchayat Bodies especially the Gram Panchayats to,

- understand the issues relating to public health in their respective area,

- prepare a baseline on various parameters on the situation obtaining in the Gram Panchayat,
- set a time bound target for improving the status of the deficiencies identified during thé baseline, and
- prepare an action plan for reaching the targets.

METHODOLOGY

• The lowest tier of the PRIs, i.e. the Gram Panchayats (GPs) have been made the nodal agency for implementing the initiative.

• Self-help Groups (SHGs) members, because of their socio-economic conditions, represent both—beneficiaries as well as ambassadors of CHCMI.

• The ANWs, SHG members, members of various voluntary organisations, CBO/NGOs, Government staff, etc. under the leadership of the Gram Panchayat and co-ordination support from PRIs in Block and District levels and other administrative set-ups and institutions work in tandem to implement CHCMI through various process interventions like capacity building, networking, data building and updating, awareness generation, **community** monitoring, etc.

PROCESS AND PLANNING INTERVENTIONS

- Collection of information on the health status and health care practices in the area by the communities with the help of SHG members, health workers, anganwadi workers,
- Spreading awareness on safe motherhood and safe childbirth.
- Bringing all pregnant women and children into complete immunisation coverage
- Ensuring all births taking place under direct supervision of either a doctor or a trained health worker or by trained birth attendents .
- Regular checking of pregnant and lactating women and the newborn.
- Spreading awareness to counter malnutrition, monitoring growth of children.
- Ensuring safe potable water, sanitary latrines, smokeless chulas, soak pits.
- Spreading awareness amongst the **community** on preventable diseases like diarrhoea, RTI, malaria, etc.
- Spreading awareness about the health services.
- Development of awareness against superstitions and bad practices in relation to the diseases and the treatment.
- Development of awareness about birth control and family welfare measures.

- Assisting panchayats in registration of births and deaths and documentation of marriages.

MANAGEMENT STRUCTURE

- PRDD-HFWD-WCDSWD COMBINE (with SPHC of PRDD as its arm)
- ZP JANASWASTHYA O PARIVESH SS (with DPHC and DLTT and DRT as its arms)
- PS JANASWASTHYA O PARIVESH SS (with BLTT as its arm)
- GP JANASWASTHYS-O-SIKSHA US (with GPFT as its arm)
- GRAM UNNAYAN SAMITI (with its Functional Committee)
- SELF-HELP GROUP

Monitoring mechanism-Fourth Saturday meeting

- For awareness generation, stocktaking and preparing action plans, all GPs conduct Last Saturday meetings on a regular basis.
- Health Supervisor, ICDS Supervisor, field level functionaries remain present
- Deliberate on health related issues in the GP area.
- This is now being held in almost all the GPs.
- A chart is filled up by the GPs alongwith the proforma reports and displayed in the office for public viewing.
- Similar meetings are also to be held at the Block and the District level.

Baseline Survey undertaken by the SHGs

- Aim is to understand the basic public health scenario.
- Self-help Groups (SHGs), particularly those belonging to the economically weaker section because of their socio-economic conditions, can represent both—beneficiaries as well as ambassadors of CHCMI.
- SHGs have been sensitised and have conducted the household survey.
- SHGs to practice the good habits and shun the bad practices in their families and to encourage the **community** in this field.

Pilot Activities

- 6 districts of Uttar Dinajpur, Dakshin Dinajpur, Malda, Murshidabad, Purulia and Birbhum having the worst health indicators were selected.

- At least 6 GPs selected per district and intensive capacity exercises for the PRIs and the SHGs were undertaken.
- Baseline surveys conducted, data compiled by PRIs and situation was analysed.
- PRIs identified the problems and **community**-based health action plans were prepared in those 51 GPs.

GP Level Planning and interventions

- 51 GPs have prepared a Public Health Plan based on the data collected from the baseline survey.
- Spending on Public Health from GP fund has increased greatly.
- Some GPs are organising referral transport for pregnant mothers from their own fund.
- GPs are monitoring the EDD of pregnant mothers to facilitate institutional delivery.
- GPs and PSs organising Health camps and financing supplementary food for the malnourished children.

Suggestions of IDS Kolkata after Evaluation of CHCMI (1st Phase)

- Main challenge is to motivate PRI functionaries who are yet to take active interest.
- *General capacity building* is as important as sensitisation workshops.
- Orientation workshops should be strengthened by *experienced motivators* .
- Sensitisation alone cannot be effective unless it is combined with incentives.
- Small number of feasible and observable targets may be set-up and GPs may be rewarded if they are attained.

Suggestions of IDS Kolkata after Evaluation of CHCMI (1st Phase)

- To institutionalize, adequate financial provisioning is necessary; resources have so far been managed from sources other than earmarked Govt budgetary sources—grossly inadequate.
- Some stated goals of NRHM are in line with CHCMI's; while NRHM has made substantial financial allocation to achieve stated goals, CHCMI provides a kind of blueprint for working towards these goals.
- Obvious complementarities between the two.

Suggestions of IDS Kolkata after Evaluation of CHCMI (1st Phase)

- Money is needed for additional manpower to build capacity at various levels.

- Money is also needed to sustain motivation of SHGs; an honorium, however small, is a symbol of recognision.
- Not by money alone: Feeling of pride and self-respect in SHG members has to be nurtured by GP leadership.
- For DLTT, the district coordinators should be encouraged to invite people who are known for their abilities to motivate.

NATIONAL RURAL HEALTH MISSION (NRHM) AND PANCHAYATI RAJ INSTITUTIONS (PRIs)

- NRHM prescribed constitution of Village Health and Sanitation Committee at the village level under the PRIs to address various **community** level issues relating to health and nutrition.
- Gram Unnayan Samitis have been set-up at the village/Gram Sansad level as statutory committees under the WB Panchayats Act, and they have been empowered to plan and implement all development activities within the village.
- It has been decided that Gram Unnayan Samitis shall act as the Village Health and Sanitation Committee in the state.
- P&RD Department is issuing instructions for setting up a Functional Committee on Health and Sanitation by the Gram Unnayan Samiti.

Composition of Functional Committee on Health and Sanitation

- Elected representative from the Gram Sansad—Chairman.
- Person who secured the second highest vote in the last election to the Gram Panchayat from the Sansad area concerned.
- At least three women members to be selected by the Gram Unnayan Samiti from among its members.
- Three members to be elected from among the Secretaries and Treasurers of the women Self Help Groups from that Gram Sansad area.
- ANM and AWW working in the Gram Sansad area concerned)
- ASHA or link volunteer if any functioning in the Gram Sansad area.

Functions of the Functional Committee

- Prepare and implement a Health and Sanitation Plan for the Gram Sansad area on the following activities.
- *Awareness Generation.*
- Generating awareness for countering early marriage and early motherhood.
- Generating awareness for family planning.
- Generating awareness on exclusive breastfeeding through SHGs.

- Awareness generation and taking necessary steps through SHGs for Antenatal Care.
- Generating Awareness and take necessary steps through SHGs for antenatal Care.
- Ensure institutional delivery or at least delivery under trained hands.
- Generating awareness for prevention of HIV/AIDS as also social anathema about the disease.

Nutrition

- Take promotive and remedial steps for improving the nutritional status of women and children and reducing the incidence of malnutrition.
- Spread awareness on nutrition among women and children, Preparation and increasing the use of nutritional supplements through the SHG.
- Preparation of nutritional supplement can be introduced as a livelihood option for selected SHGs.

Immunization

Awareness and motivation for complete immunization of mothers and children including measles and TT for pregnant women.

Behavior Change communication

Undertake motivation for Behavior Change Communication for developing hygienic habits.

Other Activities

- Arrange for safe drinking water, sanitation and drainage.
- Communicate information of outbreaks of any disease to the Health system functionaries.
- Take up de-worming as a part of the school health programme in the primary schools along with arrangement for health check ups, to the possible extent.
- Providing basic equipments like weighing machine, etc. to the SHGs and AWWs for regular monitoring of child health, etc.
- Providing referral transport for the people to avail health care facilities.

Monitoring the indicators—Selection of SHGs

- One SHG of the Gram Sansad area, as selected by the Functional Committee shall be given the responsibility for effective monitoring and evaluation of the activities related to health and sanitation.

- The SHGs will be chosen on the basis of the following criteria:
  - (i) The group should have passed the Grade-I
  - (ii) At least one member should be Class-VIII pass.
  - (iii) Should be local people, conscious about the local problems and should be acceptable in the locality.
  - (iv) Preferably have previous experiences in health sector related activities.

Role of SHGs

- The activities, which may be taken up by the SHGs, are as follows;
- Conduct a survey for preparation of Baseline for identification of families.
- The survey may aim at identifying adolescent girls, pregnant mothers, children in the age group 0-5 years, the feeding habit of the children, their weights (the SHGs may weigh the babies) and eligible couples. The Health and Sanitation Plan of the Gram Sansad shall be based on the findings of the Baseline Survey. The survey findings shall be updated periodically as may be prescribed.
- Take the guidance of the ANMs and Anganwadi Workers to identify the individual requiring immediate action after completion of the survey.
- Prepare a social map based on the data generated in the survey to have knowledge of the areas and families requiring interventions

Activities by the SHGs

- Prepare a social map based on the data generated in the survey to have knowledge of the areas and families requiring interventions.
- Help the pregnant mothers to register them in the Sub Centers, avail Antenatal Checkups, to get immunized and also encourage them to take IFA tablets and encourage them to have balanced diet.
- Encourage the pregnant women and their families to make preparation for Institutional delivery.
- Visiting the nursing mothers for PNC, take the weight of the children of the targeted age group once a month and report to the ANM at a monthly meeting where the Anganwadi Workers will remain present.
- Encourage the parents of the children to take them to the AWCs

and also help the parents of identified children in need of medical attention to take them to PHCs/BPHCs.

- Ensure Awareness and motivation for complete immunization
- Spread awareness on nutrition among adolescent girls, women and children, including exclusive breastfeeding.
- Ensure consumption of prescribed doses of iron tablets by women of specified age group
- Undertake behavior change communication for developing hygienic habits.
- Communicate information of outbreaks of any disease to the Health system.
- Spread awareness against communicable diseases and promotion of healthy behavior.
- The list of activities detailed is illustrative and not exhaustive.

Monitoring and Supervision cost of the programme

- The SHGs may be paid monitoring and supervision costs out of the fund placed with the Functional committee according to their level of performances for different activities as specified below.
- For conducting the baseline survey and compilation of the data at the rate of 50 p and 25 p per family.

For calculating the supervision cost for the SHGs, the activities they will have to monitor are:

(i) Ensuring early registration of pregnant women, antenatal checkup and immunization of the pregnant women;
(ii) Ensuring consumption of IFA tablets by pregnant women and adolescent girls;
(iii) Ensuring delivery at safe hands;
(iv) Monthly weighing of children;
(v) Immunization of children.

- For monitoring 98% or above, the GUS may spend Rs. 500.00 per month, for 95-98% coverage, they may spend Rs. 400.00, for 90-95% coverage, they may spend Rs. 300.00 per month as monitoring and evaluation cost through the SHGs.

Funding and maintenance of Accounts of the Functional committee—

- The functional committee will be entitled to an annual grant of Rs. 10,000 for undertaking the activities mentioned above. The fund will be placed at the disposal of the Gram Panchayats who in turn will advance the amount to the Gram Unnayan Samiti concerned. The Accounts of the fund will be maintained according to norms prescribed by the P&RD Department.

Proposed Expenditure from Rs. 10,000

- Monitoring cost to the SHGs,
- Organisation of 3-4 meetings on specific themes,
- Water testing,
- Weighing Machine,
- Supply of soap to the primary schools and SSKs,
- Organisation of monitoring meetings with the SHGs and purchase of registers, and
- Cleaning of drains, removal of water hyacinth, wall writing (Rs. 5000-6000, Rs. 1000 , Rs. 400, Rs. 500, Rs. 500 , Rs. 600 , Rs. 1000).

Related Capacity Building Exercises

- Training of DLTT by the SPHC- ZP to identify effective members of DLTT and Resource Persons immediately.
- Sensitization of the Panchayat Samitis and the Gram Panchayats by the DLTT and district level officials and PRI members.
- Training of BLTT by the DLTT.
- Training of GPFT by BLTT and DLTT.
- Sensitization of GUSs.
- Training of members of GUS and SHGs by the GPFT and BLTT.

Appendix 2

NATIONAL HEALTH POLICY-2002

I. INTRODUCTORY

1.1 A National Health Policy was last formulated in 1983, and since then there have been marked changes in the determinant factors relating to the health sector. Some of the policy initiatives outlined in the NHP-1983 have yielded results, while, in several other areas, the outcome has not been as expected.

1.2 The NHP-1983 gave a general exposition of the policies which required recommendation in the circumstances then prevailing in the health sector. The noteworthy initiatives under that policy were:-

(i) A phased, time-bound programme for setting up a well-dispersed network of comprehensive primary health care services, linked with extension and health education, designed in the context of the ground reality that elementary health problems can be resolved by the people themselves;

(ii) Intermediation through 'Health volunteers' having appropriate knowledge, simple skills and requisite technologies;

(iii) Establishment of a well-worked out referral system to ensure that patient load at the higher levels of the hierarchy is not needlessly burdened by those who can be treated at the decentralized level; and

(iv) An integrated net-work of evenly spread speciality and super-speciality services; encouragement of such facilities through private investments for patients who can pay, so that the draw on the Government's facilities is limited to those entitled to free use.

1.3 Government initiatives in the pubic health sector have recorded some noteworthy successes over time. Smallpox and Guinea Worm Disease have been eradicated from the country; Polio is on the verge of being eradicated; Leprosy, Kala Azar, and Filariasis can be expected to be eliminated in the foreseeable future. There has been a substantial drop in the Total Fertility Rate and Infant Mortality Rate. The success of the initiatives taken in the public health field are reflected in the progressive improvement of many demographic/epidemiological/infrastructural indicators over time—(Box-I).

1.4 While noting that the public health initiatives over the years have contributed significantly to the improvement of these health indicators, it is to be acknowledged that public health indicators/disease-burden statistics

Box-I

Achievements Through The Years—1951-2000

Indicator	1951	1981	2000
Demographic Changes			
Life Expectancy	36.7	54	64.6(RGI)
Crude Birth Rate	40.8	33.9(SRS)	26.1(99 SRS)
Crude Death Rate	25	12.5(SRS)	8.7(99 SRS)
IMR	146	110	70 (99 SRS)
Epidemiological Shifts			
Malaria (cases in million)	75	2.7	2.2
Leprosy cases per 10,000 population	38.1	57.3	3.74
Small Pox (no. of cases)	>44,887	Eradicated	
Guineaworm (no. of cases)		>39,792	Eradicated
Polio		29709	265
Infrastructure			
SC/PHC/CHC (99-RHS)	725	57,363	1,63,181
Dispensaries and Hospitals (all)	9209	23,555 CBHI)	43,322 (95–96-
Beds (Pvt. and Public)	117,198	569,495 (95-96-CBHI)	8,70,161
Doctors (Allopathy)	61,800	2,68,700 (98-99-MCI)	5,03,900
Nursing Personnel	18,054	1,43,887 (99-INC)	7,37,000

are the outcome of several complementary initiatives under the wider umbrella of the developmental sector, covering Rural Development, Agriculture, Food Production, Sanitation, Drinking Water Supply, Education, etc. Despite the impressive public health gains as revealed in the statistics in Box-I, there is no gainsaying the fact that the morbidity and mortality levels in the country are still unacceptably high. These unsatisfactory health indices are, in turn, an indication of the limited success of the public health system in meeting the preventive and curative requirements of the general population.

1.5 Out of the communicable diseases which have persisted over time, the incidence of Malaria staged a resurgence in the 1980s before stabilising at a fairly high prevalence level during the 1990s. Over the years, an increasing level of insecticide-resistance has developed in the malarial vectors in many parts of the country, while the incidence of the more deadly P-Falciparum Malaria has risen to about 50 percent in the country as a whole. In respect of TB, the public health scenario has not shown any significant decline in the pool of infection amongst the community, and there has been a distressing trend in the increase of drug resistance to the type of infection prevailing in the country. A new and extremely virulent communicable disease—HIV/AIDS—has emerged on the health scene since the declaration of the NHP-1983. As there is no existing therapeutic cure or vaccine for this infection, the disease constitutes a serious threat, not merely to public health but to economic development in the country. The common water-borne infections—Gastroenteritis, Cholera, and some forms of Hepatitis—continue to contribute to a high level of morbidity in the population, even though the mortality rate may have been somewhat moderated.

1.6 The period after the announcement of NHP-83 has also seen an increase in mortality through 'lifestyle' diseases- diabetes, cancer and cardiovascular diseases. The increase in life expectancy has increased the requirement for geriatric care. Similarly, the increasing burden of trauma cases is also a significant public health problem.

1.7 Another area of grave concern in the public health domain is the persistent incidence of macro and micro nutrient deficiencies, especially among women and children. In the vulnerable sub-category of women and the girl child, this has the multiplier effect through the birth of low birth weight babies and serious ramifications of the consequential mental and physical retarded growth.

1.8 NHP-1983, in a spirit of optimistic empathy for the health needs of the people, particularly the poor and under-privileged, had hoped to provide 'Health for All by the year 2000 AD', through the universal provision of comprehensive primary health care services. In retrospect, it is observed that the financial resources and public health administrative capacity which it was possible to marshal, was far short of that necessary to achieve such an ambitious and holistic goal. Against this backdrop, it is felt that it would be appropriate to pitch NHP-2002 at a level consistent with our realistic expectations about financial resources, and about the likely increase in Public Health administrative capacity. The recommendations of NHP-2002 will, therefore, attempt to maximize the broad-based availability of health services to the citizenry of the country on the basis of realistic considerations of capacity. The changed circumstances relating to the health sector of the country since 1983 have generated a situation in which it is now necessary to review the field, and to formulate a new policy framework as the National Health Policy-2002. NHP-2002 will attempt to set out a new policy framework for the accelerated achievement of Public health goals in the socio-economic circumstances currently prevailing in the country.

2. CURRENT SCENARIO

2.1 FINANCIAL RESOURCES

2.1.1 The public health investment in the country over the years has been comparatively low, and as a percentage of GDP has declined from 1.3 percent in 1990 to 0.9 percent in 1999. The aggregate expenditure in the Health sector is 5.2 percent of the GDP. Out of this, about 17 percent of the aggregate expenditure is public health spending, the balance being out-of-pocket expenditure. The central budgetary allocation for health over this period, as a percentage of the total Central Budget, has been stagnant at 1.3 percent, while that in the States has declined from 7.0 percent to 5.5 percent. The current annual per capita public health expenditure in the country is no more than Rs. 200. Given these statistics, it is no surprise that the reach and quality of public health services has been below the desirable standard. Under the constitutional structure, public health is the responsibility of the States. In this framework, it has been the expectation that the principal contribution for the funding of public health services will be from the resources of the States, with some supplementary input from Central resources. In this backdrop, the contribution of Central resources to the overall public health funding has been limited to about 15 percent. The fiscal resources of the State Governments are known to be very inelastic. This is reflected in the declining percentage of State resources allocated to the health sector out of the State Budget. If the decentralized public health services in the country are to improve significantly, there is a need for the injection of substantial resources into the health sector from the Central Government Budget. This approach is a necessity—despite the formal Constitutional provision in regard to public health,—if the State public health services, which are a major component of the initiatives in the social sector, are not to become entirely moribund. The NHP-2002 has been formulated taking into consideration these ground realities in regard to the availability of resources.

2.2 EQUITY

2.2.1 In the period when centralized planning was accepted as a key instrument of development in the country, the attainment of an equitable regional distribution was considered one of its major objectives. Despite this conscious focus in the development process, the statistics given in Box-II clearly indicate that the attainment of health indices has been very uneven across the rural-urban divide.

Also, the statistics bring out the wide differences between the attainments of health goals in the better-performing States as compared to the low-performing States. It is clear that national averages of health indices hide wide disparities in public health facilities and health standards in different parts of the country. Given a situation in which national averages in respect of most indices are themselves at unacceptably low levels, the wide inter-State disparity implies that, for vulnerable sections of society in several States, access to public health services is nominal and health standards are grossly inadequate. Despite a thrust in the NHP-1983 for making good the unmet needs of public health services by establishing more public health institutions at a decentralized level, a large gap in

Box II

Differentials in Health Status Among States

Sector	*Population BPL (%)*	*IMR/ Per 1000 Births (1999-SRS)*	*<5Mortality per Live (NFHS II)*	*Weight For Age-1000 Children Under 3 years (<-2SD)*	*MMR/ Lakh (Annual % of Report 2000)*	*Leprosy cases per 10000 population*	*Malaria +ve Cases in year 2000 (in thousands)*
India	26.1	70	94.9	47	408	3.7	2200
Rural	27.09	75	103.7	49.6	-	-	-
Urban	23.62	44	63.1	38.4	-	-	-
Better Performing States							
Kerala	12.72	14	18.8	27	87	0.9	5.1
Maharashtra	25.02	48	58.1	50	135	3.1	138
TN	21.12	52	63.3	37	79	4.1	56
Low Performing States							
Orissa	47.15	97	104.4	54	498	7.05	483
Bihar	42.60	63	105.1	54	707	11.83	132
Rajasthan	15.28	81	114.9	51	607	0.8	53
UP	31.15	84	122.5	52	707	4.3	99
MP	37.43	90	137.6	55	498	3.83	528

facilities still persists. Applying current norms to the population projected for the year 2000, it is estimated that the shortfall in the number of SCs/ PHCs/CHCs is of the order of 16 percent. However, this shortage is as high as 58 percent when disaggregated for CHCs only. The NHP-2002 will need to address itself to making good these deficiencies so as to narrow the gap between the various States, as also the gap across the rural-urban divide.

2.2.2 Access to, and benefits from, the public health system have been very uneven between the better-endowed and the more vulnerable sections of society. This is particularly true for women, children and the socially disadvantaged sections of society. The statistics given in Box-III highlight the handicap suffered in the health sector on account of socio-economic inequity.

2.2.3 It is a principal objective of NHP-2002 to evolve a policy structure which reduces these inequities and allows the disadvantaged sections of society a fairer access to public health services.

Box III

Differentials in Health status Among Socio-Economic Groups

Indicator	Infant Mortality/ 1000	Under 5 Mortality/ 1000	% Children Underweight
India	70	94.9	47
Social Inequity			
Scheduled Castes	83	119.3	53.5
Scheduled Tribes	84.2	126.6	55.9
Other Disadvantaged	76	103.1	47.3
Others	61.8	82.6	41.1

2.3 DELIVERY OF NATIONAL PUBLIC HEALTH PROGRAMMES

2.3.1 It is self-evident that in a country as large as India, which has a wide variety of socio-economic settings, national health programmes have to be designed with enough flexibility to permit the State public health administrations to craft their own programme package according to their needs. Also, the implementation of the national health programme can only be carried out through the State Governments' decentralized public health machinery. Since, for various reasons, the responsibility of the Central Government in funding additional public health services will continue over a period of time, the role of the Central Government in designing broad-based public health initiatives will inevitably continue. Moreover, it has been observed that the technical and managerial expertise for designing large-span public health programmes exists with the Central Government in a considerable degree; this expertise can be gainfully utilized in designing national health programmes for implementation in varying socio-economic settings in the States. With this background, the NHP-2002 attempts to define the role of the Central Government and the State Governments in the public health sector of the country.

2.3.2.1 Over the last decade or so, the Government has relied upon a 'vertical' implementational structure for the major disease control programmes. Through this, the system has been able to make a substantial dent in reducing the burden of specific diseases. However, such an organisational structure, which requires independent manpower for each disease programme, is extremely expensive and difficult to sustain. Over a long time-range, 'vertical' structures may only be affordable for those diseases which offer a reasonable possibility of elimination or eradication in a foreseeable time-span.

2.3.2.2 It is a widespread perception that, over the last decade and a half, the rural health staff has become a vertical structure exclusively for the implementation of family welfare activities. As a result, for those public health programmes where there is no separate vertical structure, there is no identifiable service delivery system at all. The Policy will address this distortion in the public health system.

2.4 THE STATE OF PUBLIC HEALTH INFRA-STRUCTURE

2.4.1 The delineation of NHP-2002 would be required to be based on an objective assessment of the quality and efficiency of the existing public health machinery in the field. It would detract from the quality of the exercise if, while framing a new policy, it were not acknowledged that the existing public health infrastructure is far from satisfactory. For the outdoor medical facilities in existence, funding is generally insufficient; the presence of medical and para-medical personnel is often much less than that required by prescribed norms; the availability of consumables is frequently negligible; the equipment in many public hospitals is often obsolescent and unusable; and, the buildings are in a dilapidated state. In the indoor treatment facilities, again, the equipment is often obsolescent; the availability of essential drugs is minimal; the capacity of the facilities is grossly inadequate, which leads to over-crowding, and consequentially to a steep deterioration in the quality of the services. As a result of such inadequate public health facilities, it has been estimated that less than 20 percent of the population, which seek OPD services, and less than 45 percent of that which seek indoor treatment, avail of such services in public hospitals. This is despite the fact that most of these patients do not have the means to make out-of-pocket payments for private health services except at the cost of other essential expenditure for items such as basic nutrition.

2.5 EXTENDING PUBLIC HEALTH SERVICES

2.5.1 While there is a general shortage of medical personnel in the country, this shortfall is disproportionately impacted on the less-developed and rural areas. No incentive system attempted so far, has induced private medical personnel to go to such areas; and, even in the public health sector, the effort to deploy medical personnel in such under-served areas, has usually been a losing battle. In such a situation, the possibility needs to be examined of entrusting some limited public health functions to nurses, paramedics and other personnel from the extended health sector after imparting adequate training to them.

2.5.2 India has a vast reservoir of practitioners in the Indian Systems of Medicine and Homoeopathy, who have undergone formal training in their own disciplines. The possibility of using such practitioners in the implementation of State/Central Government public health programmes, in order to increase the reach of basic health care in the country, is addressed in the NHP-2002.

2.6 ROLE OF LOCAL SELF-GOVERNMENT INSTITUTIONS

2.6.1 Some States have adopted a policy of devolving programmes and funds in the health sector through different levels of the Panchayati Raj Institutions. Generally, the experience has been an encouraging one. The adoption of such an organisational structure has enabled need-based allocation of resources and closer supervision through the elected representatives. The Policy examines the need for a wider adoption of this mode of delivery of health services, in rural as well as urban areas, in other parts of the country.

2.7 NORMS FOR HEALTH CARE PERSONNEL

2.7.1 It is observed that the deployment of doctors and nurses, in both public and private institutions, is *ad-hoc* and significantly short of the requirement for minimal standards of patient care. This policy will make a specific recommendation in regard to this deficiency.

2.8 EDUCATION OF HEALTH CARE PROFESSIONALS

2.8.1 Medical and Dental Colleges are not evenly spread across various parts of the country. Apart from the uneven geographical distribution of medical institutions, the quality of education is highly uneven and in several instances even sub-standard. It is a common perception that the syllabus is excessively theoretical, making it difficult for the fresh graduate to effectively meet even the primary health care needs of the population. There is a general reluctance on the part of graduate doctors to serve in areas distant from their native place. NHP-2002 will suggest policy initiatives to rectify the resultant disparities.

2.8.2.1 Certain medical disciplines, such as molecular biology and gene-manipulation, have become relevant in the period after the formulation of the previous National Health Policy. The components of medical research in recent years have changed radically. In the foreseeable future such research will rely increasingly on the new disciplines. It is observed that the current under-graduate medical syllabus does not cover such emerging subjects. The Policy will make appropriate recommendations in respect of such deficiencies.

2.8.2.2 Also, certain speciality disciplines—Anesthesiology, Radiology and Forensic Medicine—are currently very scarce, resulting in critical deficiencies in the package of available public health services. This Policy will recommend some measures to alleviate such critical shortages.

2.9 NEED FOR SPECIALISTS IN 'PUBLIC HEALTH' AND 'FAMILY MEDICINE'

2.9.1 In any developing country with inadequate availability of health services, the requirement of expertise in the areas of 'public health' and 'family medicine' is markedly more than the expertise required for other clinical specialities. In India, the situation is that public health expertise is non-existent in the private health sector, and far short of requirement in the public health sector. Also, the current curriculum in the graduate/post-graduate courses is outdated and unrelated to contemporary community needs. In respect of 'family medicine', it needs to be noted that the more talented medical graduates generally seek specialization in clinical disciplines, while the remaining go into general practice. While the availability of post-graduate educational facilities is 50 percent of the total number of qualifying graduates each year, and can be considered adequate, the distribution of the disciplines in the post-graduate training facilities is overwhelmingly in favour of clinical specializations. NHP-2002 examines the possible means for ensuring adequate availability of personnel with specialization in the 'public health' and 'family medicine' disciplines, to discharge the public health responsibilities in the country.

2.10 NURSING PERSONNEL

2.10.1 The ratio of nursing personnel in the country vis-à-vis doctors/ beds is very low according to professionally accepted norms. There is also an acute shortage of nurses trained in super-speciality disciplines for deployment in tertiary care facilities. NHP-2002 addresses these problems.

2.11 USE OF GENERIC DRUGS AND VACCINES

2.11.1 India enjoys a relatively low-cost health care system because of the widespread availability of indigenously manufactured generic drugs and vaccines. There is an apprehension that globalization will lead to an increase in the costs of drugs, thereby leading to rising trends in overall health costs. This Policy recommends measures to ensure the future Health Security of the country.

2.12 URBAN HEALTH

2.12.1.1 In most urban areas, public health services are very meagre. To the extent that such services exist, there is no uniform organisational structure. The urban population in the country is presently as high as 30 percent and is likely to go up to around 33 percent by 2010. The bulk of the increase is likely to take place through migration, resulting in slums without any infrastructure support. Even the meagre public health services which are available do not percolate to such unplanned habitations, forcing people to avail of private health care through out-of-pocket expenditure.

2.12.1.2 The rising vehicle density in large urban agglomerations has also led to an increased number of serious accidents requiring treatment in well-equipped trauma centres. NHP-2002 will address itself to the need for providing this unserved urban population a minimum standard of broad-based health care facilities.

2.13 MENTAL HEALTH

2.13.1 Mental health disorders are actually much more prevalent than is apparent on the surface. While such disorders do not contribute significantly to mortality, they have a serious bearing on the quality of life of the affected persons and their families. Sometimes, based on religious faith, mental disorders are treated as spiritual affliction. This has led to the establishment of unlicensed mental institutions as an adjunct to religious institutions where reliance is placed on faith cure. Serious conditions of mental disorder require hospitalization and treatment under trained supervision. Mental health institutions are woefully deficient in physical infrastructure and trained manpower. NHP-2002 will address itself to these deficiencies in the public health sector.

2.14 INFORMATION, EDUCATION AND COMMUNICATION

2.14.1 A substantial component of primary health care consists of initiatives for disseminating to the citizenry, public health-related information. IEC initiatives are adopted not only for disseminating curative guidelines (for the TB, Malaria, Leprosy, Cataract Blindness Programmes), but also as part of the effort to bring about a behavioural change to prevent HIV/AIDS and other lifestyle diseases. Public health programmes, particularly, need high visibility at the decentralized level in order to have an impact. This task is difficult as 35 percent of our country's population is illiterate. The present IEC strategy is too fragmented, relies too heavily on the mass media and does not address the needs of this segment of the population. It is often felt that the effectiveness of IEC programmes is difficult to judge; and consequently it is often asserted that accountability, in regard to the productive use of such funds, is doubtful. The Policy, while projecting an IEC strategy, will fully address the inherent problems encountered in any IEC programme designed for improving awareness and bringing about a behavioural change in the general population.

2.14.2 It is widely accepted that school and college students are the most impressionable targets for imparting information relating to the basic principles of preventive health care. The policy will attempt to target this group to improve the general level of awareness in regard to 'health-promoting' behaviour.

2.15 HEALTH RESEARCH

2.15.1 Over the years, health research activity in the country has been very limited. In the Government sector, such research has been confined to the research institutions under the Indian Council of Medical Research, and other institutions funded by the States/Central Government. Research in the private sector has assumed some significance only in the last decade. In our country, where the aggregate annual health expenditure is of the order of Rs. 80,000 crores, the expenditure in 1998-99 on research, both public and private sectors, was only of the order of Rs. 1150 crores. It would be reasonable to infer that with such low research expenditure, it is virtually impossible to make any dramatic break-through within the country, by way of new molecules and vaccines; also, without a minimal back-up of applied and operational research, it would be difficult to assess whether the health expenditure in the country is being incurred through optimal applications and appropriate public health strategies. Medical Research in the country needs to be focused on therapeutic drugs/vaccines for tropical diseases, which are normally neglected by international pharmaceutical companies on account of their limited profitability potential. The thrust will need to be in the newly-emerging frontier areas of research based on genetics, genome-based drug and vaccine development, molecular biology, etc. NHP-2002 will address these inadequacies and spell out a minimal quantum of expenditure for the coming decade, looking to the national needs and the capacity of the research institutions to absorb the funds.

2.16 ROLE OF THE PRIVATE SECTOR

2.16.1 Considering the economic restructuring under way in the country, and over the globe, in the last decade, the changing role of the private sector in providing health care will also have to be addressed in this Policy. Currently, the contribution of private health care is principally through independent practitioners. Also, the private sector contributes significantly to secondary-level care and some tertiary care. It is a widespread perception that private health services are very uneven in quality, sometimes even sub-standard. Private health services are also perceived to be financially exploitative, and the observance of professional ethics is noted only as an exception. With the increasing role of private health care, the implementation of statutory regulation, and the monitoring of minimum standards of diagnostic centres/medical institutions becomes imperative. The Policy will address the issues regarding the establishment of a comprehensive information system, and based on that the establishment of a regulatory mechanism to ensure the maintaining of adequate standards by diagnostic centres/medical institutions, as well as the proper conduct of clinical practice and delivery of medical services.

2.16.2 Currently, non-Governmental service providers are treating a large number of patients at the primary level for major diseases. However, the treatment regimens followed are diverse and not scientifically optimal, leading to an increase in the incidence of drug resistance. This policy will address itself to recommending arrangements which will eliminate the risks arising from inappropriate treatment.

2.16.3 The increasing spread of information technology raises the possibility of its adoption in the health sector. NHP-2002 will examine this possibility.

2.17 THE ROLE OF CIVIL SOCIETY

2.17.1 Historically, it has been the practice to implement major national disease control programmes through the public health machinery of the State/Central Governments. It has become increasingly apparent that certain components of such programmes cannot be efficiently implemented merely through government functionaries. A considerable change in the mode of implementation has come about in the last two decades, with the increasing involvement of NGOs and other institutions of civil society. It is to be recognized that widespread debate on various public health issues has, in fact, been initiated and sustained by NGOs and other members of the civil society. Also, an increasing contribution is being made by such institutions in the delivery of different components of public health services. Certain disease control programmes require close inter-action with the beneficiaries for regular administration of drugs; periodic carrying out of pathological tests; dissemination of information regarding disease control and other general health information. NHP-2002 will address such issues and suggest policy instruments for the implementation of public health programmes through individuals and institutions of civil society.

2.18 NATIONAL DISEASE SURVEILLANCE NETWORK

2.18.1 The technical network available in the country for disease surveillance is extremely rudimentary and to the extent that the system exists, it extends only up to the district level. Disease statistics are not flowing through an integrated network from the decentralized public health facilities to the State/Central Government health administration. Such an arrangement only provides belated information, which, at best, serves a limited statistical purpose. The absence of an efficient disease surveillance network is a major handicap in providing a prompt and cost-effective health care system. The efficient disease surveillance network set-up for Polio and HIV/AIDS has demonstrated the enormous value of such a public health instrument. Real-time information on focal outbreaks of common communicable diseases—Malaria, GE, Cholera and JE—and the seasonal trends of diseases, would enable timely intervention, resulting in the containment of the thrust of epidemics. In order to be able to use an integrated disease surveillance network for operational purposes, real-time information is necessary at all levels of the health administration. The Policy would address itself to this major systemic shortcoming in the administration.

2.19 HEALTH STATISTICS

2.19.1 The absence of a systematic and scientific health statistics data-base is a major deficiency in the current scenario. The health statistics collected are not the product of a rigorous methodology. Statistics available from different parts of the country, in respect of major diseases, are often not obtained in a manner which make aggregation possible or meaningful.

2.19.2.1 Further, the absence of proper and systematic documentation of the various financial resources used in the health sector is another lacuna in the existing health information scenario. This makes it difficult to understand trends and levels of health spending by private and public providers of health care in the country, and, consequently, to address related policy issues and to formulate future investment policies.

2.19.2.2 NHP-2002 will address itself to the programme for putting in place a modern and scientific health statistics database as well as a system of national health accounts.

2.20 WOMEN'S HEALTH

2.20.1 Social, cultural and economic factors continue to inhibit women from gaining adequate access even to the existing public health facilities. This handicap does not merely affect women as individuals; it also has an adverse impact on the health, general well-being and development of the entire family, particularly children. This policy recognises the catalytic role of empowered women in improving the overall health standards of the community.

2.21 MEDICAL ETHICS

2.21.1 Professional medical ethics in the health sector is an area which has not received much attention. Professional practices are perceived to be grossly commercial and the medical profession has lost its elevated position as a provider of basic services to fellow human beings. In the past, medical research has been conducted within the ethical guidelines notified by the Indian Council of Medical Research. The first document containing these guidelines was released in 1960, and was comprehensively revised in 2001. With the rapid developments in the approach to medical research, a periodic revision will no doubt be more frequently required in future. Also, the new frontier areas of research—involving gene manipulation, organ/ human cloning and stem cell research—impinge on visceral issues relating to the sanctity of human life and the moral dilemma of human intervention in the designing of life forms. Besides this, in the emerging areas of research, there is the uncharted risk of creating new life forms, which may irreversibly damage the environment as it exists today. NHP-2002 recognises that this moral and religious dilemma, which was not relevant even two years ago, now pervades mainstream health sector issues.

2.22 ENFORCEMENT OF QUALITY STANDARDS FOR FOOD AND DRUGS

2.22.1 There is an increasing expectation and need of the citizenry for efficient enforcement of reasonable quality standards for food and drugs. Recognizing this, the Policy will make an appropriate policy recommendation on this issue.

2.23 REGULATION OF STANDARDS IN PARA MEDICAL DISCIPLINES

2.23.1 It has been observed that a large number of training institutions have mushroomed, particularly in the private sector, for para medical personnel with various skills—Lab Technicians, Radio Diagnosis Technicians, Physiotherapists, etc. Currently, there is no regulation/ monitoring, either of the curriculae of these institutions, or of the performance of the practitioners in these disciplines. This Policy will make recommendations to ensure the standardization of such training and the monitoring of actual performance.

2.24 ENVIRONMENTAL AND OCCUPATIONAL HEALTH

2.24.1 The ambient environmental conditions are a significant determinant of the health risks to which a community is exposed. Unsafe drinking water, unhygienic sanitation and air pollution significantly contribute to the burden of disease, particularly in urban settings. The initiatives in respect of these environmental factors are conventionally undertaken by the participants, whether private or public, in the other development sectors. In this backdrop, the Policy initiatives, and the efficient implementation of the linked programmes in the health sector, would succeed only to the extent that they are complemented by appropriate policies and programmes in the other environment-related sectors.

2.24.2 Work conditions in several sectors of employment in the country are sub-standard. As a result, workers engaged in such employment become particularly vulnerable to occupation-linked ailments. The long-term risk of chronic morbidity is particularly marked in the case of child labour. NHP-2002 will address the risk faced by this particularly vulnerable section of society.

2.25 PROVIDING MEDICAL FACILITIES TO USERS FROM OVERSEAS

2.25.1 The secondary and tertiary facilities available in the country are of good quality and cost-effective compared to international medical facilities. This is true not only of facilities in the allopathic disciplines, but also of those belonging to the alternative systems of medicine, particularly Ayurveda. The Policy will assess the possibilities of encouraging the development of paid treatment-packages for patients from overseas.

2.26 THE IMPACT OF GLOBALIZATION ON THE HEALTH SECTOR

2.26.1 There are some apprehensions about the possible adverse impact of economic globalisation on the health sector. Pharmaceutical drugs and other health services have always been available in the country at extremely inexpensive prices. India has established a reputation around the globe for the innovative development of original process patents for the manufacture of a wide-range of drugs and vaccines within the ambit of the existing patent laws. With the adoption of Trade Related Intellectual Property Rights (TRIPS), and the subsequent alignment of domestic patent laws consistent with the commitments under TRIPS, there will be a significant shift in the scope of the parameters regulating the manufacture of new drugs/vaccines. Global experience has shown that the introduction of a TRIPS-consistent patent regime for drugs in a developing country results in an across-the-board increase in the cost of drugs and medical services. NHP-2002 will address itself to the future imperatives of health security in the country, in the post-TRIPS era.

2.27 INTER-SECTORAL CONTRIBUTION TO HEALTH

2.27.1 It is well recognized that the overall well-being of the citizenry depends on the synergistic functioning of the various sectors in the socio-economy. The health status of the citizenry would, inter alia, be dependent on adequate nutrition, safe drinking water, basic sanitation, a clean environment and primary education, especially for the girl child. The policies and the mode of functioning in these independent areas would necessarily overlap each other to contribute to the health status of the community. From the policy perspective, it is therefore imperative that the independent policies of each of these inter-connected sectors, be in tandem, and that the interface between the policies of the two connected sectors, be smooth.

2.27.2 Sectoral policy documents are meant to serve as a guide to action for institutions and individual participants operating in that sector. Consistent with this role, NHP-2002 limits itself to making recommendations for the participants operating within the health sector. The policy aspects relating to inter-connected sectors, which, while crucial, fall outside the domain of the health sector, will not be covered by specific recommendations in this Policy document. Needless to say, the future attainment of the various goals set out in this policy assumes a reasonable complementary performance in these inter-connected sectors.

2.28 POPULATION GROWTH AND HEALTH STANDARDS

2.28.1 Efforts made over the years for improving health standards have been partially neutralized by the rapid growth of the population. It is well recognized that population stabilization measures and general health initiatives, when effectively synchronized, synergistically maximize the socio-economic well-being of the people. Government has separately announced the 'National Population Policy-2000'. The principal common features covered under the National Population Policy-2000 and NHP-2002, relate to the prevention and control of communicable diseases; giving priority to the containment of HIV/AIDS infection; the universal immunization of children against all major preventable diseases; addressing the unmet needs for basic and reproductive health services, and supplementation of infrastructure. The synchronized implementation of these two Policies—National Population Policy-2000 and National Health Policy-2002—will be the very cornerstone of any national structural plan to improve the health standards in the country.

2.29 ALTERNATIVE SYSTEMS OF MEDICINE

2.29.1 Under the overarching umbrella of the national health frame work, the alternative systems of medicine—Ayurveda, Unani, Siddha and Homoeopathy—have a substantial role. Because of inherent advantages, such as diversity, modest cost, low level of technological input and the growing popularity of natural plant-based products, these systems are attractive, particularly in the underserved, remote and tribal areas. The alternative systems will draw upon the substantial untapped potential of India as one of the eight important global centers for plant diversity in medicinal and aromatic plants. The Policy focuses on building up credibility for the alternative systems, by encouraging evidence-based research to determine their efficacy, safety and dosage, and also encourages certification and quality-marking of products to enable a wider popular acceptance of these systems of medicine. The Policy also envisages the consolidation of documentary knowledge contained in these systems to protect it against attack from foreign commercial entities by way of malafide action under patent laws in other countries. The main components of NHP-2002 apply equally to the alternative systems of medicines. However, the Policy features specific to the alternative systems of medicine will be presented as a separate document.

3. OBJECTIVES

3.1 The main objective of this policy is to achieve an acceptable standard of good health amongst the general population of the country. The approach would be to increase access to the decentralized public health system by establishing new infrastructure in deficient areas, and by upgrading the infrastructure in the existing institutions. Overriding importance would be given to ensuring a more equitable access to health services across the social and geographical expanse of the country. Emphasis will be given to increasing the aggregate public health investment through a substantially increased contribution by the Central Government. It is expected that this initiative will strengthen the capacity of the public health administration at the State level to render effective service delivery. The contribution of the private sector in providing health services would be much enhanced, particularly for the population group which can afford to pay for services. Primacy will be given to preventive and first-line curative initiatives at the primary health level through increased sectoral share of allocation. Emphasis will be laid on rational use of drugs within the allopathic system. Increased access to tried and tested systems of traditional medicine will be ensured. Within these broad objectives, NHP-2002 will endeavour to achieve the time-bound goals mentioned in Box-IV.

Box IV

Goals to be achieved by 2000-2015

Eradicate Polio and Yaws	2005
Eliminate Leprosy	2005
Eliminate Kala Azar	2010
Eliminate Lymphatic Filariasis	2015
Achieve Zero-level growth of HIV/AIDS	2007
Reduce Mortality by 50% on account of TB, Malaria and Other Vector and Water-borne diseases	2010
Reduce Prevalence of Blindness to 0.5%	2010
Reduce IMR to 30/1000 and MMR to 100/Lakh	2010
Increase utilization of public health facilities from current Level of <20 to >75%	2010
Establish an integrated system of surveillance, National Health Accounts and Health Statistics	2005

Increase health expenditure by Government as a % of GDP from the existing 0.9% to 2.0%	2010
Increase share of Central grants to Constitute at least 25% of total health spending	2010
Increase State Sector Health spending from 5.5% to 7% of the budget	2005
Further increase to 8%	2010

4. NHP-2002—POLICY PRESCRIPTIONS

4.1 FINANCIAL RESOURCES

4.1.1 The paucity of public health investment is a stark reality. Given the extremely difficult fiscal position of the State Governments, the Central Government will have to play a key role in augmenting public health investments. Taking into account the gap in health care facilities, it is planned, under the policy to increase health sector expenditure to 6 percent of GDP, with 2 percent of GDP being contributed as public health investment, by the year 2010. The State Governments would also need to increase the commitment to the health sector. In the first phase, by 2005, they would be expected to increase the commitment of their resources to 7 percent of the Budget; and, in the second phase, by 2010, to increase it to 8 percent of the Budget. With the stepping up of the public health investment, the Central Government's contribution would rise to 25 percent from the existing 15 percent by 2010. The provisioning of higher public health investments will also be contingent upon the increase in the absorptive capacity of the public health administration so as to utilize the funds gainfully.

4.2 EQUITY

4.2.1 To meet the objective of reducing various types of inequities and imbalances—inter-regional; across the rural—urban divide; and between economic classes—the most cost-effective method would be to increase the sectoral outlay in the primary health sector. Such outlets afford access to a vast number of individuals, and also facilitate preventive and early stage curative initiative, which are cost effective. In recognition of this public health principle, NHP-2002 sets out an increased allocation of 55 percent of the total public health investment for the primary health sector; the secondary and tertiary health sectors being targeted for 35 percent and 10 percent respectively. The Policy projects that the increased aggregate outlays for the primary health sector will be utilized for strengthening existing facilities and opening additional public health service outlets, consistent with the norms for such facilities.

4.3 DELIVERY OF NATIONAL PUBLIC HEALTH PROGRAMMES

4.3.1.1 This policy envisages a key role for the Central Government in designing national programmes with the active participation of the State Governments. Also, the Policy ensures the provisioning of financial resources, in addition to technical support, monitoring and evaluation at the national level by the Centre. However, to optimize the utilization of the public health infrastructure at the primary level, NHP-2002 envisages the gradual convergence of all health programmes under a single field administration. Vertical programmes for control of major diseases like TB, Malaria, HIV/AIDS, as also the RCH and Universal Immunization Programmes, would need to be continued till moderate levels of prevalence are reached. The integration of the programmes will bring about a desirable optimisation of outcomes through a convergence of all public health inputs. The Policy also envisages that programme implementation be effected through autonomous bodies at State and district levels. The interventions of State Health Departments may be limited to the overall monitoring of the achievement of programme targets and other technical aspects. The relative distancing of the programme implementation from the State Health Departments will give the project team greater operational flexibility. Also, the presence of State Government officials, social activists, private health professionals and MLAs/MPs on the management boards of the autonomous bodies will facilitate well-informed decision-making.

4.3.1.2 The Policy also highlights the need for developing the capacity within the State Public Health administration for scientific designing of public health projects, suited to the local situation.

4.3.2 The Policy envisages that apart from the exclusive staff in a vertical structure for the disease control programmes, all rural health staff should be available for the entire gamut of public health activities at the decentralized level, irrespective of whether these activities relate to national programmes or other public health initiatives. It would be for the Head of the District Health administration to allocate the time of the rural health staff between the various programmes, depending on the local need. NHP-2002 recognizes that to implement such a change, not only would the public health administrators be required to change their mindset, but the rural health staff would need to be trained and reoriented.

4.4 THE STATE OF PUBLIC HEALTH INFRASTRUCTURE

4.4.1.1 As has been highlighted in the earlier part of the Policy, the decentralized Public health service outlets have become practically dysfunctional over large parts of the country. On account of resource constraints, the supply of drugs by the State Governments is grossly inadequate. The patients at the decentralized level have little use for diagnostic services, which in any case would still require them to purchase therapeutic drugs privately. In a situation in which the patient is not getting any therapeutic drugs, there is little incentive for the potential beneficiaries to seek the advice of the medical professionals in the public health system. This results in there being no demand for medical services, so medical professionals and paramedics often absent themselves from their place of duty. It is also observed that the functioning of the public health service outlets in some States like the four Southern States—Kerala, Andhra Pradesh, Tamil Nadu and Karnataka—is relatively better, because some quantum of drugs is distributed through the primary health system network, and the patients have a stake in approaching the Public Health facilities. In this backdrop, the Policy envisages kick-starting the revival of the Primary Health System by providing some essential drugs under Central Government funding through the decentralized health system. It is expected that the provisioning of essential drugs at the public health service centres will create a demand for other professional services from the local population, which, in turn, will boost the general revival of activities in these service centres. In sum, this initiative under NHP-2002 is launched in the belief that the creation of a beneficiary interest in the public health system, will ensure a more effective supervision of the public health personnel through community monitoring, than has been achieved through the regular administrative line of control.

4.4.1.2 This Policy recognizes the need for more frequent in-service training of public health medical personnel, at the level of medical officers as well as paramedics. Such training would help to update the personnel on recent advancements in science, and would also equip them for their new assignments, when they are moved from one discipline of public health administration to another.

4.4.1.3 Global experience has shown that the quality of public health services, as reflected in the attainment of improved public health indices, is closely linked to the quantum and quality of investment through public funding in the primary health sector. Box-V gives statistics which clearly show that standards of health are more a function of the accurate targeting of expenditure on the decentralised primary sector (as observed in China and Sri Lanka), than a function of the aggregate health expenditure.

Box V

Public Health Spending in Select Countries

Indicator	*% Population with income of <$1 day*	*Infant Mortality Rate/ 1000*	*% Health Expenditure to GDP*	*% Public Expenditure on Health to Total Health Expenditure*
India	44.2	70	5.2	17.3
China	18.5	31	2.7	24.9
Sri Lanka	6.6	16	3	45.4
UK	-	6	5.8	96.9
USA	-	7	13.7	44.1

Therefore the Policy, while committing additional aggregate financial resources, places great reliance on the strengthening of the primary health structure for the attaining of improved public health outcomes on an equitable basis. Further, it also recognizes the practical need for levying reasonable user-charges for certain secondary and tertiary public health care services, for those who can afford to pay.

4.5 EXTENDING PUBLIC HEALTH SERVICES

4.5.1.1 This policy envisages that, in the context of the availability and spread of allopathic graduates in their jurisdiction, State Governments would consider the need for expanding the pool of medical practitioners to include a cadre of licentiates of medical practice, as also practitioners of Indian Systems of Medicine and Homoeopathy. Simple services/procedures can be provided by such practitioners even outside their disciplines, as part of the basic primary health services in under-served areas. Also, NHP-2002 envisages that the scope of the use of paramedical manpower of allopathic disciplines, in a prescribed functional area adjunct to their current functions, would also be examined for meeting simple public health requirements. This would be on the lines of the services rendered by nurse practitioners in several developed countries. These extended areas of functioning of different categories of medical manpower can be permitted, after adequate training, and subject to the monitoring of their performance through professional councils.

4.5.1.2 NHP-2002 also recognizes the need for States to simplify the recruitment procedures and rules for contract employment in order to provide trained medical manpower in under-served areas. State Governments could also rigorously enforce a mandatory two-year rural posting before the awarding of the graduate degree. This would not only make trained medical manpower available in the underserved areas, but would offer valuable clinical experience to the graduating doctors.

4.6 ROLE OF LOCAL SELF-GOVERNMENT INSTITUTIONS

4.6.1 NHP-2002 lays great emphasis upon the implementation of public health programmes through local self-government institutions. The structure of the national disease control programmes will have specific components for implementation through such entities. The Policy urges all State Governments to consider decentralizing the implementation of the programmes to such Institutions by 2005. In order to achieve this, financial incentives, over and above the resources normatively allocated for disease control programmes, will be provided by the Central Government.

4.7 NORMS FOR HEALTH CARE PERSONNEL

4.7.1 Minimal statutory norms for the deployment of doctors and nurses in medical institutions need to be introduced urgently under the provisions of the Indian Medical Council Act and Indian Nursing Council Act, respectively. These norms can be progressively reviewed and made more stringent as the medical institutions improve their capacity for meeting better normative standards.

4.8 EDUCATION OF HEALTH CARE PROFESSIONALS

4.8.1.1 In order to ameliorate the problems being faced on account of the uneven spread of medical and dental colleges in various parts of the country, this policy envisages the setting up of a Medical Grants Commission for funding new Government Medical and Dental Colleges in different parts of the country. Also, it is envisaged that the Medical Grants Commission will fund the upgradation of the infrastructure of the existing Government Medical and Dental Colleges of the country, so as to ensure an improved standard of medical education.

4.8.1.2 To enable fresh graduates to contribute effectively to the providing of primary health services as the physician of first contact, this policy identifies a significant need to modify the existing curriculum. A need-based, skill-oriented syllabus, with a more significant component of practical training, would make fresh doctors useful immediately after graduation. The Policy also recommends a periodic skill-updating of working health professionals through a system of continuing medical education.

4.8.2 The Policy emphasises the need to expose medical students, through the undergraduate syllabus, to the emerging concerns for geriatric disorders, as also to the cutting edge disciplines of contemporary medical research. The policy also envisages that the creation of additional seats for post-graduate courses should reflect the need for more manpower in the deficient specialities.

4.9 NEED FOR SPECIALISTS IN 'PUBLIC HEALTH' AND 'FAMILY MEDICINE'

4.9.1 In order to alleviate the acute shortage of medical personnel with specialization in the disciplines of 'public health' and 'family medicine', the Policy envisages the progressive implementation of mandatory norms to raise the proportion of post-graduate seats in these discipline in medical training institutions, to reach a stage wherein 1/4th of the seats are earmarked for these disciplines. It is envisaged that in the sanctioning of post-graduate seats in future, it shall be insisted upon that a certain reasonable number of seats be allocated to 'public health' and 'family medicine'. Since the 'public health' discipline has an interface with many other developmental sectors, specialization in Public health may be encouraged not only for medical doctors, but also for non-medical graduates from the allied fields of public health engineering, microbiology and other natural sciences.

4.10 NURSING PERSONNEL

4.10.1.1 In the interest of patient care, the policy emphasizes the need for an improvement in the ratio of nurses *vis-à-vis* doctors/beds. In order to discharge their responsibility as model providers of health services, the public health delivery centres need to make a beginning by increasing the number of nursing personnel. The Policy anticipates that with the increasing aspiration for improved health care amongst the citizens, private health facilities will also improve their ratio of nursing personnel vis-à-vis doctors/beds.

4.10.1.2 The Policy lays emphasis on improving the skill-level of nurses, and on increasing the ratio of degree-holding nurses *vis-à-vis* diploma-holding nurses. NHP-2002 recognizes a need for the Central Government to subsidize the setting up, and the running of, training facilities for nurses on a decentralized basis. Also, the Policy recognizes the need for establishing training courses for super-speciality nurses required for tertiary care institutions.

4.11 USE OF GENERIC DRUGS AND VACCINES

4.11.1.1 This Policy emphasizes the need for basing treatment regimens, in both the public and private domain, on a limited number of essential drugs of a generic nature. This is a pre-requisite for cost-effective public health care. In the public health system, this would be enforced by prohibiting the use of proprietary drugs, except in special circumstances. The list of essential drugs would no doubt have to be reviewed periodically. To encourage the use of only essential drugs in the private sector, the imposition of fiscal disincentives would be resorted to. The production and sale of irrational combinations of drugs would be prohibited through the drug standards statute.

4.11.1.2 The National Programme for Universal Immunization against Preventable Diseases requires to be assured of an uninterrupted supply of vaccines at an affordable price. To minimize the danger arising from the volatility of the global market, and thereby to ensure long-term national health security, NHP-2002 envisages that not less than 50% of the requirement of vaccines/sera be sourced from public sector institutions.

4.12 URBAN HEALTH

4.12.1.1 NHP-2002 envisages the setting up of an organised urban primary health care structure. Since the physical features of urban settings are different from those in rural areas, the policy envisages the adoption of appropriate population norms for the urban public health infrastructure. The structure conceived under NHP-2002 is a two-tiered one: the primary centre is seen as the first-tier, covering a population of one lakh, with a dispensary providing an OPD facility and essential drugs, to enable access to all the national health programmes; and a second-tier of the urban health organisation at the level of the Government general hospital, where reference is made from the primary centre. The Policy envisages that the funding for the urban primary health system will be jointly borne by the local self-government institutions and State and Central Governments.

4.12.1.2 The Policy also envisages the establishment of fully-equipped 'hub-spoke' trauma care networks in large urban agglomerations to reduce accident mortality.

4.13 MENTAL HEALTH

4.13.1.1 NHP-2002 envisages a network of decentralized mental health services for ameliorating the more common categories of disorders. The programme outline for such a disease would involve the diagnosis of common disorders, and the prescription of common therapeutic drugs, by general duty medical staff.

4.13.1.2 In regard to mental health institutions for in-door treatment of patients, the Policy envisages the upgrading of the physical infrastructure of such institutions at Central Government expense so as to secure the human rights of this vulnerable segment of society.

4.14 INFORMATION, EDUCATION AND COMMUNICATION

4.14.1 NHP-2002 envisages an IEC policy, which maximizes the dissemination of information to those population groups which cannot be effectively approached by using only the mass media. The focus would therefore be on the inter-personal communication of information and on folk and other traditional media to bring about behavioural change. The IEC programme would set specific targets for the association of PRIs/NGOs/Trusts in such activities. In several public health programmes, where behavioural change is an essential component, the success of the initiatives is crucially dependent on dispelling myths and misconceptions pertaining to religious and ethical issues. The community leaders, particularly religious leaders, are effective in imparting knowledge which facilitates such behavioural change. The programme will also have the component of an annual evaluation of the performance of the non-Governmental agencies to monitor the impact of the programmes on the targeted groups. The Central/State Government initiative will also focus on the development of modules for information dissemination in such population groups, who do not normally benefit from the more common media forms.

4.14.2 NHP-2002 envisages giving priority to school health programmes which aim at preventive-health education, providing regular health check-ups, and promotion of health-seeking behaviour among children. The school health programmes can gainfully adopt specially designed modules in order to disseminate information relating to 'health' and 'family life'. This is expected to be the most cost-effective intervention as it improves the level of awareness, not only of the extended family, but the future generation as well.

4.15 HEALTH RESEARCH

4.15.1 This Policy envisages an increase in Government-funded health research to a level of 1 percent of the total health spending by 2005; and thereafter, up to 2 percent by 2010. Domestic medical research would be focused on new therapeutic drugs and vaccines for tropical diseases, such as TB and Malaria, as also on the sub-types of HIV/AIDS prevalent in the country. Research programmes taken up by the Government in these priority areas would be conducted in a mission mode. Emphasis would also be laid on time-bound applied research for developing operational applications. This would ensure the cost-effective dissemination of existing/future therapeutic drugs/vaccines in the general population. Private entrepreneurship will be encouraged in the field of medical research for new molecules/vaccines, *inter alia*, through fiscal incentives.

4.16 ROLE OF THE PRIVATE SECTOR

4.16.1.1 In principle, this Policy welcomes the participation of the private sector in all areas of health activities—primary, secondary or tertiary. However, looking to past experience of the private sector, it can reasonably be expected that its contribution would be substantial in the urban primary sector and the tertiary sector, and moderate in the secondary sector. This Policy envisages the enactment of suitable legislation for regulating minimum infrastructure and quality standards in clinical establishments/medical institutions by 2003. Also, statutory guidelines for the conduct of clinical practice and delivery of medical services are targeted to be developed over the same period. With the acquiring of experience in the setting and enforcing of minimum quality standards, the Policy envisages graduation to a scheme of quality accreditation of clinical establishments/medical institutions, for the information of the citizenry. The regulatory/accreditation mechanisms will no doubt also cover public health institutions. The Policy also encourages the setting up of private insurance instruments for increasing the scope of the coverage of the secondary and tertiary sector under private health insurance packages.

4.16.1.2 In the context of the very large number of poor in the country, it would be difficult to conceive of an exclusive Government mechanism to provide health services to this category. It has sometimes been felt that a social health insurance scheme, funded by the Government, and with service delivery through the private sector, would be the appropriate solution. The administrative and financial implications of such an initiative are still unknown. As a first step, this policy envisages the introduction of a pilot scheme in a limited number of representative districts, to determine the administrative features of such an arrangement, as also the requirement of resources for it. The results obtained from these pilot projects would provide material on which future public health policy can be based.

4.16.2 NHP-2002 envisages the co-option of the non-governmental practitioners in the national disease control programmes so as to ensure that standard treatment protocols are followed in their day-to-day practice.

4.16.3 This Policy recognizes the immense potential of information technology applications in the area of tele-medicine in the tertiary health care sector. The use of this technical aid will greatly enhance the capacity for the professionals to pool their clinical experience.

4.17 THE ROLE OF CIVIL SOCIETY

4.17.1 NHP-2002 recognizes the significant contribution made by NGOs and other institutions of the civil society in making available health services to the community. In order to utilize their high motivational skills on an increasing scale, this Policy envisages that the disease control programmes should earmark not less than 10% of the budget in respect of identified programme components, to be exclusively implemented through these institutions. The policy also emphasizes the need to simplify procedures for government—civil society interfacing in order to enhance the involvement of civil society in public health programmes. In principle, the state would encourage the handing over of public health service outlets at any level for management by NGOs and other institutions of civil society, on an 'as-is-where-is' basis, along with the normative funds earmarked for such institutions.

4.18 NATIONAL DISEASE SURVEILLANCE NETWORK

4.18.1 This Policy envisages the full operationalization of an integrated disease control network from the lowest rung of public health administration to the Central Government, by 2005. The programme for setting up this network will include components relating to the installation of data-base handling hardware; IT inter-connectivity between different tiers of the network; and in-house training for data collection and interpretation for undertaking timely and effective response. This public health surveillance network will also encompass information from private health care institutions and practitioners. It is expected that real-time information from outside the government system will greatly strengthen the capacity of the public health system to counter focal outbreaks of seasonal diseases.

4.19 HEALTH STATISTICS

4.19.1.1 The Policy envisages the completion of baseline estimates for the incidence of the common diseases—TB, Malaria, Blindness—by 2005. The Policy proposes that statistical methods be put in place to enable the periodic updating of these baseline estimates through representative sampling, under an appropriate statistical methodology. The policy also recognizes the need to establish, in a longer time-frame, baseline estimates for non-communicable diseases, like CVD, Cancer, Diabetes; and accidental injuries, and communicable diseases, like Hepatitis and JE. NHP-2002 envisages that, with access to such reliable data on the incidence of various diseases, the public health system would move closer to the objective of evidence-based policy-making.

4.19.1.2 Planning for the health sector requires a robust information system, *inter-alia*, covering data on service facilities available in the private sector. NHP-2002 emphasises the need for the early completion of an accurate data-base of this kind.

4.19.2 In an attempt at consolidating the data base and graduating from a mere estimation of the annual health expenditure, NHP-2002 emphasises the need to establish national health accounts, conforming to the 'source-to-users' matrix structure. Also, the policy envisages the estimation of health costs on a continuing basis. Improved and comprehensive information through national health accounts and accounting systems would pave the way for decision-makers to focus on relative priorities, keeping in view the limited financial resources in the health sector.

4.20 WOMEN'S HEALTH

4.20.1 NHP-2002 envisages the identification of specific programmes targeted at women's health. The Policy notes that women, along with other under-privileged groups, are significantly handicapped due to a disproportionately low access to health care. The various Policy recommendations of NHP-2002, in regard to the expansion of primary health sector infrastructure, will facilitate the increased access of women to basic health care. The Policy commits the highest priority of the Central Government to the funding of the identified programmes relating to women's health. Also, the policy recognizes the need to review the staffing norms of the public health administration to meet the specific requirements of women in a more comprehensive manner.

4.21 MEDICAL ETHICS

4.21.1.1 NHP-2002 envisages that, in order to ensure that the common patient is not subjected to irrational or profit-driven medical regimens, a contemporary code of ethics be notified and rigorously implemented by the Medical Council of India.

4.21.1.2 By and large, medical research within the country in the frontier disciplines, such as gene-manipulation and stem cell research, is limited. However, the policy recognises that a vigilant watch will have to be kept so that the existing guidelines and statutory provisions are constantly reviewed and updated.

4.22 ENFORCEMENT OF QUALITY STANDARDS FOR FOOD AND DRUGS

4.22.1 NHP-2002 envisages that the food and drug administration will be progressively strengthened, in terms of both laboratory facilities and technical expertise. Also, the policy envisages that the standards of food items will be progressively tightened up at a pace which will permit domestic food handling/manufacturing facilities to undertake the necessary upgradation of technology so that they are not shut out of this production sector. The Policy envisages that ultimately food standards will be close, if not equivalent, to Codex specifications; and that drug standards will be at par with the most rigorous ones adopted elsewhere.

4.23 REGULATION OF STANDARDS IN PARAMEDICAL DISCIPLINES

4.23.1 NHP-2002 recognises the need for the establishment of statutory professional councils for paramedical disciplines to register practitioners, maintain standards of training, and monitor performance.

4.24 ENVIRONMENTAL AND OCCUPATIONAL HEALTH

4.24.1 This Policy envisages that the independently -stated policies and programmes of the environment-related sectors be smoothly interfaced with the policies and the programmes of the health sector, in order to reduce the health risk to the citizens and the consequential disease burden.

4.24.2 NHP-2002 envisages the periodic screening of the health conditions of the workers, particularly for high-risk health disorders associated with their occupation.

4.25 PROVIDING MEDICAL FACILITIES TO USERS FROM OVERSEAS

4.25.1 To capitalize on the comparative cost advantage enjoyed by domestic health facilities in the secondary and tertiary sectors, NHP-2002 strongly encourages the providing of such health services on a payment basis to service seekers from overseas. The providers of such services to patients from overseas will be encouraged by extending to their earnings in foreign exchange, all fiscal incentives, including the status of "deemed exports", which are available to other exporters of goods and services.

4.26 IMPACT OF GLOBALISATION ON THE HEALTH SECTOR

4.26.1 The Policy takes into account the serious apprehension, expressed by several health experts, of the possible threat to health security in the post-TRIPS era, as a result of a sharp increase in the prices of drugs and vaccines. To protect the citizens of the country from such a threat, this policy envisages a national patent regime for the future, which, while being consistent with TRIPS, avails of all opportunities to secure for the country, under its patent laws, affordable access to the latest medical and other therapeutic discoveries. The policy also sets out that the Government will bring to bear its full influence in all international fora—UN, WHO, WTO, etc.—to secure commitments on the part of the Nations of the Globe, to lighten the restrictive features of TRIPS in its application to the health care sector.

5. SUMMATION

5.1 The crafting of a National Health Policy is a rare occasion in public affairs when it would be legitimate, indeed valuable, to allow our dreams to mingle with our understanding of ground realities. Based purely on the clinical facts defining the current status of the health sector, we would have arrived at a certain policy formulation; but, buoyed by our dreams, we have ventured slightly beyond that in the shape of NHP-2002, which, in fact, defines a vision for the future.

5.2 The health needs of the country are enormous and the financial resources and managerial capacity available to meet them, even on the most optimistic projections, fall somewhat short. In this situation, NHP-2002 has had to make hard choices between various priorities and operational options. NHP-2002 does not claim to be a road-map for meeting all the health needs of the populace of the country. Further, it has to be recognized that such health needs are also dynamic, as threats in the area of public health keep changing over time. The Policy, while being holistic, undertakes the necessary risk of recommending differing emphasis on different policy components. Broadly speaking, NHP-2002 focuses on the need for enhanced funding and an organisational restructuring of the national public health initiatives in order to facilitate more equitable access to the health facilities. Also, the Policy is focused on those diseases which are principally contributing to the disease burden—TB, Malaria and Blindness from the category of historical diseases; and HIV/AIDS from the category of 'newly emerging diseases'. This is not to say that other items contributing to the disease burden of the country will be ignored; but only that the resources, as also the principal focus of the public health administration, will recognize certain relative priorities. It is unnecessary to labour the point that under the umbrella of the macro-policy prescriptions in this document, governments and private sector programme planners will have to design separate schemes, tailor-made to the health needs of women, children, geriatrics, tribals and other socio-economically under-served sections. An adequately robust disaster management plan has to be in place to effectively cope with situations arising from natural and man-made calamities.

5.3 One nagging imperative, which has influenced every aspect of this Policy, is the need to ensure that 'equity' in the health sector stands as an independent goal. In any future evaluation of its success or failure, NHP-2002 would wish to be measured against this equity norm, rather than any other aggregated financial norm for the health sector. Consistent with the primacy given to 'equity', a marked emphasis has been provided in the policy for expanding and improving the primary health facilities, including the new concept of the provisioning of essential drugs through Central funding. The Policy also commits the Central Government to an increased under-writing of the resources for meeting the minimum health needs of the people. Thus, the Policy attempts to provide guidance for prioritizing expenditure, thereby facilitating rational resource allocation.

5.4 This Policy broadly envisages a greater contribution from the Central Budget for the delivery of Public Health services at the State level. Adequate appropriations, steadily rising over the years, would need to be ensured. The possibility of ensuring this by imposing an earmarked health cess has been carefully examined. While it is recognized that the annual budget must accommodate the increasing resource needs of the social sectors, particularly in the health sector, this Policy does not specifically recommend an earmarked health cess, as that would have a tendency of reducing the space available to Parliament in making appropriations looking to the circumstances prevailing from time to time.

5.5 The Policy highlights the expected roles of different participating groups in the health sector. Further, it recognizes the fact that, despite all that may be guaranteed by the Central Government for assisting public health programmes, public health services would actually need to be delivered by the State administration, NGOs and other institutions of civil society. The attainment of improved health levels would be significantly dependent on population stabilisation, as also on complementary efforts from other areas of the social sectors—like improved drinking water supply, basic sanitation, minimum nutrition, etc.—to ensure that the exposure of the populace to health risks is minimized.

5.6 Any expectation of a significant improvement in the quality of health services, and the consequential improved health status of the citizenry, would depend not only on increased financial and material inputs, but also on a more empathetic and committed attitude in the service providers, whether in the private or public sectors. In some measure, this optimistic policy document is based on the understanding that the citizenry is increasingly demanding more by way of quality in health services, and the health delivery system, particularly in the public sector, is being pressed to respond. In this backdrop, it needs to be recognized that any policy in the social sector is critically dependent on the service providers treating their responsibility not as a commercial activity, but as a service, albeit a paid one. In the area of public health, an improved standard of governance is a prerequisite for the success of any health policy.

APPENDIX 3

NATIONAL HEALTH POLICY-1983

National Health Policy, Government of India, Ministry of Health and Family Welfare, New Delhi, 1983

Introduction

1. The Constitution of India envisages the establishment of a new social order based on equality, freedom, justice and the dignity of the individual. It aims at the elimination of poverty, ignorance and ill-health and directs the State to regard the raising of the level of nutrition and the standard of living of its people and the improvement of public health as among its primary duties, securing the health and strength of workers, men and women, specially ensuring that children are given opportunities and facilities to develop in a healthy manner.

1.2 Since the inception of the planning process in the country, the successive Five Year Plans have been providing the framework within which the States may develop their health services infrastructure, facilities for medical education, research, etc. Similar guidance has sought to be provided through the discussions and conclusions arrived at in the Joint Conferences of the Central Councils of Health and Family Welfare and the National Development Council. Besides, Central legislation has been enacted to regulate standards of medical education, prevention of food adulteration, maintenance of standards in the manufacture and sale of certified drugs, etc.

1.3 While the broad approaches contained in the successive Plan documents and discussion in the forums referred to in para 1.2 may have generally served the needs of the situation in the past, it is felt that an integrated, comprehensive approach towards the future development of medical education, research and health services requires to be established to serve the actual health needs and priorities of the country. It is in this context that the need has been felt to evolve a National Health Policy.

Our heritage

2. India has a rich, centuries-old heritage of medical and health sciences. The philosophy of Ayurveda and the surgical skills enunciated by Charaka and Shusharuta bear testimony to our ancient tradition in the scientific health care of our people. The approach of our ancient medical systems was of a holistic nature, which took into account all aspects of human health and disease. Over the centuries, with the intrusion of foreign influences and mingling of cultures, various systems of medicine evolved and have continued to be practised widely. However, the allopathic system of medicine has, in a relatively short period of time, made a major impact

on the entire approach to health care and pattern of development of the health services infrastructure in the country.

Progress achieved

3. During the last three decades and more, since the attainment of Independence, considerable progress has been achieved in the promotion of the health status of our people. Smallpox has been eliminated; plague is no longer a problem; mortality from cholera and related diseases has decreased and malaria brought under control to a considerable extent. The mortality rate per thousand of population has been reduced from 27.4 to 14.8 and the life expectancy at birth has increased from 32.7 to over 52. A fairly extensive network of dispensaries, hospitals and institutions providing specialised curative care has developed and a large stock of medical and health personnel, of various levels, has become available. Significant indigenous capacity has been established for the production of drugs and pharmaceuticals, vaccines, sera, hospital equipments, etc.

The existing picture

4. In spite of such impressive progress, the demographic and health picture of the country still constitutes a cause for serious and urgent concern. The high rate of population growth continues to have an adverse effect on the health of our people and the quality of their lives. The mortality rates for women and children are still distressingly high; almost one third of the total deaths occur among children below the age of 5 years; infant mortality is around 129 per thousand live births. Efforts at raising the nutritional levels of our people have still to bear fruit and the extent and severity of malnutrition continues to be exceptionally high. Communicable and non- communicable diseases have still to be brought under effective control and eradicated. Blindness, Leprosy and T.B. continue to have a high incidence. Only 31% of the rural population has access to potable water supply and 0.5% enjoys basic sanitation.

4.1. High incidence of diarrhoeal diseases and other preventive and infectious diseases, specially amongst infants and children, lack of safe drinking water and poor environmental sanitation, poverty and ignorance are among the major contributory causes of the high incidence of disease and mortality.

4.2. The existing situation has been largely engendered by the almost wholesale adoption of health manpower development policies and the establishment of curative centers based on the Western models, which are inappropriate and irrelevant to the real needs of our people and the socio-economic conditions obtaining in the country. The hospital-based disease and cure-oriented approach towards the establishment of medical services has provided benefits to the upper crusts, of society, specially those residing in the urban areas. The proliferation of this approach has been at the cost of providing comprehensive primary health care services to the entire population, whether residing in the urban or the rural areas. Furthermore, the continued high emphasis on the curative approach has led to the neglect of the preventive, promotive, public health and rehabilitative aspects of health care. The existing approach, instead of improving awareness and building up self-reliance, has tended to enhance dependency and weaken the community's capacity to cope with its problems. The prevailing policies in regard to the education and training of medical and health personnel, at various levels, has resulted in the development of a cultural gap between the people and the personnel providing care. The various health programmes have, by and large, failed to involve individuals and families in establishing a self-reliant community. Also, over the years, the planning process has become largely oblivious of the fact that the ultimate goal of achieving a satisfactory health status for all our people cannot be secured without involving the community in the identification of their health needs and priorities as well as in the implementation and management of the various health and related programmes.

Need for evolving a health policy—the revised 20-Point Programme

5. India is committed to attaining the goal of "Health for All by the Year 2000 A.D." through the universal provision of comprehensive primary health care services. The attainment of this goal requires a thorough overhaul of the existing approaches to the education and training of medical and health personnel and the re-organisation of the health services infrastructure. Furthermore, considering the large variety of inputs into health, it is necessary to secure the complete integration of all plans for health and human development with the overall national socio-economic development process, specially in the more closely health related sectors, e.g. drugs and pharmaceuticals, agriculture and food production, rural development, education and social welfare, housing, water supply and sanitation, prevention of food adulteration, maintenance of prescribed standards in the manufacture and sale of drugs and the conservation of the environment. In sum, the contours of the National Health Policy have to be evolved within a fully integrated planning framework which seeks to provide universal, comprehensive primary health care services, relevant to the actual needs and priorities of the community at a cost which the people can afford, ensuring that the planning and implementation of the various health programmes is through the organized involvement and participation of the community, adequately utilizing the services being rendered by private voluntary organisations active in the Health sector.

5.1. It is also necessary to ensure that the pattern of development of the health services infrastructure in the future fully takes into account the revised 20-Point Programme. The said Programme attributes very high priority to the promotion of family planning as a people's programme, on a voluntary basis; substantial augmentation and provision of primary health care facilities on a universal basis; control of Leprosy, T.B. and Blindness; acceleration of welfare programmes for women and children; nutrition programmes for pregnant women, nursing mothers and children, especially in the tribal, hill and backward areas. The Programme also places high emphasis on the supply of drinking water to all problem villages, improvements in the housing and environments of the weaker sections of society; increased production of essential food items; integrated rural developments; spread of universal elementary education; expansion of the public distribution system, etc.

Population stabilization

6. Irrespective of the changes, no matter how fundamental, that may be brought about in the over-all approach to health care and the restructuring of the health services, not much headway is likely to be achieved in improving the health status of the people unless success is achieved in securing the small family norm, through voluntary efforts, and moving towards the goal of population stabilization. In view of the vital importance of securing the balanced growth of the population, it is necessary to enunciate, separately, a National Population Policy.

Medical and Health Education

7. It is also necessary to appreciate that the effective delivery of health care services would depend very largely on the nature of education, training and appro- priate orientation towards community health of all categories of medical and health personnel and their capacity to function as an integrated team, each of its members performing given tasks within a coordinated action programme. It is, therefore, of crucial importance that the entire basis and approach towards medical and health education, at all levels, is reviewed in terms of national needs and priorities and the curricular and training programmes restructured to produce personnel of various grades of skill and competence, who are professionally equipped and socially motivated to effectively deal with day-to-day problems, within the existing constraints.

Towards this end, it is necessary to formulate, separately, a National Medical and Health Education Policy which (i) sets out the changes required to be brought about in the curricular contents and training programme of medical and health personnel, at various levels of functioning; (ii) takes into account the need for establishing the extremely essential inter-relations between functionaries of various grades; (iii) provides guidelines for the production of health personnel on the basis of realistically assessed manpower requirements; (iv) seeks to resolve the existing sharp regional imbalances in their availability; and (v) ensures that personnel at all levels are socially motivated towards the rendering of community health services.

Need for providing primary health care with special emphasis on the preventive, promotive and rehabilitative aspects

8. Presently, despite the constraint of resources, there is disproportionate emphasis on the establishment of curative centres—

dispensaries, hospitals, institutions for specialist treatment—the large majority of which are located in the urban areas of the country. The vast majority of those seeking medical relief have to travel long distance to the nearest curative centre, seeking relief for ailments which could have been readily and effectively handled at the community level. Also, for want of a well established referral system, those seeking curative care have the tendency to to visit various specialist centres, thus further contributing to congestions, duplication of efforts and consequential waste of resources. To put an end to the existing all-round unsatisfactory situation, it is urgently necessary to restructure the health services within the following broad approach:

(1) To provide, within a phased, time-bound programme a well dispersed network of comprehensive primary health care services, integrally linked with the extension and health education approach which takes into account the fact that a large majority of health functions can be effectively handled and resolved by the people themselves, with the organised support of volunteers, auxilliaries, para-medics and adequately trained multi-purpose workers of various grades of skill and competence, of both sexes. There are a large number of private, voluntary organisations active in the health field, all over the country. Their services and support would require to be utilised and intermeshed with the governmental efforts, in an integrated manner.

(2) To be effective, the establishment of the primary health care approach would involve large scale transfer of knowledge, simple skill and technologies to Health Volunteers, selected by the communities and enjoying their confidence. The functioning of the front line workers, selected by the community would require to be related to definitive action plans for the translation of medical and health knowledge into practical action, involving the use of simple and inexpensive interventions which can be readily implemented by persons who have undergone short periods of training. The quality of training of these health guides/workers would be of crucial importance to the success of this approach.

The success of the decentralized primary health care system would depend vitally on the organized building up of individual self-reliance and effective community participation; on the provision of organized, back-up support of the secondary and tertiary levels of the health care services, providing adequate logistical and technical assistance.

(4) The decentralization of services would require the establishment of a well worked out referral system to provide adequate expertise at the various levels of the organisational set-up nearest to the community, depending upon the actual needs and problems of the area, and thus ensure against the continuation of the existing rush towards the curative centers in the urban areas. The effective establishment of the referral system would also ensure the optimal utilization of expertise at the higher levels of the hierarchical structure. This approach would not only lead to the progressive improvement of comprehensive health care services at the

primary level but also provide for timely attention being available to those in need of urgent specialist care, whether they live in the rural or the urban areas.

(5) To ensure that the approach to health care does not merely constitute a collection of disparate health interventions but consists of an integrated package of services seeking to tackle the entire range of poor health conditions, on a broad front, it is necessary to establish a nation-wide chain of sanitary-*cum*-epidemiological stations. The location and functioning of these stations may be between the primary and secondary levels of the heirarchical structure, depending upon the local situations and other relevant considerations. Each such station would require to have suitably trained staff equipped to identify, plan and provide preventive, promotive and mental health care services. It would be beneficial, depending upon the local situations, to establish such stations at the Primary Health Centres. The district health organisation should have, as an integral part of its set-up, a well organised epidemiological unit to coordinate and superintend the functioning of the field stations. These stations would participate in the integrated action plans to eradicate and control diseases, besides tackling specific local environmental health problems.

In the urban agglomerations, the municipal and local authorities should be equipped to perform similar functions, being supported with adequate resources and expertise, to effectively deal with the local preventable public health problems. The aforesaid approach should be implemented and extended through community participation and contributions, in whatever form possible, to achieve meaningful results within a time-bound programme.

(6) The location of curative centres should be related to the populations they serve, keeping in view the densities of population, distances, topography, transport connections. These centres should function within the recommended referral system, the gamut of the general specialities required to deal with the local disease patterns being provided as near to the community as possible, at the secondary level of the hierarchical organisation. The concept of domiciliary care and the field-camps approach should be utilised to the fullest extent, to reduce the pressures on these centres, specially in efforts relating to the control and eradication of Blindness, Tuberculosis, Leprosy, etc. To maximise the utilisation of available resources, new and additional curative centres should be established only in exceptional cases, the basic attempt being towards the upgradation of existing facilities, at selected locations, the guiding principle being to provide specialist services as near to the beneficiaries as may be possible, within a well-planned network. Expenditure should be reduced through the fullest possible use of cheap locally available building materials, resort to appropriate architectural designs and engineering concepts and by economical investment in the purchase of machineries and equipments, ensuring against avoidable duplication of such acquisitions. It is also necessary to devise effective

mechanisms for the repair, maintenance and proper upkeep of all bio-medical equipments to secure their maximum utilisation.

(7) With a view to reducing governmental expenditure and fully utilising untapped resources, planned programmes may be devised, related to the local requirements and potentials, to encourage the establishment of practice by private medical professional, increased investment by non-governmental agencies in establishing curative centres and by offering organised logistical, financial and technical support to voluntary agencies active in the health field.

(8) While the major focus of attention in restructuring the existing governmental health organisations would relate to establishing comprehensive primary health care and public health services, within an integrated referral system, planned attention would also require to be devoted to the establishment of centres equipped to provide speciality and super-speciality services, through a well dispersed network of centres, to ensure that the present and future requirements of specialist treatment are adequately available within the country. To reduce governmental expenditures involved in the establishment of such centres, planned efforts should be made to encourage private investments in such fields so that the majority of such centres, within the governmental set-up, can provide adequate care and treatment to those entitled to free care, the affluent sectors being looked after by the paying clinics. Care would also require to be taken to ensure the appropriate dispersal of such centres, to remove the existing regional imbalances and to provide services within the reach of all, whether residing in the rural or the urban areas.

(9) Special, well-coordinated programmes should be launched to provide mental health care as well as medical care and the physical and social rehabilitation of those who are mentally retarded, deaf, dumb, blind, physically disabled, infirm and the aged. Also, suitably organised of various disabilities.

(10) In the establishment of the re-organised services, the first priority should be accorded to provide services to those residing in the tribal, hill and backward areas as well as to endemic disease affected populations and the vulnerable sections of the society.

(11) In the re-organised health services scheme, efforts should be made to ensure adequate mobility of personnel, at all level of functioning.

(12) In the various approaches, set out in (1) to (11) above, organised efforts would require to be made to fully utilise and assist in the enlargement of the services being provided by private voluntary organisations active in the health field. In this context, planning encouragement and support would also require to be afforded to fresh voluntary efforts, specially those which seek to serve the needs of the rural areas and the urban slums.

Re-orientation of the existing health personnel

9. A dynamic process of changes and innovation is required to be

brought about in the entire approach to health manpower development, ensuring the emergence of fully integrated bands of workers functioning within the "Health Team" approach.

Private practice by governmental functionaries

10. It is desirable for the States to take steps to phase out of system of private practice by medical personnel in government service, providing at the same tome for payment of appropriate compensatory no-practising allowance. The States would require to carefully review the existing situation, with special reference to the availability and dispersal of private practitioners, and take timely decisions in regard to this vital issue.

Practitioners of indigenous and other systems of medicine and their role in health care

11. The country has a large stock of health manpower comprising of private practitioners in various systems, for example, Ayurveda, Unany, Sidha, Homeopathy, Yoga, Naturopathy, etc. This resource has not so for been adequately utilized. The practitioners of these various systems enjoy high local acceptance and respect and consequently exert considerable influence on health beliefs and practise. It is, therefore, necessary to initiate organised measures to enable each of these various systems of medicine and health care to develop in accordance wit its genius. Simultaneously, planned efforts should be made to dovetail the functioning of the practitioners of these various systems and integrate their service, at the appropriate levels, within specified areas of responsibility and functioning, in the over-all health care delivery system, specially in regard to the preventive, primitive and public health objectives. Well considered steps would also require to be launched to move towards a meaningful phased integration of the indigenous and the modern systems.

APPENDIX 4

GUIDELINES FOR VILLAGE HEALTH AND SANITATION COMMITTEES, SUB-CENTRES, PHCS AND CHCS

Ministry of Health and Family Welfare, Government of India

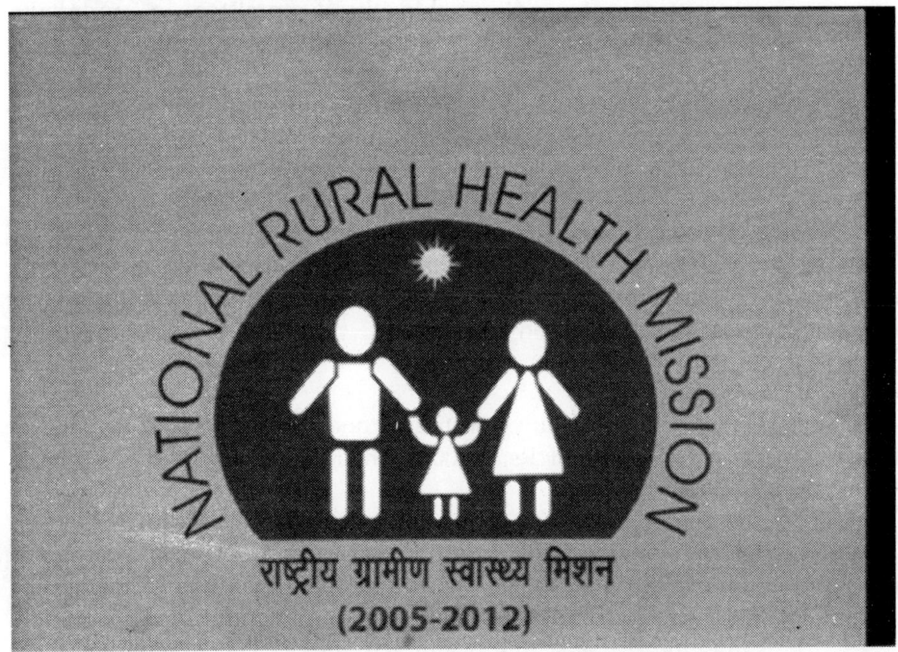

1. Guidelinrs Regarding Constitution of Village Health and Sanitation Committees and Utilisation of Untied Grants to these Committees

The detailed Implementation Framework of the National Rural Health Mission [NRHM] approved by the Union Cabinet in July, 2006 provides for the constitution and orientation of all community leaders on Village Sub Centre, Primary Health Centre and Community Health Centre Committees. The NRHM implementation has been planned within the framework of Panchayti Raj Institutions [PRIs] at various levels. The Village Health and Sanitation Committee envisaged under NRHM is also within the overall umbrella of PRI.

2. Composition of the Village Health and Sanitation Committee

To enable the Village Health and Sanitation Committee to reflect the aspirations of the local community especially of the poor households and women, it has been suggested that:

- At least 50% members on the Village Health and Sanitation Committee should be women.
- Every hamlet within a revenue village must be given due representation on the Village Health and Sanitation Committee to ensure that the needs of the weaker sections especially Scheduled Castes, Scheduled Tribes, Other Backward Classes are fully reflected in the activities of the committee.
- A provision of at least 30% representation from the Non-governmental sector.
- Representation to women's self-help group, etc. on these committees, etc. will enable the Committee to undertake women's health activities more effectively.
- Notwithstanding the above, the overall composition and nomenclature of the Village Health and Sanitation Committees is left to the State Governments as long as these committees were within the umbrella of PRIs.

3. Orientation and Training

Every Village Health and Sanitation Committee after being duly constituted by the State Governments needs to be oriented and trained to carry out the activities expected of them.

Village Health Fund

Every such committee duly constituted and oriented would be entitled to an annual untied grant of Rs. 10,000, which could be used for any of the following activities:

(i) As a revolving fund from which households could draw in times of need to be returned in installments thereafter.

(ii) For any village level public health activity like cleanliness drive, sanitation drive, school health activities, ICDS, Anganwadi level activities, household surveys, etc.

(iii) In extraordinary case of a destitute women or very poor household, the Village Health and Sanitation Committee untied grants could even be used for health care need of the poor household.

(iv) The untied grant is a resource for community action at the local level and shall only be used for community activities that involve and benefit more than one household. Nutrition, Education and Sanitation, Environmental Protection, Public Health Measures shall be key areas where these funds could be utilized.

(v) Every village is free to contribute additional grant towards the Village Health and Sanitation Committee. In villages where the community contributes financial resources to the Village Health and Sanitation Committee untied grant of Rs. 10,000, additional incentive and financial assistance to the village could be explored. The intention of this untied grant is to enable local action and to ensure that Public Health activities at the village level receive priority attention.

4. Maintenance of Bank Account

The Village Health and Sanitation Committee fund shall be credited to a bank account, which will be operated with the joint signature of ASHA/Health Link Worker/Anganwadi Worker along with the President of the Village Health and Sanitation Committee/Pradhan of the Gram Panchayat. The account maintenance of this joint account shall be the responsibility of the Village Health and Sanitation Committee especially the ASHA/AWW [wherever no ASHA]. The Village Health and Sanitation Committee, the ASHA/AWW shall maintain a register of funds received· and expenditure incurred. The register shall be available for public scrutiny and shall be inspected from time to time by the ANM/MPW/Gram Panchayat.

5. Accountability

- Every Village Health ,and Sanitation Committee needs to maintain updated Household Survey data to enable need-based interventions.
- Maintain a register where complete details of activities undertaken, expenditure incurred, etc. will be maintained for public scrutiny. This should be periodically reviewed by the ANM/Sarpanch.
- The Block level Panchayat Samiti will review the functioning and progress of activities undertaken by the VHSC.
- The District Mission in its meeting also through its members/ block facilitators supporting ASHA [wherever ASHA's are in position] elicit information on the functioning of the VHSC.
- A data base may be maintained on VHCSs by the DPMUs.

GUIDELINES FOR USE OF SUB-CENTER (SC) FUNDS UNDER NRHM

1. As part of the National Rural Health Mission, it is proposed to provide each sub-center with Rs. 10,000 as an untied fund to facilitate meeting urgent yet discrete activities that need relatively small sums of money.

2. The fund shall be kept in a joint bank account of the ANM and the Sarpanch

3. Decisions on activities for which the funds are to be spent will be approved by the Village Health Committee (VHC) and be administered by the ANM. In areas where the sub-center is not co-terminus with the Gram Panchayat (GP) and the sub center covers more than one GP, the VHC of

the Gram Panchayat where the SC is located will approve the Action Plan. The funds can be used for any of the villages, which are covered by the sub-center.

4. Untied Funds will be used only for the common good and not for individual needs, except in the case of referral and transport in emergency situations.

5. Suggested areas where Untied Funds may be used include:

- Minor modifications to sub-center-curtains to ensure privacy, repair of taps, installation of bulbs, other minor repairs, which can be done at the local level.
- Ad hoc payments for cleaning up sub-center, especially after childbirth.
- Transport of emergencies to appropriate referral centers.
- Transport of samples during epidemics.
- Purchase of consumables such as bandages in sub-center.
- Purchase of bleaching powder and disinfectants for use in common areas of the village.
- Labour and supplies for environmental sanitation, such as clearing or larvicidal measures for stagnant water.
- Payment/reward to ASHA for certain identified activities.

6. Untied funds shall not be used for any salaries, vehicle purchase, and recurring expenditures or to meet the expenses of the Gram Panchayat.

Guidelines for utilization of Untied Fund and Annual Maintenance Grant for Primary Health Centres (PHCs)

1. Health sector reforms under the National Rural Health Mission (NRHM) aims to increase functional, administrative and financial resources and autonomy to the field units under which every PHC will get Rs. 25,000 p.a. as untied grant for local health action. Similarly every PHC will get an Annual Maintenance Grant of Rs. 50,000 for improvement and maintenance of physical infrastructure. Provision of water, toilets, their use and their maintenance has to be the priorities. In addition, every PHC is being strengthened with provision of three staff nurses as against one at present and provision of two doctors (one male, one female) and Ayush practitioner.

2. Necessity of untied fund has been felt mainly due to unavailability of funds for undertaking any innovative Centre-specific need-based activity, as the allotment of funds to the States has traditionally been of the nature of tied funds for implementing a particular activity/scheme and this hardly left any funds with the public health facilities. This centralized management and schematic in-flexibility in the use of funds allotted to the States, did not provide any scope for local initiative and flexibility for local action at block and down below level. Also it has been observed that most of the Primary Health Centres have not been maintained properly due to

lack of steady fund, available locally for repair/refurbishing of infrastructure and basic facilities.

3. Since there would be substantial fund flow to the districts to be utilized for the Centres under NRHM/RCH-II and other programmes, the untied funds should not duplicate what is/can be taken up under other programmes. Each activity planned by the Centre should have clear rationale so that the impact of the untied fund can be distinctively assessed. A separate register be maintained in the PHC giving sources of funds clearly for various activities.

4. PHC untied fund shall be kept in the bank account of the concerned Rogi Kalyan Samitti (RKS)/Hospital Management Committee (HMC). PHC level Panchayat Committee/Rogi Kalyan Samiti will have the mandate to undertake and supervise the work to be undertaken from Annual Maintenance Grant. Both the funds will be spent and monitored by RKS.

5. Suggested areas where Untied Fund may be used include:

- Minor modifications to the Center-curtains to ensure privacy, repair of taps, installation of bulbs, other minor repairs, which can be done at the local level.
- Patient examination table, delivery table, DP apparatus, hemoglobin meter, copper-T insertion kit, instruments tray, baby tray, weighing scales for mothers and for newborn babies, plastic/rubber sheets, dressing scissors, stethoscopes, buckets, attendance stool, mackintosh sheet.
- Provision of running water supply.
- Provision of electricity.
- *Ad hoc* payments for cleaning up the Center, especially after childbirth.
- Transport of emergencies to appropriate referral centers.
- Transport of samples during epidemics.
- Purchase of consumables such as bandages in the Center.
- Purchase of bleaching powder and disinfectants for use in common areas.
- Under the jurisdiction of the Centre.
- Labour and supplies for environmental sanitation, such as clearing.
- Larvicidal measures for stagnant water.
- Payment/reward to ASHA for certain identified activities.
- Repair/operationalising soak pits.

6. The following nature of expenditures should not be incurred out of the untied fund:

- Purchase of Office Stationery and equipments, training-related equipments, Vehicles, etc.

- Engagement of full time or part time staff and payment of honorarium/incentives/wages of any kind.
- Purchase of drugs, consumables and furniture.
- Payments towards inserting advertisements in any Newspaper/ Journal/Magazine and IEC related expenditure.
- Organizing "Swasthya Mela" or giving stalls in any Mela for ostensible purpose of awareness generation of health schemes/ programmes.
- Payment of incentives to individuals/groups in cash/kind.
- Meeting any recurring non-plan expenditure.
- Taking up any individual-based activity except in the case of referral and transport in emergency situations.

7. The Centers are not required to take prior approval before implementing the schemes from the untied funds but shall have to send quarterly SOE and UC.

SUGGESTED GUIDELINES FOR IMPLEMENTATION OF INDIAN PUBLIC HEALTH STANDARDS (IPHS) IN SUB-CENTRES (SC), PRIMARY HEALTH CENTRES (PHC) AND COMMUNITY HEALTH CENTRES (CHC)

Although a large number of Sub-centres, Primary Health Centres and Community Health Centres have been established to provide comprehensive promotive, preventive and curative services to the rural people in the country, most of these institutions, at present are not able to function up to the level expected of them due to varied reasons. National Rural Health Mission (NRHM), launched by the Hon'ble Prime Minister on 12 April 2005, envisages to get these institutions raised to the level of optimum availability of infrastructure, manpower, logistics, etc. to improve the quality of services and the corresponding level of utilization. Through wide consultation with various stakeholders, Indian Public Health Standards (IPHS) for these centres have been framed. The key aim of the Standards is to underpin the delivery of quality services which are fair and responsive to clients' needs, which should be provided equitably and which deliver improvements in health and well-being of the population. Each PHC and CHC, as part of IPHS, is required to set-up a Rogi Kalyan Samity/Hospital Management Committee, which will bring in community control into the management of public hospitals with a purpose to provide sustainable quality care with accountability and people's participation along with total transparency.

To bring these centres to the level of Indian Public Health Standards, is no doubt, a challenge for most of the States and also may require a detailed institution specific facility survey to find out the gaps. However, considering the dynamic process of setting up of the standards and the current manpower availability, there is a need to bring these centres to IPHS in a phased manner as the existing institutions are having different level of functional status. Some are at very rudimentary stage, some are just functioning minimally and the others with little more input could come up to the level of IPHS. Taking these points into consideration, a set of guidelines has been framed to enable the States/UTs to bring these centres gradually to the IPHS level.

National Rural Health Mission (NRHM) envisages a fully functional sub-centre in coordination with the village level functionaries such as Anganwadi workers, ASHA, and the Village Health and Sanitation Committee. Similarly, all the PHCs should function as 24-hour PHCs in a gradual manner. NRHM also envisages a functional 30-bedded rural hospital at the block level providing emergency obstetric care and neonatal care in the first instance as FRU and gradually strengthen further to provide other specialists services as per the details in the IPHS. The guidelines for achieving standards for IPHS centre-wise are as below:

Sub-centre

- Conduct a facility survey and identify the gaps.
- Ensure that all the existing Sub-centres should be posted with one ANM immediately. The vacant post may be filled up on contractual basis. There should be an in-built plan to take care of vacancies arising out of retirements, long leave, and other emergency situation so that the services of ANM are available without any interruption.
- The appointment of second ANM as envisaged in the IPHS for each Sub-centre is to be made locally on contractual basis as per the demand, phase wise. The most difficult areas such as hilly and tribal areas may be given priority.
- The services of a Male Health Worker (MPW-M) is also necessary at the Sub-centre. The states should take steps to fill up the post of these MPWs (M) in a phased manner. The training capacity in the State for these MPWs also need to be enhanced.
- Utilization of untied fund for strengthening the functioning of Sub-centres.
- All the existing Sub-centres buildings should be made environment friendly, disabled friendly, with a good source of water supply, electricity/solar power/other alternative energy sources. This can be ensured with the help of Panchayat and related sectors.
- Utilization of Annual Maintenance Grant for strengthening of infrastructure and basic necessities of the Sub-centres.
- The States may declare the names and the number of existing Sub-centres that have been made functional as per the IPHS for the purpose of showing achievements under NRHM and information to the public.

Primary Health Centre (PHC)—24 Hours Service Delivery Centre with Emphasis on Institutional Delivery

NRHM envisages that all the Primary Health Centres (20,000-30,000 population) should function as a 24x7 centre in a phased manner to improve the institutional deliveries conducted at these centres. The steps that may be needed are as follows:

- Conduct an institution specific facility survey and identify the gaps.
- In order to make the PHC 24x7 delivery of services, the services of Staff Nurses are essential. It must be ensured that there should be at least 4 Staff Nurses to perform rotation duties round the clock. In order to improve the institutional deliveries, appointment of at least three Staff Nurses may be recruited on contractual basis to fill the gaps. A labour room with appropriate equipments and drugs with round the clock referral transport support either managed by the PHC or by the NGOs/CBOs for referring patients in case of emergency is essential. The States may take stock of the situation of the training capacity and the facilities available in the training institutions for turning over the required number of Staff Nurses.
- Appointment of two Medical Officers (MBBS) (preferably one lady MO), and one AYUSH practitioner, either by relocation or on contractual basis. All effort should be made, such as contractual appointment or walk-in interviews, making the District Cadre for Medical Officers and even appointment of retired MBBS doctors on contractual basis, and other incentives provided by the State government to see that all the PHCs have the Medical Officers.
- All the existing Primary Health Centres buildings as far as possible should be made environment friendly, disabled friendly, with a good source of water supply, electricity/solar power/other alternative energy sources and telephone. Rain water harvesting should also be promoted in the PHC building. This can be ensured with the help of Panchayat and related sectors such as water supply sanitation, horticulture, etc. All the proposed new buildings should have these components in their construction plan.
- Utilization of untied fund for strengthening the functioning of PHCs.
- Utilization of Annual Maintenance Grant for strengthening the infrastructure and basic necessities
- Each PHC must have a Rogi Kalyan Samity and display of the Citizens' Charter.
- Once a specific PHC has achieved the 24×7/IPHS status, the district authority/state authority should declare the institution as 24×7/IPHS.

Community Health Centre (CHC)—First Referral Unit (FRU), Assured Services

NRHM envisages a 30-bedded fully functional block level rural hospital. The greatest challenge of bringing these CHCs to FRU/IPHS is the non-availability of the specialists especially the critical ones like obstetric/gynecologist, anesthetist and pediatrician. The following steps may be taken up:

- Conduct an institution specific facility survey and identify the gaps.
- Bringing up the CHC to the level of the IPHS may be carried out in stages.

First stage: It must be ensured that all the CHCs provides 24x7 services with appropriate referral transport service. The basic requirement for making it 24x7 service delivery, there should be four General Duty Medical Officers and seven Staff Nurses, one ANM and one LHV along with other support services and physical facilities. Each CHC must be certified by the State Government/District Authority that this is functioning as a 24x7 service delivery.

Second stage: All the CHCs, declared as 24×7 may be upgraded to First Referral Units (FRUs). The Minimum requirement of FRUs including manpower, i.e. gynecologist, anesthetist, pediatrician, and round the clock services of nurses and general duty officers should be ensured. Blood storage facility and other supportive services such as laboratory, X-ray, OT, labour room, laundry, diet, waste management system, referral transport, etc. must be ensured. Each CHC should be clearly demarcated as FRU. CHCs, as FRU will provide the 24 hours delivery services including normal and assisted deliveries, emergency obstetric care including surgical intervention like cesarean section and other medical intervention, newborn care, emergency care of sick children, full range of family planning services including laparoscopic services, safe abortion services, treatment of STI/RTI, availability of blood storage unit or effective linkage facilities with blood banks, and referral transport services.

Third stage (IPHS): Once the CHCs are qualified for FRU, next step would be to post adequate number of other specialists and support manpower as per the IPHS. Once these existing gaps in relation to manpower, equipments, drugs, supplies and other support services, are filled up, the CHCs can be declared to have achieved IPHS. The CHCs declared as IPHS, apart from above mentioned services by FRU, also must provide the following services:

- Care of routine and emergency cases in surgery
- Care of routine and emergency cases in medicine
- Services of a Public Health Manager
- Delivery of all National Health Programmes including communicable and non-communicable diseases and RCH services.

Manpower

- Appointment of specialists may be made on contractual basis. All out efforts should be made, such as contractual appointment or walk-in interviews, making the specialist cadre in the State and even appointment of retired specialists on contractual basis, public-private partnership, and other incentives provided by the State government. Short-term training course on anesthesiology and emergency obstetric care to the existing serving general duty doctors may also be undertaken, to see that all the CHCs have requisite manpower depending on the bed occupancy level.
- Appointment of Public Health Programme Manager on contractual basis.
- Appointment of Eye Surgeon (one for five CHCs) on contractual basis.
- Appointment of nine Nurses Midwives/Staff Nurses on contractual basis.
- All the existing Community Health Centres buildings as far as possible should be made environment friendly, disabled friendly, with a good source of water supply, electricity/solar power/other alternative energy sources and telephone. Rain water harvesting should also be promoted in the CHC buildings. This can be ensured with the help of Panchayat and related sectors such as water supply sanitation, horticulture, etc. All the proposed new buildings should have these components in their construction plan.
- Dislocation of the existing centres for the sake of achieving the Standards may not be required, unless compulsory due to unavoidable circumstances. In that case, they could be resettled to an accessible place where the original client group could easily get the services.

As far as manpower is concerned, optimum strength should be taken into consideration.

Others

- Utilization of untied fund for strengthening the functioning of CHCs
- Utilization of Annual Maintenance Grant for strengthening the infrastructure and basic necessities
- Utilization of fund for up-gradation of CHCs to IPHS

Implementation of achieving the Standards should keep into account the linkage of the referral system right from Sub-centre to Community Health Centres and to higher up institutions from CHCs.

Appendix 5

NATIONAL POPULATION POLICY-2000

INTRODUCTION

1. The overriding objective of economic and social development is to improve the quality of lives that people lead, to enhance their well-being, and to provide them with opportunities and choices to become productive assets in society.

2. In 1952, India was the first country in the world to launch a national programme, emphasizing family planning to the extent necessary for reducing birth rates "to stabilize the population at a level consistent with the requirement of national economy." After 1952, sharp declines in death rates were, however, not accompanied by a similar drop in birth rates. The National Health Policy, 1983 stated that replacement levels of total fertility rate (TFR) should be achieved by the year 2000.

3. On 11 May, 2000 India is projected to have 1 billion (100 crore) people, i.e. 16 percent of the world's population on 2.4 percent of the globe's land area. If current trends continue, India may overtake China in 2045, to become the most populous country in the world. While global population has increased three-fold during this century, from 2 billion to 6 billion, the population of India has increased nearly five times from 238 million (23 crores) to 1 billion in the same period. India's current annual increase in population of 15.5 million is large enough to neutralize efforts to conserve the resource endowment and environment.

Box I

India's Demographic Achievement

Half a century after formulating the national family welfare programme, India has:

- reduced crude birth rate (CBR) from 40.8 (1951) to 26.4 (1998, SRS);
- halved the infant mortality rate (IMR) from 146 per 1000 live births (1951) to 72 per 1000 live births (1998, SRS);
- quadrupled the couple protection rate (CPR) from 10.4 percent (1971) to 44 percent (1999);
- reduced crude death rate (CDR) from 25 (1951) to 9.0 (1998, SRS);
- added 25 years to life expectancy from 37 years to 62 years;
- achieved nearly universal awareness of the need for and methods of family planning, and
- reduced total fertility rate from 6.0 (1951) to 3.3 (1997, SRS).

4. India's population in 1991 and projections to 2016 are as follows:

TABLE I

Population Projections for India (million)

March 1991	March 2001	March 2011	March 2016
846.3	1012.4	1178.9	1263.5

1. Milestones in the Evolution of the Population Policy are listed at Appendix II.
2. TFR: Average number of children born to a woman during her lifetime.
3. Source: Technical Group on Population Projections ,Planning Commission.

5. Stabilising population is an essential requirement for promoting sustainable development with more equitable distribution. However, it is as much a function of making reproductive health care accessible and affordable for all, as of increasing the provision and outreach of primary and secondary education, extending basic amenities including sanitation, safe drinking water and housing, besides empowering women and enhancing their employment opportunities, and providing transport and communications.

6. The National Population Policy, 2000 (NPP 2000) affirms the commitment of government towards voluntary and informed choice and consent of citizens while availing of reproductive health care services, and continuation of the target free approach in administering family planning services. The NPP 2000 provides a policy framework for advancing goals and prioritizing strategies during the next decade, to meet the reproductive and child health needs of the people of India, and to achieve net replacement levels (TFR) by 2010. It is based upon the need to simultaneously address issues of child survival, maternal health, and contraception, while increasing outreach and coverage of a comprehensive package of reproductive and child heath services by government, industry and the voluntary non-government sector, working in partnership.

OBJECTIVES

1. The immediate objective of the NPP 2000 is to address the unmet needs for contraception, health care infrastructure, and health personnel, and to provide integrated service delivery for basic reproductive and child health care. The medium-term objective is to bring the TFR to replacement levels by 2010, through vigorous implementation of inter-sectoral operational strategies. The long-term objective is to achieve a stable population by 2045, at a level consistent with the requirements of sustainable economic growth, social development, and environmental protection.

2. In pursuance of these objectives, the following National Socio-Demographic Goals to be achieved in each case by 2010 are formulated:

Box 2

National Socio-Demographic Goals for 2010

- Address the unmet needs for basic reproductive and child health services, supplies and infrastructure.
- Make school education up to age 14 free and compulsory, and reduce drop outs at primary and secondary school levels to below 20 percent for both boys and girls.
- Reduce infant mortality rate to below 30 per 1000 live births.
- Reduce maternal mortality ratio to below 100 per 100,000 live births.
- Achieve universal immunization of children against all vaccine preventable diseases.
- Promote delayed marriage for girls, not earlier than age 18 and preferably after 20 years of age.
- Achieve 80 percent institutional deliveries and 100 percent deliveries by trained persons.
- Achieve universal access to information/counseling, and services for fertility regulation and contraception with a wide basket of choices.
- Achieve 100 per cent registration of births, deaths, marriage and pregnancy.
- Contain the spread of Acquired Immunodeficiency Syndrome (AIDS), and promote greater integration between the management of reproductive tract infections (RTI) and sexually transmitted infections (STI) and the National AIDS Control Organisation.
- Prevent and control communicable diseases.
- Integrate Indian Systems of Medicine (ISM) in the provision of reproductive and child health services, and in reaching out to households.
- Promote vigorously the small family norm to achieve replacement levels of TFR.
- Bring about convergence in implementation of related social sector programs so that family welfare becomes a people centred programme.

If the NPP 2000 is fully implemented, we anticipate a population of 1107 million (110 crores) in 2010, instead of 1162 million (116 crores) projected by the Technical Group on Population Projections:

3. Population growth in India continues to be high on account of:

- The large size of the population in the reproductive age-group (estimated contribution 58 percent). An addition of 417.2 million between 1991 and 2016 is anticipated despite substantial

TABLE 2

Anticipated Growth in Population (million)

Year	*If current trends continue*		*If TFR 2.1 is achieved by 2010*
	Total Population	*Increase in population*	*Total population*
1991	846.3	—	846.3
1996	934.2	17.6	934.2
1997	949.9	15.7	949.0
2000	996.9	15.7	991.0
2002	1027.6	15.4	1013.0
2010	1162.3	16.8	1107.0

Similarly, the anticipated reductions in the birth, infant mortality and total fertility rates are:

TABLE 3

Projections of Crude Birth Rate, Infant Mortality Rate, and TFR, if the NPP 2000 is fully implemented

Year	*Crude Birth Rate*	*Infant Mortality Rate*	*Total Fertility Rate*
1997	27.2	71	3.3
1998	26.4	72	3.3
2002	23.0	50	2.6
2010	21.0	30	2.1

Source for Tables 2 and 3: Ministry of Health and Family Welfare.

reductions in family size in several states, including those which have already achieved replacement levels of TFR. This momentum of increase in population will continue for some more years because high TFRs in the past have resulted in a large proportion of the population being currently in their reproductive years. It is imperative that the reproductive age group adopts without further delay or exception the "small family norm", for the reason that about 45 percent of population increase is contributed by births above two children per family.

- Higher fertility due to unmet need for contraception (estimated contribution 20 percent). India has 168 million eligible couples, of which just 44 percent are currently effectively protected.

Urgent steps are currently required to make contraception more widely available, accessible, and affordable. Around 74 percent of the population lives in rural areas, in about 5.5 lakh villages, many with poor communications and transport. Reproductive health and basic health infrastructure and services often do not reach the villages, and, accordingly, vast numbers of people cannot avail of these services.

- High wanted fertility due to the high infant mortality rate (IMR) (estimated contribution about 20 percent). Repeated child births are seen as an insurance against multiple infant (and child) deaths and accordingly, high infant mortality stymies all efforts at reducing TFR.
- Over 50 percent of girls marry below the age of 18, the minimum legal age of marriage, resulting in a typical reproductive pattern of "too early, too frequent, too many." Around 33 percent births occur at intervals of less than 24 months, which also results in high IMR.

The country's demographic profile is given in Appendix III.

STRATEGIC THEMES

1. We identify 12 strategic themes which must be simultaneously pursued in "stand alone" or inter-sectoral programmes in order to achieve the national socio-demographic goals for 2010. These are presented below:

(i) Decentralised Planning and Programme Implementation

2. The 73rd and 74th Constitutional Amendments Act, 1992, made health, family welfare, and education a responsibility of village panchayats. The panchayati raj institutions are an important means of furthering decentralised planning and programme implementation in the context of the NPP 2000. However, in order to realize their potential, they need strengthening by further delegation of administrative and financial powers, including powers of resource mobilization.

Further, since 33 percent of elected panchayat seats are reserved for women, representative committees of the panchayats (headed by an elected woman panchayat member) should be formed to promote a gender sensitive, multi-sectoral agenda for population stabilisation, that will "think, plan and act locally, and support nationally." These committees may identify area specific unmet needs for reproductive health services, and prepare need-based, demand-driven, socio-demographic plans at the village level, aimed at identifying and providing responsive, people-centred and integrated, basic reproductive and child health care. Panchayats demonstrating exemplary performance in the compulsory registration of births, deaths, marriages, and pregnancies, universalizing the small family norm, increasing safe deliveries, bringing about reductions in infant and maternal mortality, and promoting compulsory education up to age 14, will be nationally recognized and honored.

(ii) Convergence of Service Delivery at Village Levels

3. Efforts at population stabilisation will be effective only if we direct an integrated package of essential services at village and household levels. Below district levels, current health infrastructure includes 2,500 community health centres, 25,000 primary health centres (each covering a population of 30,000), and 1.36 lakh sub-centres (each covering a population of 5,000 in the plains and 3,000 in hilly regions). Inadequacies in the existing health infrastructure have led to an unmet need of 28 percent for contraception services, and obvious gaps in coverage and outreach. Health care centres are over-burdened and struggle to provide services with limited personnel and equipment. Absence of supportive supervision, lack of training in inter-personal communication, and lack of motivation to work in rural areas, together impede citizens' access to reproductive and child health services, and contribute to poor quality of services and an apparent insensitivity to client's needs. The last 50 years have demonstrated the unsuitability of these yardsticks for provision of health care infrastructure, particularly for remote, inaccessible, or sparsely populated regions in the country like hilly and forested areas, desert regions and tribal areas. We need to promote a more flexible approach, by extending basic reproductive and child health care through mobile clinics and counseling services. Further, recognizing that government alone cannot make up for the inadequacies in health care infrastructure and services, in order to resolve unmet needs and extend coverage, the involvement of the voluntary sector and the non-government sector in partnership with the government is essential.

4. Since the management, funding, and implementation of health and education programmes has been decentralised to panchayats, in order to reach household levels, a one-stop, integrated and coordinated service delivery should be provided at village levels, for basic reproductive and child health services. A vast increase in the number of trained birth attendants, at least two per village, is necessary to universalise coverage and outreach of ante-natal, natal and post-natal health care. An equipped maternity hut in each village should be set-up to serve as a delivery room, with functioning midwifery kits, basic medication for essential obstetric aid, and indigenous medicines and supplies for maternal and new born care. A key feature of the integrated service delivery will be the registration at village levels, of births, deaths, marriage, and pregnancies. Each village should maintain a list of community midwives and trained birth attendants, village health guides, panchayat sewa sahayaks, primary school teachers and anganwadi workers who may be entrusted with various responsibilities in the implementation of integrated service delivery.

5. The panchayats should seek the help of community opinion makers to communicate the benefits of smaller, healthier families, the significance of educating girls, and promoting female participation in paid employment. They should also involve civil society in monitoring the availability, accessibility and affordability of services and supplies.

(iii) Empowering Women for Improved Health and Nutrition

6. The complex socio-cultural determinants of women's health and nutrition have cumulative effects over a lifetime. Discriminatory childcare leads to malnutrition and impaired physical development of the girl child. Undernutrition and micronutrient deficiency in early adolescence goes beyond mere food entitlements to those nutrition related capabilities that become crucial to a woman's well-being, and through her, to the well-being of children. The positive effects of good health and nutrition on the labour productivity of the poor is well documented. To the extent that women are over-represented among the poor, interventions for improving women's health and nutrition are critical for poverty reduction.

7. Impaired health and nutrition is compounded by early childbearing, and consequent risk of serious pregnancy-related complications. Women's risk of premature death and disability is highest during their reproductive years. Malnutrition, frequent pregnancies, unsafe abortions, RTI and STI, all combine to keep the maternal mortality ratio in India among the highest globally.

8. Maternal mortality is not merely a health disadvantage, it is a matter of social injustice. Low social and economic status of girls and women limits their access to education, good nutrition, as well as money to pay for health care and family planning services. The extent of maternal mortality is an indicator of disparity and inequity in access to appropriate health care and nutrition services throughout a lifetime, and particularly during pregnancy and child-birth, and is a crucial factor contributing to high maternal mortality.

9. Programmes for Safe Motherhood, Universal Immunisation, Child Survival and Oral Rehydration have been combined into an Integrated Reproductive and Child Health Programme, which also includes promoting management of STIs and RTIs. Women's health and nutrition problems can be largely prevented or mitigated through low cost interventions designed for low income settings.

10. The voluntary non-government sector and the private corporate sector should actively collaborate with the community and government through specific commitments in the areas of basic reproductive and child health care, basic education, and in securing higher levels of participation in the paid work force for women.

(iv) Child Health and Survival

11. Infant mortality is a sensitive indicator of human development. High mortality and morbidity among infants and children below 5 years occurs on account of inadequate care, asphyxia during birth, premature birth, low birth weight, acute respiratory infections, diarrhoea, vaccine preventable diseases, malnutrition and deficiencies of nutrients, including Vitamin A. Infant mortality rates have not significantly declined in recent years.

12. Our priority is to intensify neo-natal care. A National Technical Committee should be set-up, consisting principally of consultants in

obstetrics, pediatrics (neonatologists), family health, medical research and statistics from among academia, public health professionals, clinical practitioners and government. Its terms of reference should include prescribing perinatal audit norms, developing quality improvement activities with monitoring schedules and suggestions for facilitating provision of continuing medical and nursing education to all perinatal health care providers. Implementation at the grass-roots must benefit from current developments in the fields of perinatology and neonatology. The baby friendly hospital initiative (BFHI) should be extended to all hospitals and clinics, up to sub-centre levels. Additionally, besides promoting breast-feeding and complementary feeds, the BFHI should include updating of skills of trained birth attendants to improve new born care practices to reduce the risks of hypothermia and infection. Essential equipment for the new born must be provided at sub-centre levels.

13. Child survival interventions, i.e. universal immunisation, control of childhood diarrhoeas with oral rehydration therapies, management of acute respiratory infections, and massive doses of Vitamin A and food supplements have all helped to reduce infant and child mortality and morbidity. With intensified efforts, the eradication of polio is within reach. However, the decline in standards, outreach and quality of routine immunisation is a matter of concern. Significant improvements need to be made in the quality and coverage of the routine immunisation programme.

(v) Meeting the Unmet Needs for Family Welfare Services

14. In both rural and urban areas there continue to be unmet needs for contraceptives, supplies and equipment for integrated service delivery, mobility of health providers and patients, and comprehensive information. It is important to strengthen, energise and make accountable the cutting edge of health infrastructure at the village, sub-centre and primary health centre levels, to improve facilities for referral transportation, to encourage and strengthen local initiatives for ambulance services at village and block levels, to increase innovative social marketing schemes for affordable products and services and to improve advocacy in locally relevant and acceptable dialects.

(vi) Under-Served Population Groups

(a) Urban Slums

15. Nearly 100 million people live in urban slums, with little or no access to potable water, sanitation facilities, and health care services. This contributes to high infant and child mortality, which in turn perpetuate high TFR and maternal mortality. Basic and primary health care, including reproductive and child health care, needs to be provided. Coordination with municipal bodies for water, sanitation and waste disposal must be pursued, and targeted information, education and communication campaigns must spread awareness about the secondary and tertiary facilities available.

(b) Tribal Communities, Hill Area Populations and Displaced and Migrant Populations

16. In general, populations in remote and low density areas do not have adequate access to affordable health care services. Tribal populations often have high levels of morbidity arising from poor nutrition, particularly in situations where they are involuntarily displaced or resettled. Frequently, they have low levels of literacy, coupled with high infant, child, and maternal mortality. They remain under-served in the coverage of reproductive and child health services. These communities need special attention in terms of basic health, and reproductive and child health services. The special needs of tribal groups which need to be addressed include the provision of mobile clinics that will be responsive to seasonal variations in the availability of work and income. Information and counseling on infertility, and regular supply of standardised medication will be included.

(c) Adolescents

17. Adolescents represent about a fifth of India's population. The needs of adolescents, including protection from unwanted pregnancies and sexually transmitted diseases (STD), have not been specifically addressed in the past. Programmes should encourage delayed marriage and child-bearing, and education of adolescents about the risks of unprotected sex. Reproductive health services for adolescent girls and boys is especially significant in rural India, where adolescent marriage and pregnancy are widely prevalent. Their special requirements comprise information, counseling, population education, and making contraceptive services accessible and affordable, providing food supplements and nutritional services through the ICDS, and enforcing the Child Marriage Restraint Act, 1976.

(d) Increased Participation of Men in Planned Parenthood

18. In the past, population programmes have tended to exclude menfolk. Gender inequalities in patriarchal societies ensure that men play a critical role in determining the education and employment of family members, age at marriage, besides access to and utilisation of health, nutrition, and family welfare services for women and children. The active involvement of men is called for in planning families, supporting contraceptive use, helping pregnant women stay healthy, arranging skilled care during delivery, avoiding delays in seeking care, helping after the baby is born and, finally, in being a responsible father. In short, the active cooperation and participation of men is vital for ensuring programme acceptance. Further, currently, over 97 percent of sterilisations are tubectomies and this manifestation of gender imbalance needs to be corrected. The special needs of men include re-popularising vasectomies, in particular noscalpel vasectomy as a safe and simple procedure, and focusing on men in the information and education campaigns to promote the small family norm.

(vii) Diverse Health Care Providers

19. Given the large unmet need for reproductive and child health services, and inadequacies in health care infrastructure it is imperative to increase the numbers and diversify the categories of health care providers. Ways of doing this include accrediting private medical practitioners and assigning them to defined beneficiary groups to provide these services; revival of the system of licensed medical practitioner who, after appropriate certification from the Indian Medical Association (IMA), could provide specified clinical services.

(viii) Collaboration with and Commitments from Non-Government Organisations and the Private Sector

20. A national effort to reach out to households cannot be sustained by government alone. We need to put in place a partnership of non-government voluntary organisations, the private corporate sector, government and the community. Triggered by rising incomes and institutional finance, private health care has grown significantly, with an impressive pool of expertise and management skills, and currently accounts for nearly 75 percent of health care expenditures. However, despite their obvious potential, mobilising the private (profit and non-profit) sector to serve public health goals raises governance issues of contracting, accreditation, regulation, referral, besides the appropriate division of labour between the public and private health providers, all of which need to be addressed carefully. Where government interventions or capacities are insufficient, and the participation of the private sector unviable, focused service delivery by NGOs may effectively complement government efforts.

(ix) Mainstreaming Indian Systems of Medicine and Homeopathy

21. India's community supported ancient but living traditions of indigenous systems of medicine has sustained the population for centuries, with effective cures and remedies for numerous conditions, including those relating to women and children, with minimal side effects. Utilisation of ISMH in basic reproductive and child health care will expand the pool of effective health care providers, optimise utilisation of locally based remedies and cures, and promote lowcost health care. Guidelines need to be evolved to regulate and ensure standardisation, efficacy and safety of ISMH drugs for wider entry into national markets.

22. Particular challenges include providing appropriate training and raising awareness and skill development in reproductive and child health care to the institutionally qualified ISMH medical practitioners. The feasibility of utilising their services to fill in gaps in manpower at village levels, and at sub-centres and primary health centres may be explored. ISMH institutions, hospitals and dispensaries may be utilised for reproductive and child health care programmes. At village levels, the services of the ISMH "barefoot doctors", after appropriate training, may be utilised for advocacy and counseling, for distributing supplies and

equipment, and as depot holders. ISMH practices may be applied at village maternity huts, and at household levels, for ante-natal, natal and post-natal care, and for nurture of the new born.

(x) Contraceptive Technology and Research on Reproductive and Child Health

23. Government must constantly advance, encourage, and support medical, social science, demographic and behavioural science research on maternal, child and reproductive health care issues. This will improve medical techniques relevant to the country's needs, and strengthen programme and project design and implementation. Consultation and frequent dialogue by Government with the existing network of academic and research institutions in allopathy and ISMH, and with other relevant public and private research institutions engaged in social science, demography and behavioural research must continue. The International Institute of Population Sciences, and the population research centres which have been set-up to pursue applied research in population related matters, need to be revitalised and strengthened.

24. Applied research relies upon constant monitoring of performance at the programme and project levels. The National Health and Family Welfare Survey provides data on key health and family welfare indicators every five years. Data from the first National Family Health Survey (NFHS-1), 1992-93, has been updated by NFHS-2, 1998-99, to be published shortly. Annual data is generated by the Sample Registration Survey, which, *inter alia*, maps at state levels the birth, death and infant mortality rates. Absence of regular feedback has been a weakness in the family welfare progamme. For this reason, the Department of Family Welfare is strengthening its management information systems (MIS) and has commenced during 1998, a system of ascertaining impacts and outcomes through district surveys and facility surveys. The district surveys cover 50% districts every year, so that every 2 years there is an update on every district in the country. The facility surveys ascertain the availability of infrastructure and services up to primary health centre level, covering one district per month. The feedback from both these surveys enable remedial action at district and sub-district levels.

(xi) Providing for the Older Population

25. Improved life expectancy is leading to an increase in the absolute number and proportion of persons aged 60 years and above, and is anticipated to nearly double during 1996-2016, from 62.3 million to 112.9 million. When viewed in the context of significant weakening of traditional support systems, the elderly are increasingly vulnerable, needing protection and care. Promoting old age health care and support will, over time, also serve to reduce the incentive to have large families.

26. The Ministry of Social Justice and Empowerment has adopted in January 1999 a National Policy on Older Persons. It has become important to build in geriatric health concerns in the population policy. Ways of

doing this include sensitising, training and equipping rural and urban health centres and hospitals for providing geriatric health care; encouraging NGOs to design and implement formal and informal schemes that make the elderly economically self-reliant; providing for and routinising screening for cancer, osteoporosis, and cardiovascular conditions in primary health centres, community health centres, and urban health care centres at primary, secondary and tertiary levels; and exploring tax incentives to encourage grown-up children to look after their aged parents.

(xii) Information, Education, and Communication

27. Information, education and communication (IEC) of family welfare messages must be clear, focused and disseminated everywhere, including the remote corners of the country, and in local dialects. This will ensure that the messages are effectively conveyed. These need to be strengthened and their outreach widened, with locally relevant, and locally comprehensible media and messages. On the model of the total literacy campaigns which have successfully mobilised local populations, there is need to undertake a massive national campaign on population-related issues, via artists, popular film stars, doctors, vaidyas, hakims, nurses, local midwives, women's organisations, and youth organisations.

LEGISLATION, PUBLIC SUPPORT AND NEW STRUCTURES

LEGISLATION

As a motivational measure, in order to enable state governments to fearlessly and effectively pursue the agenda for population stabilisation contained in the National Population Policy, 2000, one legislation is considered necessary. It is recommended that the 42nd Constitutional Amendment that freezes till 2001, the number of seats to the Lok Sabha and the Rajya Sabha based on the 1971 Census be extended up to 2026.

PUBLIC SUPPORT

Demonstration of strong support to the small family norm, as well as personal example, by political, community, business, professional and religious leaders, media and film stars, sports personalities, and opinion-makers, will enhance its acceptance throughout society. The government will actively enlist their support in concrete ways.

NEW STRUCTURES

The NPP 2000 is to be largely implemented and managed at panchayat and nagarpalika levels, in coordination with the concerned state/Union Territory administrations. Accordingly, the specific situation in each state/UT must be kept in mind. This will require comprehensive and multisectoral coordination of planning and implementation between health and family welfare on the one hand, along with schemes for education, nutrition, women and child development, safe drinking water, sanitation, rural roads, communications, transportation, housing, forestry development, environmental protection, and urban development. Accordingly, the following structures are recommended:

(i) National Commission on Population

A National Commission on Population, presided over by the Prime Minister, will have the Chief Ministers of all states and UTs, and the Central Minister in charge of the Department of Family Welfare and other concerned Central Ministries and Departments, for example Department of Woman and Child Development, Department of Education, Department of Social Justice and Empowerment in the Ministry of HRD, Ministry of Rural Development, Ministry of Environment and Forest, and others as necessary, and reputed demographers, public health professionals, and NGOs as members. This Commission will oversee and review implementation of policy. The Commission Secretariat will be provided by the Department of Family Welfare.

(ii) State/UT Commissions on Population

Each state and UT may consider having a State/UT Commission on Population, presided over by the Chief Minister, on the analogy of the National Commission, to likewise oversee and review implementation of the NPP 2000 in the state/UT.

(iii) Coordination Cell in the Planning Commission

The Planning Commission will have a Coordination Cell for inter-sectoral coordination between Ministries for enhancing performance, particularly in States/UTs needing special attention on account of adverse demographic and human development indicators.

(iv) Technology Mission in the Department of Family Welfare

To enhance performance, particularly in states with currently below average socio-demographic indices that need focused attention, a Technology Mission in the Department of Family Welfare will be established to provide technology support in respect of design and monitoring of projects and programmes for reproductive and child health, as well as for IEC campaigns.

FUNDING, PROMOTIONAL AND MOTIVATIONAL MEASURES FOR ADOPTION OF THE SMALL FAMILY NORM

FUNDING

The programmes, projects and schemes premised on the goals and objectives of the NPP 2000, and indeed all efforts at population stabilisation, will be adequately funded in view of their critical importance to national development. Preventive and promotive services such as ante-natal and post-natal care for women, immunisation for children, and contraception will continue to be subsidised for all those who need the services. Priority in allocation of funds will be given to improving health care infrastructure at the community and primary health centres, sub-centre and village levels. Critical gaps in manpower will be remedied through redeployment, particularly in under-served and inaccessible areas, and referral linkages will be improved. In order to implement immediately the Action Plan, it would be necessary to double the annual budget of the Department of Family Welfare to enable government to address the shortfall in unmet needs for health care infrastructure, services and supplies (in Appendix IV).

Even though the annual budget for population stabilisation activities assigned to the Department of Family Welfare has increased over the years, at least 50 percent of the budgetary outlay is deployed towards non-plan activities (recurring expenditures for maintenance of health care infrastructure in the states and UTs, and towards salaries). To illustrate, of the annual budget of Rs. 2920 crores for 1999-2000, nearly Rs. 1500 crores is allocated towards non-plan activities. Only the remaining 50 percent becomes available for genuine plan activities, including procurement of supplies and equipment. For these reasons, since 1980 the Department of Family Welfare has been unable to revise norms of operational costs of health infrastructure, which in turn has impacted directly the quality of care and outreach of services provided.

PROMOTIONAL AND MOTIVATIONAL MEASURES FOR ADOPTION OF THE SMALL FAMILY NORM

The following promotional and motivational measures will be undertaken:

(i) Panchayats and Zila Parishads will be rewarded and honoured for exemplary performance in universalising the small family norm, achieving reductions in infant mortality and birth rates, and promoting literacy with completion of primary schooling.

(ii) The Balika Samridhi Yojana run by the Department of Women and Child Development, to promote survival and care of the girl child, will continue. A cash incentive of Rs. 500 is awarded at the birth of the girl child of birth order 1 or 2.

(iii) Maternity Benefit Scheme run by the Department of Rural Development will continue. A cash incentive of Rs. 500 is awarded to mothers who have their first child after 19 years of age, for birth of the first or second child only. Disbursement of the cash award will in future be linked to compliance with ante-natal check up, institutional delivery by trained birth attendant, registration of birth and BCG immunisation.

(iv) A Family Welfare-linked Health Insurance Plan will be established. Couples below the poverty line, who undergo sterilisation with not more than two living children, would become eligible (along with children) for health insurance (for hospitalisation) not exceeding Rs. 5000, and a personal accident insurance cover for the spouse undergoing sterilisation.

(v) Couples below the poverty line, who marry after the legal age of marriage, register the marriage, have their first child after the mother reaches the age of 21, accept the small family norm, and adopt a terminal method after the birth of the second child, will be rewarded.

(vi) A revolving fund will be set-up for income-generating activities by village-level self-help groups, who provide community-level health care services.

(vii) Crèches and child care centres will be opened in rural areas and urban slums. This will facilitate and promote participation of women in paid employment.

(viii) A wider, affordable choice of contraceptives will be made accessible at diverse delivery points, with counseling services to enable acceptors to exercise voluntary and informed consent.

(ix) Facilities for safe abortion will be strengthened and expanded.

(x) Products and services will be made affordable through innovative social marketing schemes.

(xi) Local entrepreneurs at village levels will be provided soft loans and encouraged to run ambulance services to supplement the existing arrangements for referral transportation.

(xii) Increased vocational training schemes for girls, leading to self-employment will be encouraged.

(xiii) Strict enforcement of Child Marriage Restraint Act, 1976.

(xiv) Strict enforcement of the Pre-Natal Diagnostic Techniques Act, 1994.

(xv) Soft loans to ensure mobility of the ANMs will be increased.

(xvi) The 42nd Constitutional Amendment has frozen the number of representatives in the Lok Sabha (on the basis of population) at 1971 Census levels. The freeze is currently valid until 2001, and has served as an incentive for State Governments to fearlessly pursue the agenda for population stabilisation. This freeze needs to be extended until 2026.

CONCLUSION

In the new millennium, nations are judged by the well-being of their peoples; by levels of health, nutrition and education; by the civil and political liberties enjoyed by their citizens; by the protection guaranteed to children and by provisions made for the vulnerable and the disadvantaged.

The vast numbers of the people of India can be its greatest asset if they are provided with the means to lead healthy and economically productive lives. Population stabilisation is a multisectoral endeavour requiring constant and effective dialogue among a diversity of stakeholders, and coordination at all levels of the government and society. Spread of literacy and education, increasing availability of affordable reproductive and child health services, convergence of service delivery at village levels, participation of women in the paid work force, together with a steady, equitable improvement in family incomes, will facilitate early achievement of the socio-demographic goals. Success will be achieved if the Action Plan contained in the NPP 2000 is pursued as a national movement.

National Socio-Demographic Goals for 2010

- Address the unmet needs for basic reproductive and child health services, supplies and infrastructure.
- Make school education up to age 14 free and compulsory, and reduce drop outs at primary and secondary school levels to below 20 percent for both boys and girls.
- Reduce infant mortality rate to below 30 per 1000 live births.
- Reduce maternal mortality ratio to below 100 per 100,000 live births.
- Achieve universal immunization of children against all vaccine preventable diseases.
- Promote delayed marriage for girls, not earlier than age 18 and preferably after 20 years of age.
- Achieve 80 percent institutional deliveries and 100 percent deliveries by trained persons.
- Achieve universal access to information/counseling, and services for fertility regulation and contraception with a wide basket of choices.
- Achieve 100 per cent registration of births, deaths, marriage and pregnancy.
- Contain the spread of Acquired Immunodeficiency Syndrome (AIDS), and promote greater integration between the management of reproductive tract infections (RTI) and sexually transmitted infections (STI) and the National AIDS Control Organisation.
- Prevent and control communicable diseases.
- Integrate Indian Systems of Medicine (ISM) in the provision of reproductive and child health services, and in reaching out to households.
- Promote vigorously the small family norm to achieve replacement levels of TFR.
- Bring about convergence in implementation of related social sector programs so that family welfare becomes a people centred programme.

If the NPP 2000 is fully implemented, we anticipate a population of 1107 million (110 crores) in 2010, instead of 1162 million (116 crores) projected by the Technical Group on Population Projections:

Population growth in India continues to be high on account of:

- The large size of the population in the reproductive age-group (estimated contribution 58 percent). An addition of 417.2 million between 1991 and 2016 is anticipated despite substantial reductions in family size in several states, including those which have already achieved replacement levels of TFR. This momentum of increase in population will continue for some more years because high TFRs in the past have resulted in a large proportion of the population being currently in their reproductive years. It is imperative that the reproductive age group adopts without further delay or exception the "small family norm", for the reason that about 45 percent of population increase is contributed by births above two children per family.
- Higher fertility due to unmet need for contraception (estimated contribution 20 percent). India has 168 million eligible couples, of which just 44 percent are currently effectively protected. Urgent steps are currently required to make contraception more widely available, accessible, and affordable. Around 74 percent of the population lives in rural areas, in about 5.5 lakh villages, many with poor communications and transport. Reproductive health and basic health infrastructure and services often do not reach the villages, and, accordingly, vast number of people cannot avail of these services.
- High wanted fertility due to the high infant mortality rate (IMR) (estimated contribution about 20 percent). Repeated child births are seen as an insurance against multiple infant (and child) deaths and accordingly, high infant mortality stymies all efforts at reducing TFR.
- Over 50 percent of girls marry below the age of 18, the minimum legal age of marriage, resulting in a typical reproductive pattern of "too early, too frequent, too many." Around 33 percent births occur at intervals of less than 24 months, which also results in high IMR.

ACTION PLAN

OPERATIONAL STRATEGIES

(i) and (ii) Converge Service Delivery at Village Levels

1. Utilise village self-help groups to organise and provide basic services for reproductive and child health care, combined with the ongoing Integrated Child Development Scheme (ICDS). Village self-help groups are in existence through centrally sponsored schemes of: (a) Department of Women and Child Development, Ministry of HRD, (b) Ministry of Rural Development, and (c) Ministry of Environment and Forests. Organise

neighbourhood acceptor groups, and provide them with a revolving fund that may be accessed for income generation activities. The groups may establish rules of eligibility, interest rates, and accountability for which capital may be advanced, usually to be repaid in installments within two years. The repayments may be used to fund another acceptor group in a nearby community, who would exert pressure to ensure timely repayments. Two trained birth attendants and the anganwadi worker (AWW) should be members of this group.

2. Implement at village levels a one-stop integrated and coordinated service delivery package for basic health care, family planning and maternal and child health-related services, provided by the community and for the community. Train and motivate the village self-help acceptor groups to become the primary contact at household levels. Once every fortnight, these acceptor groups will meet, and provide at one place 6 different services for (i) registration of births, deaths, marriage and pregnancy; (ii) weighing of children under 5 years, and recording the weight on a standard growth chart; (iii) counseling and advocacy for contraception, plus free supply of contraceptives; (iv) preventive care, with availability of basic medicines for common ailments: antipyretics for fevers, antibiotic ointments for infections, ORT/ORS1 for childhood diarrhoeas, together with standardised indigenous medication and homeopathic cures; (v) nutrition supplements; and (vi) advocacy and encouragement for the continued enrolment of children in school up to age 14. One health staff, appointed by the panchayat, will be suitably trained to provide guidance. Clustering services for women and children at one place and time at village levels will promote positive interactions in health benefits and reduce service delivery costs.

3. Wherever these village self-help groups have not developed for any reason, community midwives, practitioners of ISMH, retired school teachers and ex-defence personnel may be organised into neighbourhood groups to perform similar functions.

4. At village levels, the anganwadi centre may become the pivot of basic health care activities, contraceptive counseling and supply, nutrition education and supplementation, as well as pre-school activities. The aanganwadi centres can also function as depots for ORS/basic medicines and contraceptives.

5. A maternity hut should be established in each village to be used as the village delivery room, with storage space for supplies and medicines. It should be adequately equipped with kits for midwifery, ante-natal care, and delivery; basic medication for obstetric emergency aid; contraceptives, drugs and medicines for common ailments; and indigenous medicines/ supplies for maternal and new-born care. The panchayat may appoint a competent and mature midwife, to look after this village maternity hut. She may be assisted by volunteers.

6. Trained birth attendants as well as the vast pool of traditional dais should be made familiar with emergency and referral procedures. This will

greatly assist the Auxiliary Nurse Midwife (ANM) at the sub-centres to monitor and respond to maternal morbidity/emergencies at village levels.

7. Each village may maintain a list of community mid-wives, village health guides, panchayat sewa sahayaks, trained birth attendants, practitioners of indigenous systems of medicine, primary school teachers and other relevant persons, as well as the nearest institutional health care facilities that may be accessed for integrated service delivery. These persons may also be helpful in involving civil society in monitoring availability, quality and accessibility of reproductive and child health services; in disseminating education and communication on the benefits of smaller and healthier families, with emphasis on education of the girl child; and female participation in the work force.

8. Provide a wider basket of choices in contraception, through innovative social marketing schemes to reach household levels.

Comment: Meaningful decentralisation will result only if the convergence of the national family welfare programme with the ICDS programme is strengthened. The focus of the ICDS programme on nutrition improvement at village levels and on pre-school activities must be widened to include maternal and child health care services. Convergence of several related activities at service delivery levels with, in particular, the ICDS programme, is critical for extending outreach and increasing access to services. Intersectoral coordination with appropriate training and sensitisation among field functionaries will facilitate dissemination of integrated reproductive and child health services to village and household levels. People will willingly cooperate in the registration of births, deaths, marriages and pregnancies if they perceive some benefit. At the village level, this community meeting every fortnight, may become their most convenient access to basic health care, both for maternal and child health, as well as for common ailments. Households may participate to receive integrated service delivery, along with information about ongoing micro-credit and thrift schemes. Government and non-government functionaries will be expected to function in harmony to ensure integrated service delivery. The panchayat will promote this coordination and exercise effective supervision.

(iii) Empowering Women for Improved Health and Nutrition

1. Create an enabling environment for women and children to benefit from products and services disseminated under the reproductive and child health programme. Cluster services for women and children at the same place and time. This promotes positive interactions in health benefits and reduces service delivery costs.

2. As a measure to empower women, open more child care centres in rural areas and in urban slums, where a woman worker may leave her children in responsible hands. This will encourage female participation in paid employment, reduce school drop-out rates, particularly for the girl child, and promote school enrolment as well. The anganwadis provide a partial solution.

3. To empower women, pursue programmes of social afforestation to facilitate access to fuelwood and fodder. Similarly, pursue drinking water schemes for increasing access to potable water. This will reduce long absences from home, and the need for large number of children to perform such tasks.

4. In any reward scheme intended for household levels, priority may be given to energy saving devices such as solar cookers, or provision of sanitation facilities, or extension of telephone lines. This will empower households, in particular women.

5. Improve district, sub-district and panchayat-level health management with coordination and collaboration between district health officer, sub-district health officer and the panchayat for planning and implementation activities. There is need to:

- Strengthen the referral network between the district health office, district hospital and the community health centres, the primary health centres and the sub-centres in management of obstetric and neo-natal complications.
- Strengthen community health centres to provide comprehensive emergency obstetric and neo-natal care. These may function as clinical training centres as well. Strengthen primary health centres to provide essential obstetric and neo-natal care. Strengthen sub-centres to provide a comprehensive range of services, with delivery rooms, counseling for contraception, supplies of free contraceptives, ORS and basic medicines, together with facilities for immunisation.
- Establish rigorous problem identification mechanisms through maternal and peri-natal audit, from village level upwards.

6. Ensure adequate transportation at village level, sub-centre levels, zila parishads, primary health centres and at community health centres. Identifying women at risk is meaningful only if women with complications can reach emergency care in time.

7. Improve the accessibility and quality of maternal and child health services through:

- Deployment of community mid-wives and additional health providers at village levels; cluster services for women and children at the same place and time, from village level upwards, e.g. ante-natal and post-partum care, monitoring infant growth, availability of contraceptives and medicine kits; and routinised immunisations at sub-centre levels.
- Strengthen the capacity of primary health centres to provide basic emergency obstetric and neo-natal health care.
- Involve professional agencies in developing and disseminating training modules for standard procedures in the management of

obstetric and neo-natal cases. The aim should be to routinise these procedures at all appropriate levels.

- Improve supervision by developing guidance and supervision checklists.

8. Monitor performance of maternal and child health services at each level by using the maternal and child health local area monitoring system, which includes monitoring the incidence and coverage of ante-natal visits, deliveries assisted by trained health care personnel and post-natal visits, among other indicators. The ANM at the sub-centre should be responsible and accountable for registering every pregnancy and child birth in her jurisdiction, and for providing universal ante-natal and post-natal services.

9. Improve technical skills of maternal and child health care providers by:

Strengthening skills of health personnel and health providers through classroom and on-the-job training in the management of obstetric and neo-natal emergencies. This should include training of birth attendants and community midwives at district-level hospitals in life-saving skills, such as management of asphyxia and hypothermia.

Training on integrated management of childhood illnesses for infants (1 week—2 months).

10. Support community activities such as dissemination of IEC material, including leaflets and posters, and promotion of folk jatras, songs and dances to promote healthy mother and healthy baby messages, along with good management practices to ensure safe motherhood, including early recognition of danger signs.

11. Programme development comprising:

Partnership in family health and nutrition. The anganwadi worker will identify women and children in the villages who suffer from malnutrition and/or micro-nutritional deficiencies, including iron, vitamin A, and iodine deficiency; provide nutritional supplements and monitor nutritional status.

Convergence, strengthening, and universalisation of the nutritional programmes of the Department of Family Welfare and the ICDS run by the Department of Women and Child Development, ensuring training and timely supply of food supplements and medicines.

Include STD/RTI and HIV/AIDS prevention, screening and management, in maternal and child health services.

Provide quality care in family planning, including information, increased contraceptive choices for both spacing and terminal methods, increase access to good quality and affordable contraceptive supplies and services at diverse delivery points, counseling about the safety, efficacy and possible side effects of each method, and appropriate follow-up.

12. Develop a health package for adolescents.

13. Expand the availability of safe abortion care. Abortion is legal, but there are barriers limiting women's access to safe abortion services. Some

operational strategies are:

Community-level education campaigns should target women, household decision-makers and adolescents about the availability of safe abortion services and the dangers of unsafe abortion.

Make safe and legal abortion services more attractive to women and household decision-makers by (i) increasing geographic spread; (ii) enhancing affordability; (iii) ensuring confidentiality, and (iv) providing compassionate abortion care, including post-abortion counseling.

Adopt updated and simple technologies that are safe and easy, e.g. manual vacuum extraction not necessarily dependant upon anaesthesia, or non-surgical techniques which are non-invasive.

Promote collaborative arrangements with private sector health professionals, NGOs and the public sector, to increase the availability and coverage of safe abortion services, including training of mid-level providers.

Eliminate the current cumbersome procedures for registration of abortion clinics. Simplify and facilitate the establishment of additional training centres for safe abortions in the public, private, and NGO sectors. Train these health care providers in provision of clinical services for safe abortions.

Formulate and notify standards for abortion services. Strengthen enforcement mechanisms at district and sub-district levels to ensure that these norms are followed.

Follow norms-based registration of service provision centres, and thereby switch the onus of meticulous observance of standards onto the provider.

Provide competent post-abortion care, including management of complications and identification of other health needs of post-abortion patients, and linking with appropriate services. As part of post-abortion care, physicians may be trained to provide family planning counseling and services such as sterilisation, and reversible modern methods such as IUDs, as well as oral contraceptives and condoms.

Modify syllabus and curricula for medical graduates, as well as for continuing education and in-house learning, to provide for practical training in the newer procedures.

Ensure services for termination of pregnancy at primary health centres and at community health centres.

14. Develop maternity hospitals at sub-district levels and at community health centres to function as FRUs for complicated and life-threatening deliveries.

15. Formulate and enforce standards for clinical services in the public, private, and NGO sectors.

16. Focus on distribution of non-clinical methods of contraception (condoms and oral contraceptive pills) through free supply, social marketing as well as commercial sales.

17. Create a national network consisting of public, private and NGO centres, identified by a common logo, for delivering reproductive and child

health services free to any client. The provider will be compensated for the service provided, on the basis of a coupon, duly counter-signed by the beneficiary, and paid for by a system to be devised. The compensation will be identical to providers across all sectors. The end-user will choose the provider of the service. A group of management experts will devise checks and balances to prevent misuse.

(iv) Child Health and Survival

1. Support community activities, from village level upwards to monitor early and adequate ante-natal, natal and post-natal care. Focus attention on neo-natal health care and nutrition.

2. Set-up a National Technical Committee on neo-natal care, to align programme and project interventions with newly emerging technologies in neo-natal and peri-natal care.

3. Pursue compulsory registration of births in coordination with the ICDS Programme.

4. After the birth of a child, provide counseling and advocacy about contraception, to encourage adoption of a reversible or a terminal method. This will also contribute to the health and well-being of both mother and child.

5. Improve capacities at health centres in basic midwifery services, essential neo-natal care, including the management of sick neo-nates outside the hospital.

6. Sensitise and train health personnel in the integrated management of childhood illnesses. Standard case management of diarrhoea and acute respiratory infections must be provided at sub-centres and primary health centres, with appropriate training, and adequate equipment. Besides, training in this sector may be imparted to health care providers at village levels, especially in indigenous systems.

7. Strengthen critical interventions aimed at bringing about reductions in maternal malnutrition, morbidity and mortality, by ensuring availability of supplies and equipment at village levels, and at sub centres.

8. Pursue rigorously the pulse polio campaign to eradicate polio.

9. Ensure 100 percent routine immunisation for all vaccine preventable diseases, in particular tetanus and measles.

10. As a child survival initiative, explore promotional and motivational measures for couples below the poverty line who marry after the legal age of marriage, to have the first child after the mother reaches the age of 21, and adopt a terminal method of contraception after the birth of the second child.

11. Children form a vulnerable group and certain sub-groups merit focused attention and intervention, such as street children and child labourers. Encourage voluntary groups as well as NGOs to formulate and implement special schemes for these groups of children.

12. Explore the feasibility of a national health insurance covering hospitalisation costs for children below 5 years, whose parents have

adopted the small family norm, and opted for a terminal method of contraception after the birth of the second child.

13. Expand the ICDS to include children between 6-9 years of age, specifically to promote and ensure 100 percent school enrolment, particularly for girls. Promote primary education with the help of anganwadi workers, and encourage retention in school till age 14. Education promotes awareness, late marriages, small family size and higher child survival rates.

14. Provide vocational training for girls. This will enhance perception of the immediate utility of educating girls, and gradually raise the average age of marriage. It will also increase enrolment and retention of girls at primary school, and likely also at secondary school levels. Involve NGOs, the voluntary sector and the private sector, as necessary, to target employment opportunities.

(v) Meeting the Unmet Needs for Family Welfare Services

1. Strengthen, energise and make publicly accountable the cutting edge of health infrastructure at the village, sub-centre and primary health centre levels.

2. Address on priority the different unmet needs detailed in Appendix IV, in particular, an increase in rural infrastructure, deployment of sanctioned and appropriately trained health personnel, and provisioning of essential equipment and drugs.

3. Formulate and implement innovative social marketing schemes to provide subsidised products and services in areas where the existing coverage of the public, private and NGO sectors is insufficient in order to increase outreach and coverage.

4. Improve facilities for referral transportation at panchayat, zilla parishad and primary health centre levels. At sub-centres, provide ANMs with soft loans for purchase of mopeds, to enhance their mobility. This will increase coverage of ante-natal and post natal check-ups, which, in turn, and will bring about reductions in maternal and infant mortality.

5. Encourage local entrepreneurs at village and block levels to start ambulance services through special loan schemes, with appropriate vehicles to facilitate transportation of persons requiring emergency as well as essential medical attention.

6. Provide special loan schemes and make site allotments at village levels to facilitate the starting of chemist shops for basic medicines and provision for medical first aid.

(vi) Under-Served Population Groups

(a) Urban Slums

1. Finalise a comprehensive urban health care strategy.

2. Facilitate service delivery centres in urban slums to provide comprehensive basic health, reproductive and child health services by NGOs and private sector organisations, including corporate houses.

3. Promote networks of retired government doctors and para-medical and non-medical personnel who may function as health care providers for clinical and non-clinical services on remunerative terms.

4. Strengthen social marketing programmes for non-clinical family planning products and services in urban slums.

5. Initiate specially targeted information, education and communication campaigns for urban slums on family planning, immunization, ante-natal, natal and post-natal check-ups and other reproductive health care services. Integrate aggressive health education programmes with health and medical care programmes, with emphasis on environmental health, personal hygiene and healthy habits, nutrition education and population education.

6. Promote inter-sectoral coordination between departments/ municipal bodies dealing with water and sanitation, industry and pollution, housing, transport, education and nutrition, and women and child development, to deal with unplanned and uncoordinated settlements.

7. Streamline the referral systems and linkages between the primary, secondary and tertiary levels of health care in the urban areas.

8. Link the provision of continued facilities to urban slum-dwellers with their observance of the small family norm.

(b) Tribal Communities, Hill Area Populations and Displaced and Migrant Populations

1. Many tribal communities are dwindling in numbers, and may not need fertility regulation. Instead, they may need information and counseling in respect of infertility.

2. The NGO sector may be encouraged to formulate and implement a system of preventive and curative health care that responds to seasonal variations in the availability of work, income and food for tribal and hill area communities and migrant and displaced populations. To begin with, mobile clinics may provide some degree of regular coverage and outreach.

3. Many tribal communities are dependent upon indigenous systems of medicine which necessitates a regular supply of local flora, fauna and minerals, or of standardised medication derived from these. Husbandry of such local resources and of preparation and distribution of standardised formulations should be encouraged.

4. Health care providers in the public, private and NGOs sectors should be sensitised to adopt a "burden of disease" approach to meet the special needs of tribal and hill area communities.

(c) Adolescents

1. Ensure for adolescents access to information, counseling and services, including reproductive health services, that are affordable and accessible. Strengthen primary health centres and sub-centres, to provide counseling, both to adolescents and also to newly weds (who may also be adolescents). Emphasise proper spacing of children.

2. Provide for adolescents the package of nutritional services available under the ICDS programme.

Comment: Improvements in health status of adolescent girls has an inter-generational impact. It reduces the risk of low birth weight and minimizes neo-natal mortality. Malnutrition is a problem that seriously impairs the health of adolescent and adult women and has its roots in early childhood. The causal linkages between anaemia and low birth weight, prematurity, perinatal mortality, and maternal mortality has been extensively studied and established.

3. Enforce the Child Marriage Restraint Act, 1976, to reduce the incidence of teenage pregnancies. Preventing the marriage of girls below the legally permissible age of 18 should become a national concern.

Comment: It will promote higher retention of girls at schools, and is also likely to encourage their participation in the paid work force.

4. Provide integrated intervention in pockets with unmet needs in the urban slums, remote rural areas, border districts and among tribal populations.

(d) Increased Participation of Men in Planned Parenthood

1. Focus attention on men in the information and education campaigns to promote the small family norm, and to raise awareness by emphasising the significant benefits of fewer children, better spacing, better health and nutrition, and better education.

2. Currently, over 97 percent of the sterilisations are tubectomies. Repopularise vasectomies, in particular the noscalpel vasectomy, as a safe, simple, painless procedure, more convenient and acceptable to men.

3. In the continuing education and training at all levels, there is need to ensure that the noscalpel vasectomy, and all such emerging techniques and skills are included in the syllabi, together with abundant practical training. Medical graduates, and all those participating in "in-service" continuing education and training, will be equipped to handle this intervention.

(vii) Diverse Health Care Providers

1. At district and sub-district levels, maintain block-wise data base of private medical practitioners whose credentials may be certified by the Indian Medical Association (IMA). Explore the possibility of accrediting these private practitioners for a year at a time, and assign to each a satellite population, not exceeding 5,000 (depending upon distances and spread), for whom they may provide reproductive and child health services. The private practitioners would be compensated for the services rendered through designated agencies. Renewal of contracts after one year may be guided by client satisfaction. This will serve as an incentive to expand the coverage and outreach of high quality health care. Appropriate checks and balances will safeguard misuse.

2. Revive the earlier system of the licensed medical practitioners who,

after appropriate certification from the IMA, may participate in the provision of clinical services.

3. Involve the non-medical fraternity in counseling and advocacy so as to demystify the national family welfare effort, such as retired defence personnel, retired school teachers and other persons who are active and willing to get involved.

4. Modify the under/post-graduate medical, nursing, and paramedical professional course syllabi and curricula, in consultation with the Medical Council of India, the Councils of ISMH, and the Indian Nursing Council, in order to reflect the concepts and implementation strategies of the reproductive and child health programme and the national population policy. This will also be applied to all in-service training and educational curricula.

5. Ensure the efficient functioning of the First Referral Units, i.e. 30 bed hospitals at block levels which provide emergency obstetric and child health care, to bring about reductions in Maternal Mortality Ratio (MMR) and Infant Mortality Rate (IMR). In many states, these FRUs are not operational on account of an acute shortage of specialists, i.e. gynaecologist/obstetrician, anaesthetist and pediatrician. Augment the availability of specialists in these three disciplines, by increasing seats in medical institutions, and simultaneously enable and facilitate the acquisition of in-service post-graduate qualifications through the National Board of Medical Examination and open universities like IGNOU in larger numbers. As an incentive, seats will be reserved for those in-service medical graduates who are willing to abide by a bond to serve for 5 years at First Referral Units after completion of the course. States would need to sanction posts of Specialists at the FRUs. Further, these specialists should be provided with clear promotion channels.

(viii) *(a) Collaboration with and Commitments from the Non-Government Sector*

1. There remain innumerable hurdles that inhibit genuine long-term collaboration between the government and non-government sectors. A forum of representatives from government, the non-government organisations and the private sector may identify these hurdles and prepare guidelines that will facilitate and promote collaborative arrangements.

2. Collaboration with and commitments from NGOs to augment advocacy, counseling and clinical services, while accessing village levels. This will require increased clinic outlets as well as mobile clinics.

3. Collaboration between the voluntary sector and the NGOs will facilitate dissemination of efficient service delivery to village levels. The guidelines could articulate the role and responsibility of each sector.

4. Encourage the voluntary sector to motivate village-level self-help groups to participate in community activities.

5. Specific collaboration with the non-government sector in the social marketing of contraceptives to reach village levels will be encouraged.

(b) Collaboration with and Commitments from Industry

1. The corporate sector and industry could, for instance, take on the challenge of strengthening the management information systems in the seven most deficient states, at primary health centre and sub-centre levels. Introduce electronic data entry machines to lighten the tedious work load of ANMs and the multi-purpose workers at sub-centres and the doctors at the primary health centres, while enabling wider coverage and outreach.

2. Collaborate with non-government sectors in running professionally sound advertisement and marketing campaigns for products and services, targeting all segments of the population, from village level upwards, in other words, strengthen advocacy and IEC, including social marketing of contraceptives.

3. Provide markets to sustain the income-generating activities from village levels upwards. In turn, this will ensure consistent motivation among the community for pursuing health and education-related community activities.

4. Help promote transportation to remote and inaccessible areas up to village levels. This will greatly assist the coverage and outreach of social marketing of products and services.

5. The social responsibility of the corporate sector in industry must, at the very minimum, extend to providing preventive reproductive and child health care for its own employees (if >100 workers are engaged).

6. Create a national network consisting of voluntary, public, private and non-government health centres, identified by a common logo, for delivering reproductive and child health services, free to any client. The provider will be compensated for the service provided, on the basis of a coupon system, duly counter-signed by the beneficiary and paid for by a system that will be fully articulated. The compensation will be identical to providers, across all sectors. The end user exercises choices in the source of service delivery. A committee of management experts will be set-up to devise ways of ensuring that this system is not abused.

7. Form a consortium of the voluntary sector, the non-government sector and the private corporate sector to aid government in the provision and outreach of basic reproductive and child health care and basic education.

8. In the area of basic education, set-up privately run/managed primary schools for children up to age 14-15. Alternately, if the schools are set-up/managed by the panchayat, the private corporate sector could provide the mid-day meals, the text-books and/or the uniforms.

(ix) Mainstreaming Indian Systems of Medicine and Homeopathy

1. Provide appropriate training and orientation in respect of the RCH programme for the institutionally qualified ISMH medical practitioners (already educated in midwifery, obstetrics and gynaecology over 5-1/2 years), and utilise their services to fill in gaps in manpower at appropriate levels in the health infrastructure, and at sub-centres and primary health centres, as necessary.

2. Utilise the ISMH institutions, dispensaries and hospitals for health and population-related programmes.

3. Disseminate the tried and tested concepts and practices of the indigenous systems of medicine, together with ISMH medication at village maternity huts and at household levels for ante-natal and post-natal care, besides nurture of the newborn.

4. Utilise the services of ISMH 'barefoot doctors' after appropriate training and orientation towards providing advocacy and counseling for disseminating supplies and equipment, and as depot holders at village levels.

(x) Contraceptive Technology and Research on RCH

1. Government will encourage, support and advance the pursuit of medical and social science research on reproductive and child health, in consultation with ICMR and the network of academic and research institutions.

2. The International Institute of Population Sciences and the Population Research Centres will continue to review programme and monitoring indicators to ensure their continued relevance to strategic goals.

3. Government will restructure the Population Research Centres, if necessary.

4. Standards for clinical and non-clinical will be issued and regularly reviewed.

5. A constant review and evaluation of the community needs assessment approach will be pursued to align programme delivery with good management practices and with newly emerging technologies.

6. A committee of international and Indian experts, voluntary and non-government organisations and government may be set-up to regularly review and recommend specific incorporation of the advances in contraceptive technology and, in particular, the newly emerging techniques, into programme development.

(xi) Providing for the Older Population

1. Sensitize, train and equip rural and urban health centres and hospitals towards providing geriatric health care.

2. Encourage NGOs and voluntary organisations to formulate and strengthen a series of formal and informal avenues that make the elderly economically self-reliant.

3. Tax benefits could be explored as an encouragement for children to look after their aged parents.

(xii) Information Education and Communication

1. Converge IEC efforts across the social sectors. The two sectors of Family Welfare and Education have coordinated a mutually supportive IEC strategy. The Zila Saksharta Samitis design and deliver joint IEC campaigns in the local idiom, promoting the cause of literacy as well as family welfare.

Optimal use of folk media has served to successfully mobilize local populations. The state of Tamil Nadu made exemplary use of the IEC strategy by spreading the message through every possible media, including public transport, on milestones on national high ways as well as through advertisement and hoardings on roadsides, along city/rural roads, on billboards, and through processions, films, school dramas, public meetings, local theatre and folk songs.

2. Involve departments of rural development, social welfare, transport, cooperatives, education with special reference to schools, to improve clarity and focus of the IEC effort, and to extend coverage and outreach. Health and population education must be inculcated from the school levels.

3. Fund the nagarpalikas, panchayats, NGOs and community organisations for interactive and participatory IEC activities.

4. Demonstration of support by elected leaders, opinion-makers, and religious leaders with close involvement in the reproductive and child health programme greatly influences the behaviour and response patterns of individuals and communities. This serves to enthuse communities to be attentive towards the quality and coverage of maternal and child health services, including referral care. Public leaders and film stars could spread widely the messages of the small family norm, female literacy, delayed marriages for women, fewer babies, healthier babies, child immunization and so on. The involvement and enthusiastic participation of elected leaders will ensure dedicated involvement of administrators at district and sub-district levels. Demonstration of strong support to the small family norm, as well as personal example, by political, community, business, professional, and religious leaders, media and film stars, sports personalities and opinion-makers, will enhance its acceptance throughout society.

5. Utilise radio and television as the most powerful media for disseminating relevant socio-demographic messages. Government could explore the feasibility of appropriate regulations, and even legislation, if necessary, to mandate the broadcast of social messages during prime time.

6. Utilise dairy cooperatives, the public distribution systems, other established networks at district and sub-district levels for IEC and for distribution of contraceptives and basic medicines to target infant/childhood diarrhoeas, anaemia and malnutrition among adolescent girls and pregnant mothers. This will widen outreach and coverage.

7. Sensitise the field level functionaries across diverse sectors (education, rural development, forest and environment, women and child development, drinking water mission, cooperatives) to the strategies, goals and objectives of the population stabilisation programmes.

8. Involve civil society for disseminating information, counseling and spreading education about the small family norm, the need for fewer but healthier babies, higher female literacy and later marriages for women. Civil society could also be of assistance in monitoring the availability of contraceptives, vaccines and drugs in rural areas and in urban slums.

Index